Lippincott's
Illustrated Reviews:
Immunology

Lippincott's Illustrated Reviews: Immunology

Thao Doan, MD
Senior Medical Director
Abbott Laboratories
Waukegan, Illinois

Roger Melvold, Ph.D.
Professor and Chair, Department of Microbiology and Immunology
University of North Dakota School of Medicine and Health Sciences
Grand Forks, North Dakota

Susan Viselli, PhD
Associate Professor, Department of Biochemistry
Midwestern University
Downers Grove, Illinois

Carl Waltenbaugh, PhD
Professor, Department of Microbiology-Immunology
Feinberg School of Medicine
Northwestern University
Chicago, Illinois

Wolters Kluwer Health | Lippincott Williams & Wilkins

Philadelphia · Baltimore · New York · London
Buenos Aires · Hong Kong · Sydney · Tokyo

Editor: Betty Sun
Developmental Editor: Kathleen H. Scogna
Marketing Manager: Jennifer Kuklinski
Associate Production Manager: Kevin P. Johnson
Designer: Doug Smock
Compositor: Hearthside Publishing Services

9 8 7 6 5 4 3 2 1

Library of Congress Cataloging-in-Publication Data

ISBN: 0-7817-9543-5 / 978-0-7817-9543-2

DISCLAIMER

Care has been taken to confirm the accuracy of the information present and to describe generally accepted practices. However, the authors, editors, and publisher are not responsible for errors or omissions or for any consequences from application of the information in this book and make no warranty, expressed or implied, with respect to the currency, completeness, or accuracy of the contents of the publication. Application of this information in a particular situation remains the professional responsibility of the practitioner; the clinical treatments described and recommended may not be considered absolute and universal recommendations.

The authors, editors, and publisher have exerted every effort to ensure that drug selection and dosage set forth in this text are in accordance with the current recommendations and practice at the time of publication. However, in view of ongoing research, changes in government regulations, and the constant flow of information relating to drug therapy and drug reactions, the reader is urged to check the package insert for each drug for any change in indications and dosage and for added warnings and precautions. This is particularly important when the recommended agent is a new or infrequently employed drug.

Some drugs and medical devices presented in this publication have Food and Drug Administration (FDA) clearance for limited use in restricted research settings. It is the responsibility of the health care provider to ascertain the FDA status of each drug or device planned for use in their clinical practice.

To purchase additional copies of this book, call our customer service department at **(800) 638-3030** or fax orders to **(301) 223-2320**. International customers should call **(301) 223-2300**.

Visit Lippincott Williams & Wilkins on the Internet: http://www.lww.com. Lippincott Williams & Wilkins customer service representatives are available from 8:30 am to 6:00 pm, EST.

This book is dedicated to
our students who constantly inspire us to
reexamine our immunologic concepts

Acknowledgments

We thank Kathleen Scogna, Senior Developmental Editor, for her efficient guidance in this project. In addition, we thank Betty Sun, Executive Editor, for her encouragement. We extend special thanks the Matt Chansky, Illustrator Coordinator, whose artistic talent was invaluable. Thanks also to Anne Seitz and Diane Geesey, Production Editors, and the staff at Lippincott Williams & Wilkins for their expertise and assistance. We thank Dr. Roger H. Kobayashi and Jan Lips for their advice, particularly with respect to the Clinical Applications. Finally, we appreciate our families and friends for their continued support.

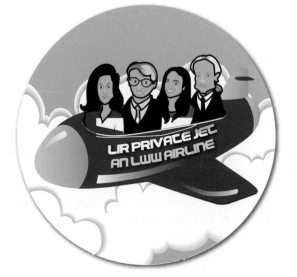

Contents

UNIT I
Sense of Being: The Concept of Self and Self/Nonself Recognition

ΓΝΩΘΙ ΣΑΥΤΟΝ *("Know thyself")*
Words originally inscribed in gold on the pronaus of the
Temple of Apollo at Delphi

This dictum—short in length but deep in meaning—encapsulates a basic need for all forms of life.

In a way, most organisms in our world live alone. They are composed of single cells or particles, and as such, their need to distinguish themselves is seemingly simple. Their single cell or particle is "*I*," and all else is "*them*." They need to sense which of "*them*" is appropriate to mate with or perhaps to congregate with, but otherwise their version of self is limited by their own membrane.

Multicellular organisms faced a new problem as they evolved. They gave up some of their independence to reap the advantages of being part of a greater whole—an organism composed of multiple semi-independent units. Initially, any such unit was pretty much like every other one within the greater structure, so extending the concept of self to include others that were essentially identical was perhaps a relatively small leap. "*I*" became "*us*" but only as multiples of "*I*." As organisms became more complex and the different cells within a single organism began to engage in a division of labor, they generated an array of cells with different forms and functions. Distinguishing "*I*" or "*us*" from "*them*" became increasingly complex: *Is that adjoining cell, which seems so different from "I," really a part of "us," or is it an intruder from "them"?*

The development of commensal arrangements between organisms (e.g., moss and fungi combining to form lichens, humans and normal bacterial flora in the gut and on the skin) required yet more questions: *If there is an intruder, does it represent a threat or can it safely be ignored? If it represents a threat, what should be done to eliminate it?*

These questions are the starting points from which the immune system operates. The human immune system utilizes a variety of methods to ask and answer these questions. Some of these methods have been widely used for eons; others have been developed more recently by more restricted groups of organisms. This unit introduces how the human immune system deals with these questions.

The Need for Self Recognition

1

I. OVERVIEW

A wide variety of organisms and their associated molecules pose a constant threat to the human body. The human immune system—the defensive mechanisms that identify and neutralize these threats—is able to distinguish "**nonself**" organisms and molecules from "**self**," that which belongs within the body (Fig. 1.1). Threats may enter the body from the outside (e.g., infectious organisms or toxic agents) or may arise from potentially harmful changes occurring within the body (e.g., the malignant transformation of a previously normal cell into a cancer cell). Fortunately, the immune system consists of three layers of defense (Fig. 1.2). The first line of defense is provided by a set of mechanical, chemical, and biologic barriers that protect the body. If these barriers are breached, the second and third lines of protective systems are activated: first the innate immune system and then the adaptive immune system.

The innate and adaptive immune systems utilize cell-surface and soluble receptors to sense potential threats. These receptors of the innate and adaptive systems are generated in different ways, however, providing a major distinction between the two systems (Fig. 1.3).

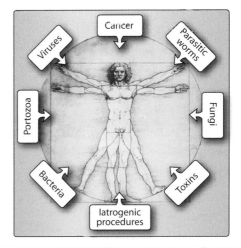

Figure 1.1
Threats to the individual. The body is continuously exposed to many infectious agents, cancerous cells, toxic molecules, and even therapeutic drugs.

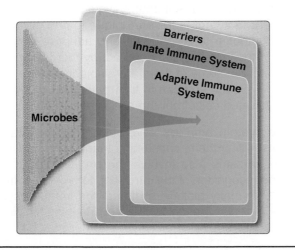

Figure 1.2
Protection from and response to microbial invasion. Initial protection is provided by a set of barriers. When breached, invading microbes trigger the innate immune system and, if necessary, the adaptive immune system.

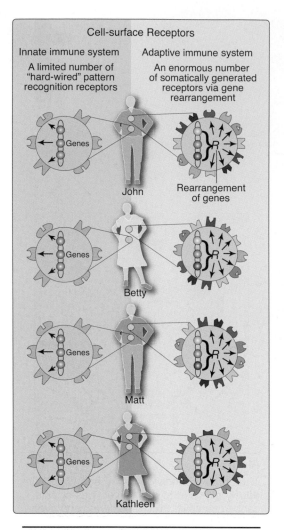

Figure 1.3
Innate pattern recognition receptors and adaptive somatically generated receptors. Each individual expresses pattern recognition receptors (innate immune system) and somatically generated receptors (adaptive immune system).

Some receptors recognize and bind to self molecules. Other receptors recognize and bind to nonself molecules. Some receptors for nonself are limited in number and are "hard-wired" in the genome, common to all normal individuals. They specifically detect molecules produced by a wide variety of other organisms (e.g., molecules commonly found on bacterial cells but not on human cells). These "common" receptors, called **pattern recognition receptors** (PRRs), number perhaps a hundred or so and are part of the **innate immune system**, the second line of defense (Fig. 1.4A). Cells and molecules of the innate immune system respond rapidly to a microbial invasion and are often sufficient for defense.

The **adaptive immune system** (Fig. 1.4B), with its unique cells and molecules, is the third level of defense against these potential threats to the body, following the barriers and the innate immune system. Bone marrow-derived and thymus-derived lymphocytes (B cells and T cells, respectively) generate distinct receptors during development. Each lymphocyte randomly generates a unique receptor through the rearrangement and rejoining of a relatively small number of genes into a "combination gene" encoding the receptor. These receptors, called **somatically generated receptors**, are generated randomly prior to any contact with self or nonself; the process is described in detail in Chapter 8. By combining multiple genes, therefore, each individual can generate enormous numbers of B and T cells, each with a unique receptor. A subsequent process, in which the receptors are uniquely vetted by each individual, results in the retention of a set of receptors that is individualized to that particular self and his or her nonself environment. In addition, the initial responses of the cells of the adaptive immune system to a given threat or stimulus can lead to enhanced or depressed responses during subsequent encounters with the same threat or stimulus. This ability to modify the immune response to substances encountered on multiple occasions is the basis for **immunologic memory**, one of the hallmarks distinguishing the adaptive from the innate immune system.

Both the innate and adaptive immune systems involve a variety of molecules and cells. Some of these are unique to one or the other system, while some contribute to both innate and adaptive responses. For example, cells of the innate system can act by themselves to resist infectious organisms. But some of them are also critical for activation of cells in the adaptive system and can in turn have their activity elevated and directed by activated cells from the adaptive system.

The immune system employs several defense mechanisms against foreign agents: killing them, consuming them, and isolating them. Many of these mechanisms also involve the proliferation of relevant host cells, following recognition of the intruders, to provide sufficient numbers for defense. Like many biologic systems, the immune system employs redundancy—multiple mechanisms with overlapping functions—to ensure that if one mechanism is not effective, another may be.

Through time, hosts and microbes have repeatedly changed their tactics. Some microbes have developed means of evading some immune responses. Hosts, in return, have developed additional defensive strategies. These strategies could eventually be evaded by some microbes. These new microbial innovations again drive development

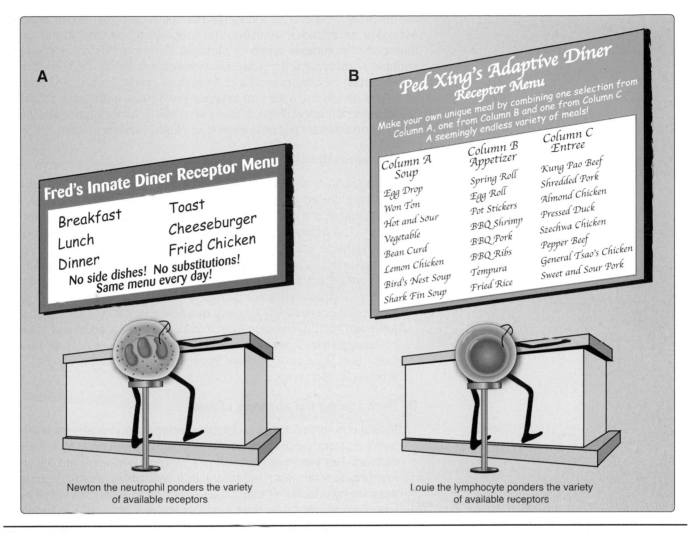

Figure 1.4
Diversity of receptors of the innate and adaptive immune systems. **A.** Receptors of the innate immune system (pattern recognition receptors) are limited in number and diversity and are consistent from one normal individual to another. **B.** The somatically generated receptors of lymphocytes in the adaptive immune system use random combinations of genes to assemble a very large number of different receptors.

of yet additional defensive mechanisms, and so on. Thus the relationship between host and microbe is essentially an ever-spiraling arms race.

II. THE IMMUNOLOGIC CONCEPT OF SELF

If you were to describe what makes you unique as an individual, you might list the attributes you possess (e.g., eye, hair, and skin color, blood type). You might also list or imply the attributes you would never have (e.g., lipopolysaccharides, hemagglutinins, feathers, scales, wings). The immune system makes similar distinctions. For example, the hardwired receptors of the innate immune system have been selected over evolutionary time only to recognize nonself molecules whose presence indicates an intruder, such as the lipopolysaccharides found on the surfaces of numerous types of bacteria. On the other hand, the highly variable receptors of the adaptive immune response, generated anew within certain somatic cells of each individual, recognize both self and nonself. As a result, the cells that express them must undergo a process of selection or "education" first to learn what self is for that particular individual, then to consider (by default) that all other elements constitute nonself.

A. Recognizing self

Recognition of self is used by the body's cells to determine whether an encountered molecule or cell has the appropriate structures to show that it is a part of the body. This is important for several purposes. The ability to recognize self enables the cells of multicellular organisms to know whether other cells with which they come into contact actually belong to the same organism and whether interactions with them are safe. In many immune functions, recognition of such self structures among cells is absolutely critical to their ability to interact successfully to carry out some function. These self structures are normally absent from invasive microbial cells and may also be absent from some abnormal cells of the body (e.g., some cancer cells) and from cells of other individuals of the same species (e.g., a transplanted graft).

B. Recognizing the absence of self

In addition to permitting productive interaction, the absence of such self indicators can trigger an attack upon any cells that lack these indicators. For example, certain cells (natural killer cells) of the innate immune system bear receptors that recognize stress signals expressed by infected or cancerous cells. Using a second set of receptors, natural killer cells then examine the stressed cells to determine whether they possess sufficient levels of a particular set of cell surface molecules called MHC I that should be present on every normal nucleated cell of the body. Cells that become abnormal owing to cancer or certain viral infections may greatly reduce (or eliminate entirely) the expression of these molecules. Natural killer cells can detect this decreased MHC I expression and destroy the abnormal cells.

C. Recognizing nonself

The ability to recognize something that is nonself and has not yet been encountered represents a significant biologic challenge. The immune system meets this challenge through two approaches utilizing the pattern recognition receptors and the somatically generated receptors that were mentioned previously (see Fig. 1.3). The first is a genetically stable set of receptors that has been evolutionarily selected to recognize and bind structures that are produced by distantly related organisms (e.g., microbes) or are produced by host cells in response to stress (e.g., infection or injury). The extremely variable somatically generated receptors of lymphocytes are based on a relatively small number of genes that are routinely transmitted from one generation to the next but are then rearranged somatically within each lymphocyte of each individual to construct a vast and randomly generated set of receptors, some of which will be capable of recognizing and binding to nonself.

1. **Via pattern recognition receptors:** PRRs are designed to recognize and bind to only nonself structures that are not normally present within the body but are abundant in the microbial world. The structures of these receptors are directly encoded (hardwired) in the genome. Thus they are transmitted across generations and expressed in each individual within a species in an essentially identical form. This type of recognition is characteristic of the innate immune system. PRRs identify structures that are typically associated with microbes but not with host cells. Some PRRs (e.g., the toll-like receptors) are found on the membranes of various cell types, while others (e.g., complement molecules) exist in a soluble form. The role of PRRs is introduced in more detail in Chapters 2 and 5 concerning the innate immune response.

2. **Via somatically generated receptors:** A subset of white blood cells, the T and B lymphocytes, are the only cells capable of producing somatically generated receptors of the adaptive immune system. Each T or B cell utilizes the rearrangement of DNA (and in some cases, somatic mutation) to develop an enormous number of different receptors. While each cell produces only a single type of receptor able to recognize only a single structure, the total number of such cells undergoing this process permits the development of a pool of receptors capable of recognizing more than 10^{10} different structures. Because each such cell generates its receptor in a random manner, some cells develop structures capable of recognizing self, and others develop receptors capable of recognizing nonself. As a result, T and B lymphocytes undergo processes ("education") to remove those bearing receptors that could potentially recognize and attack normal structures within the body. In addition, some lymphocytes develop receptors that are not capable of properly interacting with other cells within the body, and these are eliminated as well. Once activated, the remaining T and B lymphocytes can launch powerful and lethal immune responses designed to eliminate nonself cells and molecules.

III. IMMUNOLOGIC MEMORY

Cells and molecules of the innate immune system treat each encounter with a particular microbial invader as if they were meeting it for the first time. The adaptive system, on the other hand, has the capacity to use the initial encounter with a particular stimulus (e.g., a specific microbe) to modify or adapt its response(s) to any subsequent encounters with that same stimulus (Fig. 1.5). This **immunologic memory** allows the adaptive immune system to tailor its responses to cells or molecules that it encounters on multiple occasions. In some cases, as in common microbes, subsequent responses may be increasingly rapid and vigorous to speedily eliminate the microbes, often before their presence can be detected by other means. In other cases, immune responses may be depressed against other commonly encountered nonself entities, such as harmless cells and molecules present on our skin, in the air we

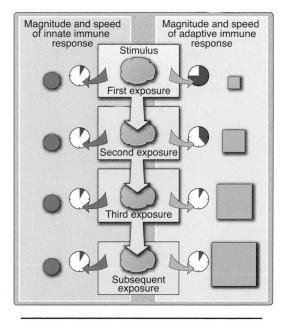

Figure 1.5

Immunologic memory. The innate immune system reacts to a given stimulus with a consistent intensity, regardless of how many times it has been exposed to that stimulus. The adaptive immune system can adapt and modify its response after each exposure to a given stimulus

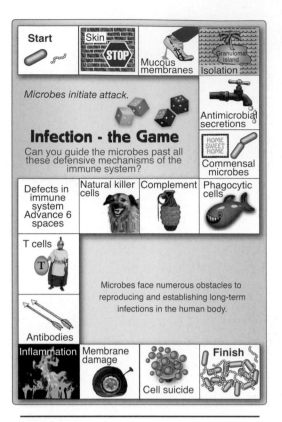

Figure 1.6
Immune defense mechanisms. The immune system utilizes an arsenal of protective mechanisms to inhibit or destroy invading microbes. The illustration presented includes some of them, and their sequence can vary.

breathe, or in the food and water we consume. Immunologic memory thus provides the body with an ability to deal differently with threatening or nonthreatening nonself.

IV. DEFENSE MECHANISMS

The immune system is, along with the nervous system and the endocrine system, one of the great communication systems of the body. Most immune responses require successful interactions between multiple cells and molecules.

Once the immune system decides to eliminate a particular threat, it relies on three general approaches. The threat may be isolated, it may be disrupted, or it may be ingested and consumed; or some combination of these actions may be used. Within these general categories, many types of mechanisms are available (Fig. 1.6) to inhibit the spread or growth of microbial intruders or to kill them. Mechanical barriers (e.g., skin and mucous membranes), chemical barriers (e.g., microcidal molecules), and biologic barriers (e.g., the presence of commensal microbes) resist the initial entry of microbes into the body. Invasive microbes may be walled off within structures (e.g., granulomas) to restrict their ability to spread to other parts of the body. Disruption of nonself cells may occur through physical damage inflicted on their membranes or by inducing them to undergo a process of programmed suicide (**apoptosis**) in which they destroy their own nucleic acids. **Phagocytic** cells capture and ingest microbes and cellular debris. The ingestion and subsequent degradation of microbes or cellular debris also triggers some phagocytic cells to secrete molecules that selectively activate other elements of the immune system. Natural killer cells can detect and destroy host cells that display certain abnormal characteristics (e.g., stemming from viral infection). Antibodies (produced by B lymphocytes) and complement molecules can attach to microbes and initiate their destruction, while T lymphocytes can directly or indirectly attack microbes and infected cells. Many cells of the immune system also proliferate rapidly upon perceiving the presence of a threat to ensure sufficient numbers to cope with that threat.

Chapter Summary

- The immune system distinguishes cells and molecules that belong within the body (**self**) from those that do not (**nonself**), using the **innate** and **adaptive** immune systems.
- Both the innate and adaptive immune systems use cell-surface and soluble receptors to sense potential threats.
- Cells and molecules of the innate immune system respond rapidly to a microbial invasion and are often sufficient for defense.
- Recognition of self is used by cells to determine whether an encountered molecule or cell has the appropriate structures to show that it is a part of the body.
- The recognition of something that is nonself and has not yet been encountered is achieved through pattern recognition receptors and somatically generated receptors.
- **Immunologic memory** allows the adaptive immune system to tailor its responses to things that it encounters on multiple occasions.
- The immune system can eliminate threats by **isolation**, **disruption**, or **ingestion** (consumption) or by a combination of these actions.

Study Questions

1.1 Immune recognition of molecules belonging to self is important to

   A. activate natural killer cells of the innate immune system.
   B. determine the safety of interacting with the molecule.
   C. induce somatic generation of a B or T lymphocyte receptor for the molecule.
   D. stimulate binding by pattern recognition receptors.
   E. trigger an attack upon the cell expressing the self molecule.

The correct answer is B. Identification of self tells the immune system that the cell or molecule recognized is not a foe. Natural killer cells use this mechanism of self recognition to halt their attack on cells that they perceive to be abnormal. Receptor generation by B and T cells occurs independently of initial encounter with self molecules. Pattern recognition receptors, on the other hand, are genetically programmed to recognize nonself. By triggering an attack upon a cell expressing the self molecule, an immune recognition molecule violates its "nonaggression pact" with the cells and molecules of the host and establishes an internal coup known as autoimmunity.

1.2 Natural killer cells assess whether other cells are abnormal by detecting types and levels of surface-associated

   A. MHC I molecules.
   B. nonself molecules.
   C. pathogen-associated molecular patterns.
   D. pattern recognition receptors.
   E. somatically generated cell surface receptors

The correct answer is A. MHC class I molecules are self-identification molecules found on all nucleated host cells. Natural killer cells, after making contact with cells expressing stress signals, make the decision whether to kill them or not by assessing whether they express the appropriate types and levels of MHC I molecules. Although they are members of the innate immune system, natural killer cells do not recognize nonself, pathogen-associated molecular patterns or pattern recognition receptors. Natural killer cells are unable to recognize somatically generated cell surface receptors.

1.3 Pattern recognition receptors bind to

    A. B and T lymphocytes.
    B. host cell-associated molecules.
    C. MHC I molecules.
    D. natural killer cells.
    E. pathogen-associated molecular patterns.

> The correct answer is E. Pattern recognition receptors (PRRs) are genomically determined to bind to molecules widely expressed by microbes but not by host cells. Consequently, PRRs cannot recognize host-associated molecules such as MHC class I molecules or cells of host origin such as B, T, or natural killer lymphocytes.

1.4 Somatically generated receptors found on B and T lymphocytes are

    A. bound only to MHC I molecules.
    B. encoded in the germline to recognize pathogen-associated molecular patterns.
    C. first produced after an initial encounter with nonself.
    D. identical among individuals.
    E. randomly generated during development.

> The correct answer is E. Bone marrow-derived (B) and thymus-derived (T) lymphocytes somatically generate receptors during development. Unlike natural killer cells, B cells and T cells are unable to assess the quantity of MHC class I molecules on nucleated cells. Unlike innate immune system receptors, B and T lymphocyte somatic receptors are randomly generated and vary greatly between individuals. B and T lymphocytes receptors are formed prior to antigen stimulation.

1.5 Immunologic memory refers to

    A. activation of phagocytic cells to ingest microbial invaders.
    B. changes in adaptive immune responses with subsequent encounters with antigen.
    C. constancy of the response of the innate immune response to a particular microbe.
    D. recognition of pathogen-associated molecular patterns by pattern recognition receptors.
    E. stimulating a defective host cell with reduced MHC I molecules to commit suicide.

> The correct answer is B. A hallmark of the adaptive immune system is that it progressively alters its response upon reexposure to an antigenic stimulus, and in doing so, it must recall the previous exposure, a process known as memory. Although they are members of the innate immune system and do not possess immunologic memory, phagocytes may be influenced by the adaptive immune system. Consistency in immune response from initial to subsequent encounters is a hallmark of the innate immune response. Immunologic memory of the adaptive immune system is not passed genetically from one generation of individuals to the next. Detection of diminished MHC class I expression is a function of natural killer cells, members of the innate immune system.

1.6 Influenza viruses infect humans and elicit an immune response that is often insufficient to protect the individual from sickness or death. Which of the following structures are on influenza viruses, allowing them to be recognized by the human immune system?

    A. MHC I molecules
    B. MHC II molecules
    C. pathogen-associated molecular patterns
    D. pattern recognition receptor
    E. somatically generated receptors

> The correct answer is C. The molecules on the virus that are not on host cells are the pathogen-associated molecular patterns. The pattern recognition receptors are found on host cells and molecules. MHC I and II molecules are present on all nucleated host cells but not on viruses. The somatically generated receptors are on host T and B lymphocytes.

Antigens and Receptors

2

I. OVERVIEW

Immune responses are initiated by the interaction between a **receptor** and a **ligand** (a molecule that interacts with a receptor). These interactions are what trigger the activation of leukocytes or white blood cells. The shapes of the ligand and its receptor are critical. The effectiveness of interaction often increases with the **affinity** or strength of interaction between ligand and receptor (Fig. 2.1). Receptors may be displayed on cell surfaces (e.g., cell-surface receptors) or may be soluble molecules (e.g., secreted products of leukocytes). Ligands may be expressed by cells as cell-surface molecules (e.g., on microbes) or as soluble molecules (e.g., the secreted products of cells).

Several factors influence the binding of a ligand to a cell-surface receptor: The shape and charge affect binding **affinity**, the collective affinities where multiple receptors may be involved (**avidity**), the intracellular signals that are triggered, and the presence of other receptors

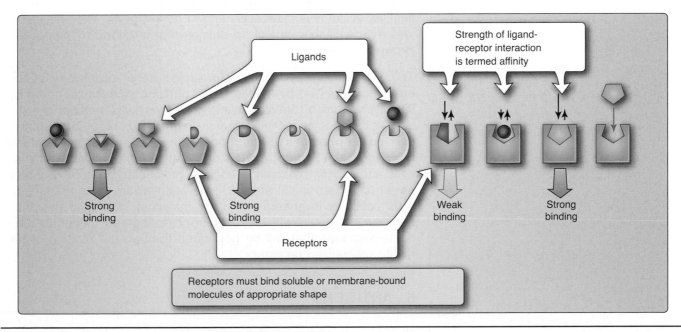

Figure 2.1
Receptor-ligand interactions. Receptors bind molecules or ligands that may be either soluble or bound to membranes. If the binding is sufficient, the receptor is able to provide a signal to the cell.

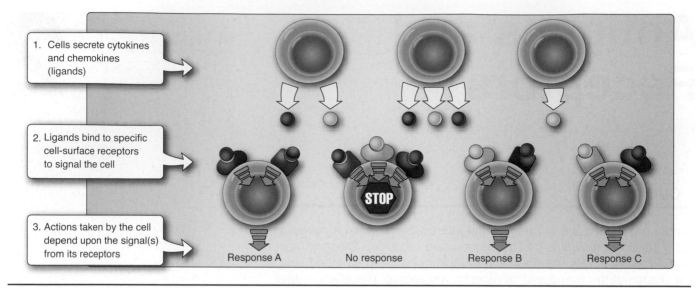

1. Cells secrete cytokines and chemokines (ligands)

2. Ligands bind to specific cell-surface receptors to signal the cell

3. Actions taken by the cell depend upon the signal(s) from its receptors

Response A   No response   Response B   Response C

Figure 2.2
Receptor-ligand context influences outcome. A cell integrates messages coming from multiple receptors to determine what action it ultimately takes.

that may also influence the action in question. The context in which cells receive signals can influence whether they respond to those signals (Fig. 2.2). Cells must often correlate information from multiple activated receptors, some providing positive signals and others providing negative signals, to determine what action they will ultimately take. A grouping of ligands that may be recognized by cells of both the innate and adaptive immune systems is collectively known as **antigens**. The smallest individually identifiable part of an antigen that is bound by a receptor is known as an **epitope**.

The innate immune system employs a limited set of receptors to recognize epitopes expressed by a wide range of microorganisms. The adaptive immune system, on the other hand, generates a vast number of epitope-specific lymphocyte receptors that are expressed only by **bone marrow-derived lymphocytes** (**B lymphocytes** or **B cells**) and **thymus-derived lymphocytes (T lymphocytes** or **T cells**). Different receptors on B cells and T cells precisely recognize molecular features of epitopes as an important initial step in generating an immune response. As with receptors in general, both the molecular nature of the antigen and how it interacts with leukocyte receptors greatly influence the immune response that will be generated through the binding of these highly specialized receptors.

II. ANTIGENS

Classically, an antigen is defined as an organism, a molecule, or part of a molecule that is recognized by the immune system. Antigens may be simple or complex, protein, carbohydrate, or synthetic in origin. Often, the term is associated primarily with those molecules recognized by the extremely diverse receptors found on T and B lymphocytes. We will follow this usage and reserve the terms "antigen" and "epitope" for the substances that are recognized and bound by these somatically generated B and T cell receptors. It must be noted, however, that molecules designated as antigens in this context may also be bound by other types of receptors on other cells.

A. Epitopes: the basic recognition unit

Antigen receptors recognize discrete regions of molecules called **antigenic determinants** or epitopes, the smallest part of an antigen that is "seen" by somatically generated B and T cell receptors (Fig. 2.3). Different lymphocytes, each with a unique set of receptors, may recognize different epitopes on the same antigen. Some receptors (e.g., those of B cells) can recognize their specific epitopes whether they are part of free soluble molecules, surface-bound molecules, or even degraded (proteolytic) fragments of antigens. Other receptors (e.g., T cell receptors) can bind only to epitopes that are on small fragments affixed to specialized host cell surface molecules that display them to the T cells. Depending upon the nature of the immune responses they trigger, antigens/epitopes are divided into three broad functional types: immunogens, haptens, and tolerogens.

B. Immunogens

Immunogens contain epitopes that both induce an immune response and are the targets of that response (Table 2.1). The strength of the immune response by the innate system is the same no matter how many times it encounters the same immunogen. In contrast, reexposure of the adaptive immune system to the same immunogen usually increases the intensity of the epitope-specific immune response. Although epitopes on antigens may bind to soluble or cell-surface receptors, not all antigens are immunogens. Unfortunately, the terms "antigen" and "immunogen" are often used interchangeably. In this text, we use the term "immunogen" to mean a substance or antigen that evokes a specific, positive immune response and the term "antigen" to mean a molecule or cell recognized by the immune system. Some nonimmunogenic molecules (e.g., haptens) can be bound to an immunogen. In this context, the immunogen is referred to as a **carrier**.

C. Haptens

Haptens are small, normally nonimmunogenic, molecules, usually of nonbiologic origin, that behave like synthetic epitopes. Haptens are antigens and can bind to immune receptors but cannot by themselves induce a specific immune response and hence are not immunogenic. However, when a hapten is chemically bound to an immunogen (also called a **carrier**), immune responses may be generated against both the hapten and the epitopes on the immunogen (see Table 2.1).

D. Tolerogens

During development of the immune **repertoire** (the sum of all of the epitopes for which a given individual has generated immunologic receptors), **tolerance** to self molecules and cells develops first. Therefore a lack of immune response to self antigens exists in the

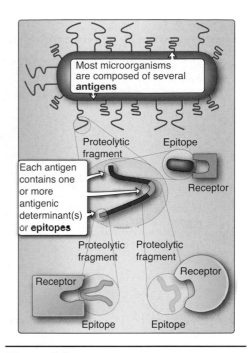

Figure 2.3
Epitopes and antigens: degrees of complexity. Complex antigens may contain large numbers of different epitopes.

Table 2.1
IMMUNOGENS, HAPTENS, AND TOLEROGENS

Injection with	Structure	Response to protein epitope	Response to hapten	Comment
Immunogen or carrier	Protein / Epitope	Yes	Not applicable	An injected protein (sometimes called a carrier) that elicits an immune response is called an immunogen
Synthetic epitope or hapten	Tyr / NO$_2$ / NO$_2$	Not applicable	No	Injection of a synthetic molecule, in this case 2,4-dinitrophenyltyrosine, by itself does not elicit an immune response and is called a hapten
Hapten–Carrier conjugate	NO$_2$ / NO$_2$	Yes	Yes	Injection of a hapten chemically bound to a carrier elicits an immune response to both carrier epitope(s) and to the hapten
Hapten NOT conjugated to carrier	Tyr / NO$_2$ / NO$_2$ +	Yes	No	Injection of unconjugated hapten and carrier does not elicit a response

normal, healthy state. Nonself antigens are subsequently recognized as foreign. Tolerance can also develop later in life, for example to antigens that are administered orally. **Tolerogens** induce adaptive immune unresponsiveness. However, unlike immunogens, exposure to a tolerogen results in a diminished response rather than an enhanced one (see Table 2.1).

E. Immunogenicity

Although there are no firm rules for predicting whether a substance is an immunogen prior to exposure to the immune system, there are several guidelines:

- **Size:** Proteins greater than 10 kDa are usually more immunogenic.
- **Complexity:** Complex proteins with numerous, diverse epitopes are more likely to induce an immune response than are simple peptides that contain only one or a few epitopes.

- **Conformation and accessibility:** Epitopes must be "seen by" and be accessible to the immune system.
- **Chemical properties:** A protein immunogen has to be enzymatically cleavable by phagocytes. For example, L-amino acid-containing polypeptides are generally good immunogens, while D-amino acid-containing polypeptides are poor immunogens, because proteolytic enzymes are able to cleave only the L-forms of amino acids. Many carbohydrates, steroids, and lipids tend to be poor immunogens. Amino acids and haptens are, by themselves, not immunogenic (Fig. 2.4).

III. RECEPTORS

The immune system depends upon receptors, and the ligands that are bound by them, for its function. The engagement of receptors provides the initiating event that can lead to a wide variety of activities, depending upon the particular receptor and ligand and upon the type of cell or molecules that the receptor is associated with. Some receptors are designed to bind molecules that then generate signals between cells. Others sample the environment to detect the presence of intruders. Yet others examine their neighbors to be sure that they belong to self and do not present a threat.

A. Preformed receptors

The initial defense to an infectious agent comes from elements of the innate immune system that contain preformed receptors that allow a quick response. This response confers some protection while the adaptive immune system prepares to respond.

1. **Pattern recognition receptors:** Receptors of the innate immune system recognize broad structural **motifs** (similarities in design) that are generally not present within the host but are instead found on microbes. These receptors, **pattern recognition receptors** (PRRs), are present in soluble forms (e.g., complement proteins, which comprise a particular kind of immune defense system discussed later in the chapter) or on host cell surfaces. They recognize **pathogen-associated molecular patterns** (PAMPs), which include combinations of sugars, some proteins, lipids, and nucleic acids broadly associated with microbes (Fig. 2.5). PRR binding to PAMPs triggers various forms of inflammation intended to destroy the pathogens.

2. **Toll-like receptors:** In humans, PRRs also include **toll-like receptors** (TLRs) that are present on a variety of host cells (Table 2.2). When triggered by binding to a PAMP on an infectious organism, TLRs mediate the generation of defensive responses that include transcriptional activation, synthesis and secretion of **cytokines** (immune chemicals secreted by immune cells) to promote inflammation, and the attraction of macrophages, neutrophils, **natural killer** (NK) cells, and dendritic cells to the site of infection.

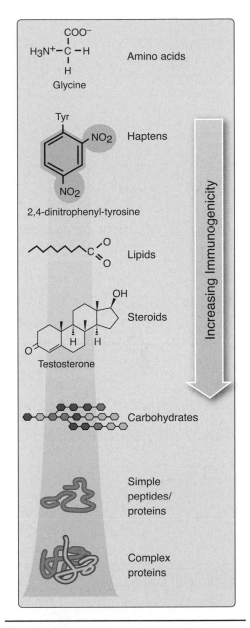

Figure 2.4
Factors governing immunogenicity. In general, the greater the size and complexity of the antigen, the greater the variety of possible epitopes and the greater the immunogenicity.

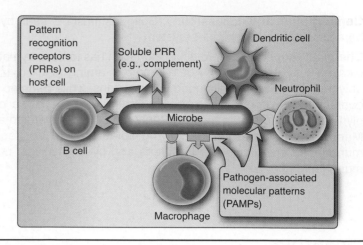

Figure 2.5
Pattern-recognition receptors (PRRs). Pattern recognition receptors detect and bind pathogen-associated molecular patterns (PAMPs).

3. **Killer activation receptors:** NK cells are part of the lymphocyte lineage that do not express the extremely variable types of antigen-specific receptors found on B cells and T cells. Nevertheless, they do bear receptors that are able to detect alterations in host cells that have been infected by pathogens, particularly viruses. **Killer activation receptors** (KARs) on NK cells allow them to recognize the presence of stress-related molecules (called **MICA** and **MICB** molecules in humans) expressed by host cells that are unhealthy or abnormal for various reasons, including being infected. Binding of MICA or MICB molecules by the NK cell's KARs induces the NK cell to attach and destroy the targeted (e.g., infected) host cell (Fig. 2.6). This process, and its important role in innate immunity, is discussed in greater detail in Chapter 4.

4. **Killer inhibition receptors:** Another set of receptors, the **killer inhibition receptors** (KIRs), is used by NK cells to monitor **major histocompatibility complex** (MHC) class I molecules normally displayed on the cell surfaces of all nucleated cells in the body (see Fig. 2-6). By scrutinizing MHC class I molecules, NK cells have a second means to determine the normality of host cells. Many processes, including some cancers and some types of viral infection, decrease the number of MHC class I molecules displayed on the surface of the affected cell. Once bound to a target cell via its KARs, the NK cells use their KIRs to assess the expression of MHC class I molecules on that cell. If NK cells determine that the level is subnormal, they proceed to kill the target cell. If they determine that normal levels are present, the killing process is terminated and the target cell is released unharmed.

5. **Complement receptors:** The **complement system** is a complex set of soluble molecules that generate a variety of reactions that attract immune cells to the site of infection and lead to destruction

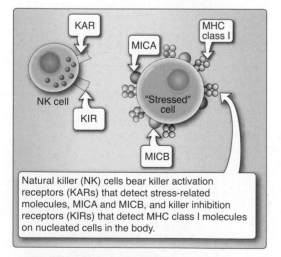

Natural killer (NK) cells bear killer activation receptors (KARs) that detect stress-related molecules, MICA and MICB, and killer inhibition receptors (KIRs) that detect MHC class I molecules on nucleated cells in the body.

Figure 2-6
Killer-cell activation receptors (KARs) and killer-cell inhibition receptors (KIRs).

Table 2.2
TOLL-LIKE RECEPTORS (TLRS)

TLR	Expressed on	Recognizes and Binds	Found on
TLR1	Monocytes/macrophages Dendritic cell subset B lymphocytes	Multiple tri-acyl lipopeptides	Bacteria
TLR2	Monocytes/macrophages Subset of dendritic cells Mast cells	Multiple glycolipids Multiple lipopeptides Multiple lipoproteins Lipotechonic acid Peptidoglycan HSP70 Zymosan Numerous other molecules	Bacteria Bacteria Bacteria Bacteria Gram-positive bacteria Host cells Fungi
TLR3	Dendritic cells B lymphocytes	Viral DNA (double stranded)	Viruses
TLR4	Monocytes/macrophages Dendritic cell subset Mast cells Intestinal epithelium	Lipopolysaccharide Several heat shock proteins Fibrinogen (host cell product) Heparan sulfate fragments Hyaluronic acid fragments Numerous other molecules	Gram-negative bacteria Bacterial and host cells Host cells Host cells Host cells
TLR5	Monocytes/macrophages Dendritic cell subset Intestinal epithelium	Flagellin	Bacteria
TLR6	Monocytes/macrophages Mast cells B lymphocytes	Multiple lipopeptides (di-acyl)	Mycoplasma
TLR7	Monocytes/macrophages Dendritic cell subset B lymphocytes	Imidezoquinoline Loxoribine Bropirimine	Synthetic compound Synthetic compound Synthetic compound
TLR8	Monocytes/macrophages Dendritic cell subset Mast cells	Unknown	Unknown
TLR9	Monocytes/macrophages Dendritic cell subset B lymphocytes	CgG motif of bacterial DNA	Bacteria
TLR10	Monocytes/macrophages B lymphocytes	Unknown	Unknown
TLR11	Macrophages and liver Kidney Bladder epithelial cells	Unknown	Uropathogenic bacteria

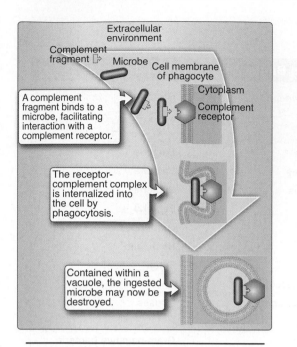

Figure 2.7
Complement receptors. Binding by complement receptors on phagocytic cells facilitates binding, ingestion, and destruction of microbes.

of microbes. Some of these activities are accomplished by the binding of certain complement components or their fragments to microbial surfaces and "tagging" that microbe for destruction by other elements of the immune system. Cell-surface-bound **complement receptors** on phagocytic cells and B cells recognize these bound complement fragments and facilitate the binding, ingestion, and internal degradation of the tagged microbes (Fig. 2.7).

6. **Fc receptors: Immunoglobulins** (including those epitope-binding immunoglobulins termed **antibodies**) are classified as IgA (immunoglobulin A), IgD, IgE, IgG, and IgM based upon their structure. Although the structural and functional details of immunoglobulins are discussed in detail in Chapters 8 and 9, the important point for our purposes here is that epitope binding by IgA, IgG, or IgM antibodies triggers a conformational change in the "tail" or **Fc portion** of the antibody. **Fc receptors** (FcRs) are expressed on the surfaces of phagocytic cells (see Fig. 2.8). Phagocytic cells recognize and bind epitope-engaged antibodies (recognizable by the altered conformation of the Fc region), which leads to the phagocytosis of the epitope-antibody-FcR complex. Antibodies that have not bound one or more epitopes do not bind to FcRs, and in this way, an antibody that has not bound to an epitope remains in circulation. The Fc receptor that binds IgE is the exception, which binds IgE molecules that have not yet encountered their epitopes; intracellular signaling does not occur until the IgE antibody binds the appropriate antigen.

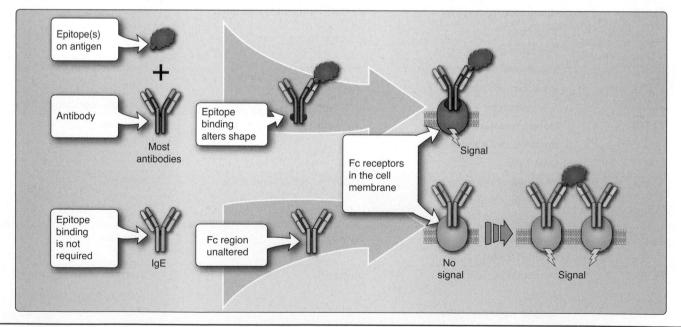

Figure 2.8
Fc Receptors. Like complement receptors, Fc receptors permit phagocytes to identify and ingest microbes and molecules that antibodies have previously "tagged" for destruction. The receptor for IgE is an exception, however. It binds free IgE and no cellular signalling occurs prior to the binding of antigen to the IgE.

B. Somatically generated receptors

The preformed receptors of the innate immune system (e.g., PRRs, TLRs, and complement) are encoded in the germline and passed on intact from one generation to the next. In contrast, the specialized receptors of B cells and T cells of the adaptive immune system are regenerated anew in the lymphocytes of each individual through random somatic chromosomal rearrangements and mutations. The result is a vast array of receptors specific for precise molecular details found in unique epitopes that may be encountered in the future.

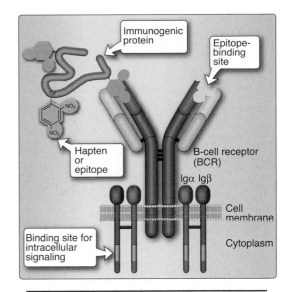

1. **B cell receptors:** B cell receptors (BCRs) are composed of monomeric immunoglobulin (see Chapter 8) associated with disulfide-linked heterodimers called Igα and Igβ (Fig. 2.9). When a BCR binds an epitope, the specialized cytoplasmic tails of Igα and Igβ initiate an intracellular signaling cascade that may lead to B cell activation. In addition, some activated B cells terminally differentiate into **plasma cells**, which secrete immunoglobulins that have the same epitope-binding specificity as their BCR. The structure and function of immunoglobulins are described in greater detail in Chapters 8 and 9.

Figure 2.9

Immunoglobulins serve as B-cell receptors (BCRs). B cells bear receptors that arc composed of two identical large (heavy) chains and two identical smaller (light) chains. Molecules such as Igα and Igβ are associated with BCRs and help provide a signal to the cell when the BCR binds an epitope.

2. **T cell receptors:** Structurally similar to immunoglobulin molecules, **T cell receptors** (TCRs) are heterodimers, consisting of either an αβ or a γδ chain pair (an αβ receptor is shown in Figure 2.10; γδ receptors have similar structures). TCRs are always membrane bound and recognize antigen combined with MHC molecules. They are associated with the **cluster of differentiation 3** or **CD3 complex** of transmembrane surface molecules. The CD3 complex functions much like the Igα and Igβ of BCRs in that it links the TCR with intracellular signaling molecules. An additional accessory molecule (CD4 or CD8) is also present to serve as a type of coreceptor for the TCR. The structure and function of the T cell receptors are described in greater detail in Chapters 8 and 9.

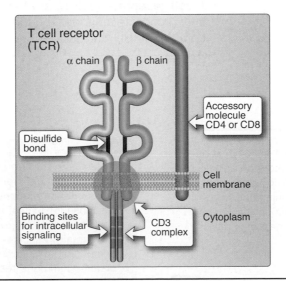

Figure 2.10

αβ T cell receptors (TCRs). T cells bear receptors that are composed of two chains, either an α-β combination (shown) or a γ-δ combination. The CD3 complex is associated with the TCR and facilitates cell signalling (see Chapter 10).

Chapter Summary

- Antigens contain one or more **epitopes** or antigenic determinants, the basic units recognized by immune receptors.

- Antigens may be classified as **immunogens** if they stimulate an immune response, as **haptens** if they induce an immune response only when coupled to an immunogenic carrier molecule, or as **tolerogens** if they cause cells of the immune system to become selectively unresponsive to reexposure to these same molecules.

- Preformed receptors on cells of the **innate immune system** allow a rapid host response to a pathogen. The **adaptive immune system** uses somatically generated receptors.

- **Pattern recognition receptors** (PRRs) bind **pathogen-associated molecular patterns** (PAMPs), which are combinations of sugars, proteins, lipids, and nucleic acids on pathogens, resulting in inflammation with the goal of destroying the pathogen.

- **Toll-like receptors** (TLRs) mediate cytokine production to promote inflammation and trafficking of immune cells to the site.

- **Natural killer** (NK) cells use **killer activated receptors** (KARs) to identify abnormal host cells and **killer inhibitor receptor**s (KIRs) to inhibit their destruction when not appropriate.

- **Complement receptors** (CRs) are displayed on phagocytic cells and B cells that allow for recognition of microbes and immune complexes.

- **Fc receptors** (FcRs) bind epitope-antibody complexes and stimulate phagocytosis.

- Monomeric immunoglobulins serve as epitope-specific **B cell receptors** (BCRs); B cells upon maturation differentiate into **plasma cells** that secrete immunoglobin with a specificity identical to that of the membrane-bound BCR.

- **T cell receptors** (TCRs) exist solely in membrane-bound forms and recognize epitopes bound by **major histocompatibility complex** (MHC) molecules.

Study Questions

2.1 Dansyl (5-dimethylaminonaphthalene-1-sulfonyl) is a synthetic molecule that binds to receptors on certain B cells but does not stimulate them to produce dansyl-specific antibodies unless it is first conjugated to a larger, immunogenic molecule such as bovine serum albumin. These findings indicate that dansyl is a(n):

   A. adjuvant.
   B. carrier.
   C. hapten.
   D. immunogen.
   E. tolerogen.

The answer is C. Dansyl is a hapten in that it meets three criteria: It is a synthetic molecule; by itself, it does not stimulate an immune response; and when it is coupled to an immunogenic molecule, an immune response is stimulated toward both dansyl and the immunogen. An adjuvant increases the intensity of an immune response. A carrier molecule is also an immunogen. An immunogen is a substance that stimulates an immune response. A tolerogen causes unresponsiveness.

2.2 Which of the following is most likely to induce the greatest adaptive immune response in a 25-year-old-man?

    A. 250,000-Da plasma protein from the same 25-year-old human male

    B. 150,000-Da toxin produced by bacteria

    C. 500-Da plasma protein from a chimpanzee

    D. 400-Da cholesterol molecule from an unrelated human female

    E. 200-Da carbohydrate molecule common to all species

The answer is B. Bacterial toxins are often very immunogenic. An individual should normally not make adaptive immune responses against her or his own plasma proteins. A 500-Da plasma protein from a chimpanzee is small enough to "fall under the radar" of the adaptive immune system, most likely because it lacks sufficient numbers of epitopes. A cholesterol molecule is most likely not immunogenic irrespective of size. Immune responses in normal individuals will not be directed against carbohydrates that their tissues or fluids express.

2.3 During an early part of its development, the binding of a lymphocyte's antigen receptor to its specific epitope may result in the inactivation or death of that cell. Under these circumstances, the epitope in question would be described as a(n)

    A. adjuvant.

    B. carrier.

    C. hapten.

    D. immunogen.

    E. tolerogen.

The answer is E. A tolerogen is a molecule that selectively causes unresponsiveness by the adaptive immune system. In contrast, an adjuvant serves to increase immunogenicity. A carrier and an immunogen induce adaptive immune responses. A hapten cannot induce an immune response unless it is chemically bound to an immunogen.

2.4 Natural killer cells lyse Epstein-Barr virus–infected B cells with deficient MHC I expression. The NK receptors that initiate the lytic activity are

    A. complement receptors.

    B. Fc receptors.

    C. killer activation receptors.

    D. killer inhibition receptors

    E. T cell receptors.

The answer is C. Natural killer (NK) cells scrutinize nucleated cells using killer activation receptors (KARs) that detect stress molecules (MICA and MICB) expressed on cells in response to intracellular infection. Epstein-Barr virus infection causes cells to display stress molecules and at the same time decrease their expression of MHC class I molecules. Engagement of KAR triggers the lytic activity by the NK cells. Killing of the target cells will proceed unless killer inhibition receptors (recognizing MHC class I molecules on the targets cells) are appropriately engaged. If KIR are not engaged at a sufficient level, the KAR-initiated lysis proceeds. Complement receptors bind activated fragments of complement that occur in the extracellular environment. Fc receptors bind antibodies that engage extracellular environment antigens. NK cells do not express T cell receptors.

2.5 Antibody mediated recruitment of macrophages occurs through action of

    A. complement receptors.

    B. Fc receptors.

    C. killer activation receptors.

    D. pattern recognition receptors.

    E. toll-like receptors.

The answer is B. Binding to an epitope causes a conformation change in the Fc portion of the antibody molecule. Fc receptors (FcRs) recognize and bind to the conformationally altered antibody molecule, and this engagement of epitope-bound antibody by FcRs stimulates phagocytosis of cells and molecules "tagged" by antibodies for destruction. Complement receptors bind and facilitate the phagocytosis of cells and molecules tagged by complement components or fragments. Killer activation receptors, pattern recognition receptors, and toll-like receptors do not recognize antigen-antibody complexes.

2.6 A 7-year-old girl has a history of peanut allergy with symptoms that include generalized itching and hives after eating peanuts. Her symptoms became more severe with subsequent accidental exposures to peanuts. For this child, a peanut is most likely a(n)

A. adjuvant.
B. hapten.
C. immunogen.
D. innate immune system antigen.
E. tolerogen.

The answer is C. Repeated exposure to peanuts intensifies the immune reaction, indicating that the child most likely has developed an adaptive immune response to a peanut protein. A tolerogen would serve to diminish the immune response upon repeated exposure. It is unlikely that an adjuvant is present that would intensify her allergic response to peanuts. Peanuts by themselves induced this response, but a hapten will not induce an immune response. The fact that the immune response intensifies upon repeated exposure effectively rules out an innate immune response.

2.7 Epitope binding before Fc receptor engagement is not required for

A. carrier molecules.
B. hapten-carrier conjugates.
C. haptens.
D. IgE.
E. IgG.

The answer is D. Fc receptors only engage the "tail" or Fc portion of immunoglobulin (Ig) molecules. Only IgE is bound to the appropriate Fc receptor prior to epitope binding. Fc receptor binding is not required for haptens, carriers, or their conjugates.

2.8 Cells of the immune system are triggered by the binding of surface receptors. In general, the action taken is determined by

A. a single receptor per cell.
B. a single type of receptor found on all cells.
C. the integration of signals generated by multiple receptors on single cells.
D. multiple receptors that bind soluble ligands only.
E. nonspecific receptors capable of binding a wide array of ligands.

The answer is C. Cells bear many types of receptors, each capable of specifically binding a different ligand. The signals generated by the binding of various combinations of receptors on the surface of a given cell are integrated by that cell and used to determine the action to be taken.

UNIT II
The Innate Immune System

Our initial immune defenses rely on types of cells and molecules that have performed admirably for hundreds of millions of years. Early in the history of life, organisms developed mechanisms to ask whether a particular cell was "self or nonself" and "friend or foe." As life diversified, different groups of organisms developed specialized molecules with restricted distribution. For example, bacteria expressed molecules that were not expressed by protozoa or by algae—or by trees or by humans. Over time, these group-specific markers enabled one type (e.g., multicellular animals) to encode and synthesize receptors able to recognize and bind molecules that are characteristic of other groups (e.g., bacteria). As a result, organisms encoded within their genomes a series of "hard-wired" receptors capable of a type of self-nonself distinction.

Some of these hard-wired receptors functioned as soluble molecules. Upon recognizing and binding to a nonself intruder, they could initiate a series of enzymatic reactions that might directly destroy the intruder or at least render it more susceptible to some other means of destruction. Other receptors were placed on the surface of certain host cells that moved around in the body. These cells, generically termed phagocytes, often have janitorial duties: clearing the body of debris. But when, in the course of their duties, their receptors detect the presence of nonself, phagocytes undergo a change of personality. They become angry and aggressive. Like a mild-mannered Clark Kent, they "step into a telephone booth" and emerge as Superman, with powers to attack and destroy the intruders they have intercepted. It is upon these soluble and membrane-bound hard-wired receptors that the human innate immune system is built.

Barriers to Infection

3

I. OVERVIEW

We live in a microbial world. Our bodies are constantly surrounded by astronomical numbers of microbes (Table 3.1). In addition to the microbes themselves, the molecules they produce and some molecules from other environmental sources (e.g., venoms) can also injure body cells and tissues. The body has several mechanical, chemical, and biologic **barriers** that provide the first line of defense against the entry of microbes into the aseptic, nutrient-rich environment of our tissues. These barriers can be thought of as the moats and thick walls that provided the initial protection to the inhabitants of castles under enemy attack.

II. PHYSICAL BARRIERS

The initial mechanical barriers that protect the body against invasive microbes include the epidermis and keratinocytes of the skin; the epithelium of the mucous membranes of the gastrointestinal, respiratory, and urogenital tracts; and the cilia in the respiratory tract (Fig. 3.1). These mechanical barriers also incorporate a number of chemical and biologic barriers that minimize or prevent entry of potential pathogenic organisms into the body.

A. Skin

The epidermis or outer layer of skin varies in thickness from 0.05 to 1.5 mm depending upon location (Fig. 3.2). The outermost of the five layers of the epidermis, or *stratum corneum*, is composed of dead, tightly layered, and cornified squamous cells. Produced by **keratinocytes** of the lower four layers, cells of the stratum corneum provide a water-tight barrier that both prevents our dehydration and provides a microbe-inhospitable dry environment on the surface of our skin. Continuously dividing keratinocytes and constant sloughing of the superficial epidermal layer removes microbes attached to cutaneous surfaces.

B. Mucous membranes

The epithelium of mucous membranes lines all of the body's cavities that come into contact with the environment, such as the respiratory, gastrointestinal, and urogenital tracts (Fig. 3.3). This epithelium contains goblet cells that secrete mucus. It is estimated that 4 liters of mucus are secreted within the gastrointestinal tract alone on a daily basis (although much of it is resorbed in the large intestine). In the

Table 3.1
OUR MICROBIAL ENVIRONMENT

Location	Bacterial Load	
Skin	10^3 per cm^2	10^{12} total
Scalp	10^6 per cm^2	
Nasal mucus	10^7 per gram	
Saliva	10^8 per gram	
Mouth	—	10^{10} total
Feces	$>10^8$ per gram	
Alimentary tract	—	10^{14} total

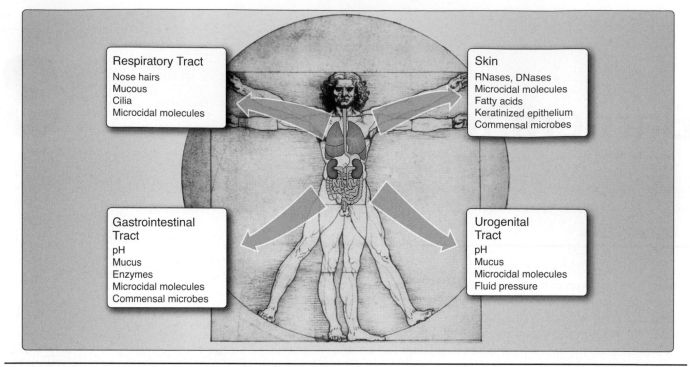

Figure 3.1
Protective barriers of the body. The barriers of the body represent the first line of defense and prevent or retard the entry cells and molecules into the body.

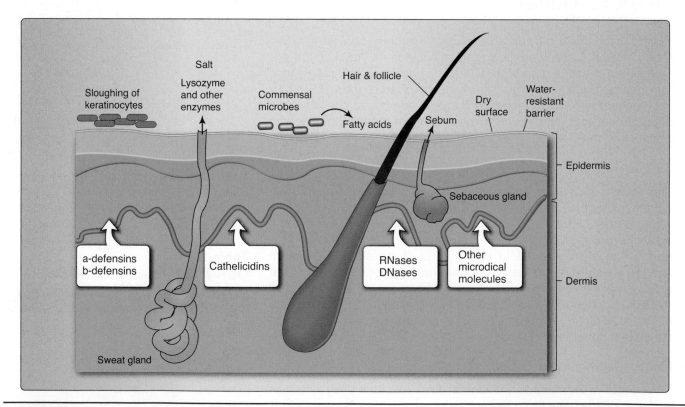

Figure 3.2
Skin contains a variety of defense mechanisms. The epidermis provides a dry, watertight barrier continually sloughing dead cells (keratinocytes). Dermal glands bathe the epidermis with microcidal molecules as well as with sebum and sweat producing an acidic pH and deposit salt on the surface of the skin. The dermis contains additional defense molecules and phagocytic molecules (e.g., neutrophils, macrophages) that attack invaders. Commensal microbes secrete fatty acids that inhibit colonization by other microbes.

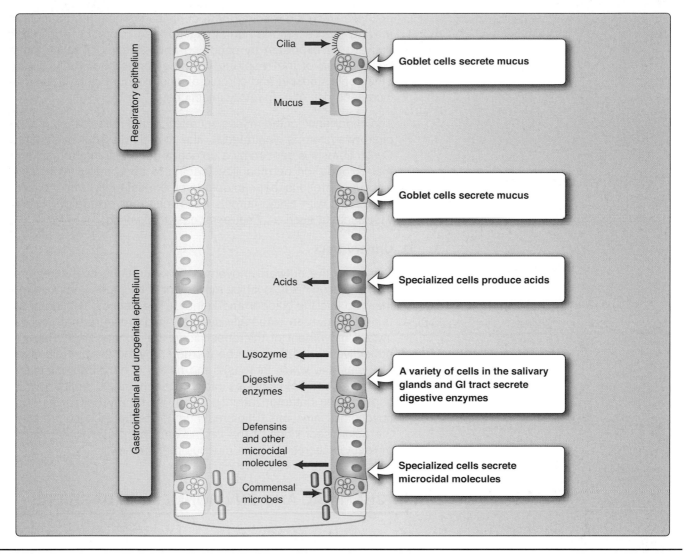

Figure 3.3
Defense mechanisms of the mucous membranes. Mucus entraps microbes and particulate matter (which, in the respiratory tract, is swept out by cilia). Protective commensal microbes are present, and numerous microcidal molecules, enzymes, and acids are produced.

respiratory tract, the mucus traps inhaled bacteria, fungi, and other particles. In the gastrointestinal tract, the mucus and mucous membranes help to protect the epithelial cells and underlying tissues from damage by digestive enzymes and to propel ingested matter through the tract. Mucosal surfaces of the moist epithelium facilitate the exchange of molecules with the environment while also resisting microbial invasion. Additionally, the sloughing of the intestinal epithelial cells has a protective effect similar to that from the sloughing of keratinocytes in the skin.

C. Respiratory tract

Air turbulence caused by hairs within the nostrils deposits particles larger than 10 μm in the nasal mucosa. The hairlike **cilia** of the epithelia lining the respiratory tract passages help the tract clean by moving the secretions containing trapped microbes and particles outward for expulsion by coughing and sneezing. The rhythmically beating cilia of the respiratory epithelium is commonly disrupted by chronic smoking and chronic alcohol consumption, leading to an increased risk of respiratory infections.

The importance of the mucus secreted by the membranes of the respiratory system is illustrated by the genetic disorder cystic fibrosis. Cystic fibrosis is caused by a defective gene that interferes with normal chloride ion permeability, leading to abnormally thickened and viscous secretions that can obstruct the respiratory tract. As a result, individuals with cystic fibrosis have recurrent respiratory infections with bacteria such as *Pseudomonas aeruginosa.*

D. Urinary tract

Similar to the outward movement of secretions of the respiratory tract, urination helps to inhibit movement of microbes from the environment up into the bladder and kidneys. The periodic voiding of sterile urine provides an externally directed fluid pressure that inhibits the inward movement of microbes along the urinary tract. This simple protective mechanism can be disrupted by the therapeutic insertion of a catheter, which increases the risk of urinary tract infections by facilitating entry of microbes into the urinary tract. Urinary tract infections due to catheterization account for nearly half of all hospital nosocomial infections. The female urogenital tract is also protected by the acidic secretions of the vagina and the presence of microcidal molecules secreted by the mucous membranes.

III. CHEMICAL AND ENVIRONMENTAL BARRIERS

The acidic pH of the skin, stomach, and vagina serves as a chemical barrier against microbes. Microcidal molecules, such as α-defensins, β-defensins, cathelicidin, RNases, DNases, and lysozyme, which are secreted by a variety of cell types, also provide protective environment barriers.

A. pH

Most pathogens are very sensitive to an acidic environment, where an acid pH (less than 6) inhibits the growth of potential pathogens.

1. **Skin:** The skin contains oil and sweat glands (sebaceous and sudoriferous glands, respectively), some of whose products are slightly acidic. In general, the skin has a pH of about 5.5. **Sebum** is a mix of lipids produced by the sebaceous glands. Excessive sebum secretion is often associated with oily skin and acne, particularly in adolescents, as it can clog skin pores (entrapping and retaining microbes) and create less favorable pH levels.

2. **Stomach:** Compared to the colon, the stomach has very few bacteria because of the highly acidic environment (normal pH of 1.0 to 3.0). The acidic environment of the stomach prevents the colonization of the intestines by ingested microbes.

3. **Vagina:** The acidic environment of the vagina and cervical os in healthy women is normally pH 4.4 to 4.6. This acidic environment is the result of lactic acid production by the commensal bacteria *Lactobacilli* spp. (see Section IV).

B. Microcidal action of secreted molecules

Several tissues that are in contact with the environment synthesize and secrete a variety of **microcidal molecules** that act to inhibit or kill microbes that are attempting to colonize. A few of the primary microcidal molecules are discussed here.

1. **Skin:** The skin is protected in part by several antimicrobial peptides secreted by a variety of cell types found within the skin. Among these are α-defensins, β-defensins, and cathelicidin. All are able to inhibit microbial growth by direct action upon the microbes, perhaps by damaging the microbial membranes and causing lysis. They can also act as chemoattractants for cells of the innate immune system and facilitate the ingestion and destruction of microbes by phagocytes. Fatty acids released by some of the commensal microbes that are present on the skin also act to inhibit growth by some other bacteria.

   Other molecules with enzymatic activity are present in the skin as well. Sweat contains **lysozyme**, an enzyme that breaks down peptidoglycan (a constituent of most bacterial cell walls). Also present in the skin are molecules that act on the RNA and DNA of a wide range of microbes. **RNases** and **DNases**, in fact, are powerful enough to require the wearing of protective gloves while performing molecular biology procedures—not to protect the hands, but to protect the material that is being manipulated from destruction by the enzymes on the skin. Finally, the evaporation of sweat creates a slightly salty environment that inhibits growth of many bacteria.

2. **Respiratory tract:** To protect the mucosal surfaces of the lungs, some cells of the respiratory epithelium secrete microcidal molecules such as β-defensins. These and other molecules in the respiratory tract can attach to microbes and make them more susceptible to ingestion and destruction by phagocytic cells.

3. **Gastrointestinal tract:** The gastrointestinal tract defends against pathogens in many ways. In addition to the low pH of the stomach, some epithelial cells secrete microcidal molecules such as α-defensins and cryptidin that help to destroy many potential pathogens. Approximately 22 different digestive enzymes are released from the salivary glands, stomach, and small intestine. Among these is lysozyme found in saliva. These enzymes help the digestive process but are also effective in killing and degrading many potential pathogens that may be ingested.

4. **Lacrimal secretions:** Lacrimal glands are small almond-shaped structures, located above the outer corner of the eye, that produce tears. As part of protecting the eyes, the secretions of lacrimal glands contain lysozyme.

IV. BIOLOGIC BARRIERS: COMMENSAL MICROBES

Commensal microbes are those that exist in a symbiotic relationship with the body. The skin and the gastrointestinal tract are colonized by over 500 commensal bacterial and other microbial species that are estimated to make up over 95% of the cells present in a normal human body (Table 3.2). Commensal microbes colonizing the skin and gastrointestinal tracts "defend" their territory and inhibit the establishment of other potentially pathogenic microbes. In the gastrointestinal tract, these microbes also assist in the digestive process.

Commensal microbes are not pathogenic (disease-causing) except under special circumstances. For example, commensal microbes can cause disease in people who are immunocompromised (i.e., their immune systems do not function effectively). The introduction of medical devices, such as catheters, into the body can also cause commensal bacteria from the skin to enter areas of the body that are normally sterile. Any disruption of the normal flora of the body may lead to disease. Pseudomembranous colitis is a condition caused by *Clostridium difficile,* a pathogenic bacterium that produces a toxin that damages the gastrointestinal tract and causes watery diarrhea, abdominal cramps, and fever. The condition may occur after a course of broad-spectrum antibiotic therapy. One explanation for the condition is that use of antibiotics reduces the levels of normal commensal bacteria of the gastrointestinal tract, thus permitting the establishment and overgrowth by *Clostridium difficile.*

Chapter Summary

- The body has several mechanical, chemical, and biologic **barriers** that provide the first line of defense against the entry of microbes and toxic molecules.

- The initial mechanical barriers that protect the body against invasive microbes include the epidermis and keratinocytes of the skin; the epithelium of mucous membranes of the gastrointestinal, respiratory, and urogenital tracts; and the cilia in respiratory tract.

- The slightly acidic **pH** of the skin and vagina is inhibitory to microbial growth. The high acidity of the stomach is highly inhibitory.

- **Microcidal molecules** inhibit microbial growth. Present in the skin are molecules such as RNases and DNases, defensins, and cathelicidin. Some cells of the respiratory epithelium secrete β-defensins; some epithelial cells secrete α-defensins and cryptidins.

- **Commensal microbes** are those that exist in a symbiotic relationship with the body. Commensal microbes colonizing the skin and gastrointestinal tracts inhibit the establishment of other potentially pathogenic microbes.

Table 3.2
COMMENSAL MICROBES

Body Area		Common Organisms (Bacterial unless Otherwise Noted)
Skin		*Acinetobacter* spp.
		Staphylococcus spp.
	Scalp	*Malassezia* spp. (fungus)
	Oil glands	*Propionibacterium* spp.
Mouth/throat		*Actinomyces* spp.
		Fusobacterium spp.
		Lactobacillus spp.
		Leptotrichia spp.
		Mycoplasma spp.
		Neisseria spp.
		Staphylococcus spp.
		Streptococcus spp.
Nasal cavity/pharynx		*Corynebacterium* spp.
		Haemophilus influenzae
		Neisseria meningitidis
		Staphylococcus spp.
		Streptococcus spp.
Stomach		*Helicobacter pylori*
Small/large intestine		*Bacteroides* spp.
		Bifidobacterium spp. (breast-fed infants)
		Candida albicans (fungus)
		Clostridium spp.
		Enterobacter spp.
		Escherichia coli
		Klebsiella spp.
		Lactobacillus spp. (bottle-fed infants)
		Proteus spp.
		Pseudomonas aeruginosa
		Streptococcus spp.
Upper respiratory tract		*Corynebacterium catarrhalis*
		Neisseria meningitidis
		Streptococcus spp. (α-hemolytic)
Urogenital tract	Urethral opening	*Corynebacterium* spp.
		Enterococcus faecalis
		Staphylococcus epidermidis
	Vagina	*Candida albicans* (fungus)
		Corynebacterium spp.
		Lactobacillus spp.
		Streptococcus spp.
Eye	Surface	*Staphylococcus* spp.
		Streptococcus spp.
		Branhamella catarrhalis

Study Questions

3.1 A 30-year-old female developed vaginal candidiasis (a fungal infection) after receiving antibiotic therapy for a sinus infection. One possible explanation for the fungal infection is antibiotic-induced reduction in vaginal

A. lysozyme secretion.
B. mucus secretion.
C. normal commensal bacteria.
D. pH.
E. RNases and DNases.

> The answer is C. Use of antibiotics can reduce normal commensal microbe populations, increasing the opportunity for colonization by more pathogenic microbes. Antibiotics do not alter the secretion of mucus and microcidal molecules from the mucous membranes of the vagina. The pH is likewise not reduced by antibiotic use.

3.2 People with cystic fibrosis have recurrent infections with bacteria such as *Pseudomonas aeruginosa* because of respiratory tract changes that include a/an

A. decrease in lysozyme secretion.
B. decrease in mucus secretion.
C. decrease in pH.
D. increase in thickness and viscosity of secretions.
E. increase in watery secretions.

> The answer is D. The genetic defect in cystic fibrosis causes the mucus to be thick and viscous. The mucus is not decreased in volume, pH, or enzymatic content. Nor is it increased in volume.

3.3 During a hospital stay, a catheter was placed into the urethra of a 70-year-old male, who subsequently developed cystitis (urinary bladder infection). One of the factors that most likely contributed to establishment of the infection was

A. epithelial cell facilitation of molecule exchange with the environment.
B. introduction of microbes into the urethra during placement of the catheter.
C. mucus secretion from epithelial cells lining the urinary tract.
D. pH levels in the sterile urine of the catheterized patient.
E. sebaceous and sudoriferous gland secretion of sebum and sweat.

> The answer is B. Placement of a catheter into the urethra can facilitate access of microbes from the external surface. The catheter does not itself alter urinary pH or mucus production. Nor does it affect the respiratory tract or glands of the skin.

3.4 Which of the following is an example of a normal physiologic pH barrier to microbial colonization?

A. respiratory tract pH between 9.0 and 11.0
B. skin pH of approximately 8.0
C. stomach pH between 1.0 and 3.0
D. upper gastrointestinal tract pH between 6.5 and 7.5
E. vaginal pH of approximately 7.0

> The answer is C. Normal stomach pH is between 1.0 and 3.0. The values given for the respiratory tract, skin, upper gastrointestinal tract, and vagina are abnormal.

3.5 Which of the following is a correct pairing of a soluble molecule with its microcidal action in the respiratory tract?

A. β-defensins increase microbial susceptibility to phagocytosis.
B. DNase enzymatically damages microbial membranes.
C. Fatty acids of commensal microbes degrade microbial peptidoglycan.
D. Lacrimal secretions facilitate ingestion of microbes by phagocytes.
E. Lysozyme degrades DNA and RNA produced by pathogenic microbes.

> The answer is A. Peptidoglycan is degraded not by fatty acids or DNase, but by lysozyme. Lysozyme does not act on RNA and DNA. The lacrimal fluid contains lysozyme that acts on microbial peptidoglycan, not on host phagocytes.

Cells of the Innate Immune System

4

I. OVERVIEW

White blood cells or **leukocytes** serve as sentinels and defenders against infection by patrolling the tissues and organs of the body. They move around the body via the lymphatic and blood circulatory systems and can leave and reenter the circulation to move through body tissues. As "soldiers" of the immune system, leukocytes have specialized roles in defense of the body. Leukocytes are classified by morphology, including the number of lobes that their nuclei possess and the presence or absence of microscopically visible granules in their cytoplasm (Fig. 4.1). Histologic structure is often a helpful clue to the cell's function. Some leukocytes may combat invasive organisms directly; others produce soluble molecules that serve as deterrents to microbial invasion throughout the body. Some leukocytes are autonomous, wielding lethal blows against invaders without intervention from other cells. Others are poised for "combat," awaiting "orders" from their superiors. Still others serve as field marshals by regulating the assault. Leukocytes may be found as individual cells throughout the body or as accumulations at the sites of infection or inflammation. A knowledge of the role that each leukocyte plays is important to understanding immune function.

All blood-borne cells ultimately derive from **pluripotent hematopoietic stem cells**. They are called pluripotent because each stem cell has the capacity to produce all leukocytes as well as red blood cells (erythroid lineage) and platelets (thrombocytic lineage). Pluripotent stem cells resident in the bone marrow are the source of lymphocytes and plasma cells; macrophages, monocytes, and dendritic cells; neutrophils, eosinophils, and basophils (the three types of granulocytes—see below); and erythrocytes and platelets. Cells of the **myeloid lineage**, especially those containing cytoplasmic granules (eosinophils, basophils, and neutrophils), together with agranular phagocytic cells (monocytes, macrophages, and dendritic cells) are involved in innate defenses. Other myeloid lineage–derived cells are involved in gas transport (erythrocytes or red blood cells) and in clotting (platelets). Most of the cells derived from the lymphoid lineage (lymphocytes and plasma cells) are responsible for adaptive immune responses (see Unit III). Other cells (natural killer, or NK, cells and the phagocytes) bridge both innate and adaptive immune systems.

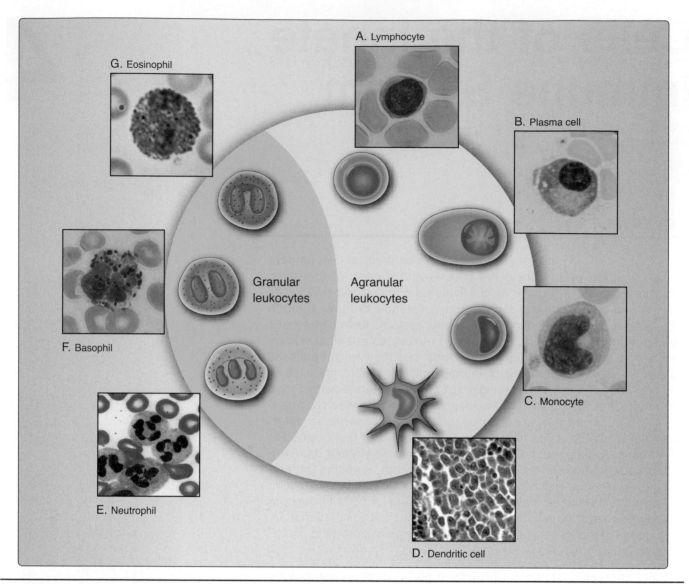

Figure 4.1

Types of leukocytes. White blood cells or leukocytes may be broadly classified by the absence (agranular) or presence (granular) of cytoplasmic inclusions or granules. **A.** Lymphocytes include T, B, and natural killer (NK) cells. **B.** B cells that enlarge and differentiate into immunoglobulin secretors are known as plasma cells. **C.** Monocytes are phagocytic cells in the circulation, and are called macrophages when they enter tissues. **D.** Dendritic cells are phagocytic cells that bear tree-like cytoplasmic processes. **E.** Neutrophils have multilobed nuclei and cytoplasmic granules that stain with neutral (pH) dyes. **F.** Basophils have bilobed nuclei and cytoplasmic granules that stain with basic (pH) dyes. **G.** Eosinophils have bilobed nuclei and cytoplasmic granules that stain with acidic (pH) dyes.

II. AGRANULAR LEUKOCYTES

White blood cells that have multilobed nuclei and contain conspicuous cytoplasmic granules are known as **granulocytes**. Others with a single, unlobed nucleus and cytoplasm that contains few or no granules are known as **agranular leukocytes**. Agranular leukocytes derive from lymphoid or myeloid lineage precursors and account for approximately 35% to 38% of the leukocytes in circulation.

A. Lymphoid lineage cells

Cells that differentiate along the lymphocytic pathways are known as **lymphocytes**. Lymphocytes may differentiate along one of several different pathways (see Fig. 4.2). **B lymphocytes** or **B cells** reside

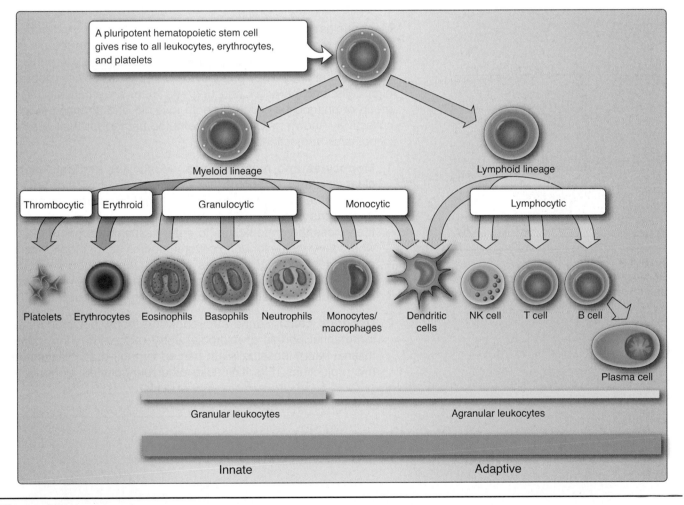

Figure 4.2
Hematopoietic lineages. Pluripotent stems cells within the bone marrow give rise to all the cells found in the blood. Cells of the myeloid lineage differentiate further into platelets, erythrocytes, eosinophils, basophils (and mast cells), neutrophils, monocytes/macrophages and some dendritic cells. Cells of the lymphoid lineage differentiate further into T and B lymphocytes, NK cells, and some dendritic cells.

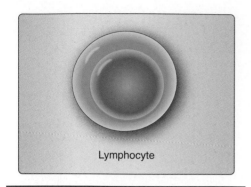

Figure 4.3
Lymphocytes. Except for differing in size
(4- to 15-μm range), lymphocytes generally
look alike, although they may vary functionally.

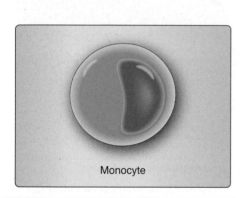

Figure 4.4
Monocytes. Circulating mononuclear phagocytes are called monocytes. When the leave
the circulation and enter tissues they are
called macrophages.

in the bone marrow and are able to synthesize immunoglobulin molecules. In fact, B cells and their further differentiated progeny, **plasma
cells**, are the only cells that are capable of immunoglobulin synthesis. Other lymphoid lineage cells of bone marrow origin migrate to,
differentiate in, and are vetted within the environment of the thymus.
Those cells (**thymocytes**) that exit the thymus are known as thymus-
derived lymphocytes or **T lymphocytes** (**T cells**). We will address
the differentiation and function of B cells, plasma cells, and T cells
and their roles in adaptive immune function in Chapters 7 to 21.

A third lymphoid lineage cell distinct from B and T cells and their
progeny is the **natural killer (NK) cell**. These large, nonphagocytic,
granular lymphocytes are named for their ability to kill abnormal
(e.g., infected or malignant) host cells (Fig. 4.3). They account for 5%
to 10% of all lymphocytes in the circulation.

B. Monocytic lineage cells

Mononuclear cells that differentiate from myeloid precursors are
known as **monocytes** in the circulation or **macrophages** once they
leave the circulation and enter the tissues. These cells are the scavengers of the body. They phagocytose, or pick up cellular debris, foreign cells, and particles and degrade them enzymatically. Another
group of phagocytic cells with both myeloid and lymphoid origins is
collectively known as **dendritic cells**, so named for their branchlike
cytoplasmic projections.

1. **Monocytes and macrophages:** Monocytes are large mononuclear cells and account for approximately 5% to 7% of the leukocytes in the peripheral blood (Fig. 4.4). Monocytes spend 1 to 2
   days in the circulation (their half-life is approximately 8.4 hours),
   then cross the endothelium to enter tissues throughout the body,
   where they reside for up to several months as macrophages. Both
   monocytes and macrophages actively sample their environment
   by phagocytosis and serve as scavengers to remove cellular debris. Ingested materials are enzymatically degraded.

2. **Dendritic cells:** Found throughout the body, but predominantly
   in potential portals of microbial entry (e.g., skin, lung, gastrointestinal tract), these cells are named for their branchlike cytoplasmic projections (Fig. 4.5). Like other phagocytes, dendritic cells

Figure 4.5
Dendritic cells. As professional
phagocytes, dendritic cells utilize
their cytoplasmic extensions to
sample their environment.

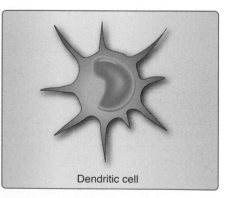

actively engulf cells and particles in their environment by phagocytosis (see Chapter 20). In addition, dendritic cells sample copi-
ous quantities of extracellular fluids by macropinocytosis, in which
their cytoplasmic projections encircle and engulf tissue fluids and
the molecules and particles contained within. Dendritic cells may
arise from either myeloid or lymphoid (also called plasmacytoid)
lineage cells. As actively phagocytic cells, dendritic cells are important in innate immune defenses.

III. GRANULAR LEUKOCYTES

Leukocytes that contain conspicuous cytoplasmic granules are known
as granulocytes. These cells have multilobed nuclei and cytoplasmic
granules that contain amines (stained by basic dyes), basic proteins
(stained with acidophilic or eosinophilic dyes), or both (neutral staining).

A. Neutrophils

Comprising approximately 60% of the peripheral blood leukocytes,
neutrophils are the most numerous leukocyte population. They are
also called **polymorphonuclear (PMN) cells** because of their variable number of nuclear segments (two to five). With a half-life of approximately 7 hours, over 100 billion neutrophils enter the circulation
daily in normal adults. It takes about two weeks for metamyelocytes
(an intermediate stage neutrophil with a kidney-shaped nucleus)
to differentiate from the juvenile or band form (with an elongating
nucleus), to the staff or stab (German, meaning "staff") form, and
then to the segmented or mature stage (Fig 4.6). Neutrophils are
very effective at killing bacteria. An increase in the number of peripheral blood neutrophils is often an indication of acute infection. As re-
serves of PMNs within the bone marrow become exhausted during
an infectious disease, the number of metamyelocytes and juvenile
forms increase in the circulation.

B. Basophils and mast cells

The acidic cytoplasmic granules of **basophils** contain vasoactive
amines (e.g., histamine) that cause smooth muscle contraction and
are readily stained with "base-loving" dyes (Fig. 4.7). These bilobed

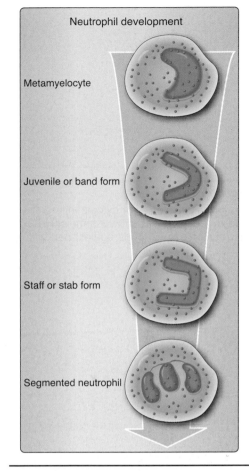

Figure 4.6
Neutrophil development. Neutrophils are the
most numerous leukocytes and play a vital
role in policing the body against microbial
invasion. They require about two weeks to
mature from metamyelocytes through intermediate stages and become mature segmented neutrophils.

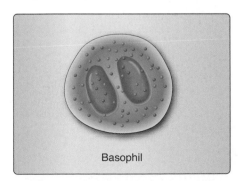

Figure 4.7
Basophils. Release of their cytoplasmic granules (degranulation)
disseminates vasoactive amines
and other molecules associated
with allergic reactions.

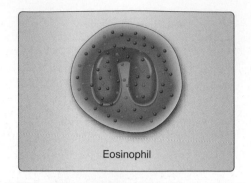

Eosinophil

Figure 4.8
Eosinophils. Release of cytoplasmic granules by eosinophiles provides molecules that are potent weapons against parasitic worms.

cells are found in low numbers in the peripheral blood (0% to 1%) or in their tissue resident form, known as **mast cells**. Both basophils and mast cells are important in allergic reactions of the adaptive immune response (discussed in Chapter 14).

C. Eosinophils

So named because of their "eosin-loving" granules (eosin is a dye used in histology), **eosinophils** are bilobed granulocytes with cytoplasmic granules that contain basic proteins. Although they comprise 0% to 5% of the peripheral blood leukocytes, eosinophils are active participants in innate and adaptive immune responses to parasitic helminth (worm) infections (Fig. 4.8).

Chapter Summary

- All blood-borne cells ultimately derive from **pluripotent hematopoietic stem cells** that have the capacity to produce all **leukocytes**, **red blood cells**, and **platelets**.

- Cells of the **myeloid lineage** (**eosinophils**, **basophils**, **neutrophils**, **monocytes**, **macrophages**, and some **dendritic cells**) are involved in innate immune defenses.

- Many of the cells derived from the **lymphoid lineage** (**lymphocytes** and **plasma cells**) are responsible for adaptive immune responses.

- **Agranular leukocytes** derive from lymphoid or myeloid lineage precursors and account for approximately 35% to 38% of the leukocytes in circulation.

- **B cells** and **plasma cells** are the only cells capable of **immunoglobulin synthesis**.

- Mononuclear cells (**monocytes** and **macrophages**) are the scavengers of the body. They phagocytose; that is, they pick up cellular debris, foreign cells, and particles and degrade them enzymatically.

- **Natural killer cells** large, nonphagocytic, granular lymphocytes that kill abnormal (e.g., infected or malignant) host cells and account for 5% to 10% of all lymphocytes in the circulation.

- Sixty percent of the peripheral blood leukocytes are **neutrophils**. These cells are very effective at killing bacteria.

Study Questions

4.1 Which of the following types of cells are notable for their presence at the sites of helminth infections?

   A. basophils
   B. eosinophils
   C. lymphocytes
   D. monocytes
   E. neutrophils

The answer is B. Eosinophils contain cytoplasmic granules that serve as potent agents against infection by parasitic worms (helminths). Basophils do not migrate to the site of an infection. Although lymphocytes, monocytes, and neutrophils will migrate to infection sites, eosinophils uniquely migrate to parasitic worm infection sites.

4.2 Natural killer cells are members of which of the following families of leukocytes?

   A. basophils
   B. eosinophils
   C. lymphocytes
   D. monocytes
   E. neutrophils

The answer is C. Natural killer (NK) cells are lymphocytes and are often described as large, granular, non-T, non-B lymphocytes. Although they do contain cytoplasmic granules, these are considerably less prominent than those found in granulocytes (basophils, eosinophils, and neutrophils). Nor are NK cells members of the monocyte family.

4.3 A 16-year-old-boy has acute appendicitis (infection of the appendix). Which of the following blood cells is most likely to increase in number as a result of his condition?

   A. basophils
   B. eosinophils
   C. lymphocytes
   D. monocytes
   E. neutrophils

The answer is E. A marked increase in blood neutrophils is a hallmark of infection. Basophils and eosinophils are rarely seen in the circulation in numbers that exceed 5% of the blood-borne leukocytes. Monocytes and lymphocytes increase in notable numbers usually only in chronic disorders.

4.4 Which of the following cells are important effector cells in allergic reactions?

   A. basophils
   B. dendritic cells
   C. lymphocytes
   D. monocytes
   E. neutrophils

The answer is A. Blood-borne basophils and tissue resident mast cells are responsible for allergic responses caused by the release of vasoactive amines within their cytoplasmic granules. Dendritic cells, lymphocytes, and monocytes all play roles in adaptive immune responses, but are not the actual effector cells in allergic reactions. Neutrophils actively destroy invasive bacteria.

4.5 Which of the following cells sample their extracellular environment by macropinocytosis?

   A. basophils
   B. dendritic cells
   C. eosinophils
   D. macrophages
   E. neutrophils

The answer is B. Dendritic cells use two mechanisms to sample their extracellular environment. One, phagocytosis, internalizes by endocytosis molecules and cells that are bound to the cell's surface receptors. The other, macrophagocytosis, involves the engulfment of extracellular fluids by cytoplasmic projections. Basophils, eosinophils, macrophages, and neutrophils do not use macrophagocytosis.

4.6 Red blood cells are derived from

   A. granulocytic lineage cells
   B. lymphocytic lineage cells
   C. monocytic lineage cells
   D. myeloid lineage cells
   E. thrombocytic lineage cells

The answer is D. Erythrocytes or red blood cells derive from myeloid lineage cells. Erythrocytes play a unique role in the blood in the transport of gases to and from lungs to the tissues. None of the other cells derived from granulocyte (basophils, eosinophils, and neutrophils), lymphocytic (B and T lymphocytes, NK cells, and plasma cells), monocytic (monocytes, macrophages, and dendritic cells), and thrombocytic (platelets) lineages produce cells responsible for gas exchange.

4.7 A subset of which of the following of these undergo
further differentiation within the thymus?

    A. basophils
    B. eosinophils
    C. lymphocytes
    D. monocytes
    E. neutrophils

> The answer is C. Thymus-derived or T cells are a subset of lymphocytes. None of the other cell types differentiate within the thymus.

4.8 Three days ago, an otherwise healthy 17-year-old boy
sustained a skin laceration during a lacrosse match.
Yesterday, he complained of mild "flulike" symptoms.
This morning, he became suddenly ill with a fever,
general muscle aches, and dizziness; then he lost
consciousness. Upon arrival in the emergency department, he had a temperature of 37.8°C and a heart
rate of 136 beats per minute. His blood leukocyte
count was 22,000 cells per μl (reference range:
4500 to 12,500 per μl). The predominant cell type(s)
in this patient's blood is/are most likely

    A. B lymphocytes.
    B. juvenile and mature neutrophils.
    C. monocytes and macrophages.
    D. natural killer cells.
    E. T lymphocytes.

> The answer is B. Numbers of circulating neutrophils (mostly segmented form) quickly increase upon an acute infection. Such numbers are recruited that some juvenile forms are pressed into the circulation prior to their maturation. B and T lymphocytes, natural killer (NK) cells, and monocytes and macrophages do not show the same rate of increase.

4.9 Lymphoid lineage cells

    A. are the most numerous leukocyte population.
    B. consist of B, T, and NK cells.
    C. contain conspicuous cytoplasmic granules.
    D. differentiate from myeloid cell precursors.
    E. phagocytose debris and foreign cells.

> The answer is B. Lymphocytes including bone-marrow derived (B cells), thymus-derived (T cells), and natural killer (NK) cells derive from lymphoid lineage cells. They account for fewer than 40% of blood leukocytes; neutrophils are the most numerous. Lymphoid lineage cells are agranular leukocytes and are also poorly phagocytic.

Innate Immune Function

5

I. OVERVIEW

If microbes should penetrate the body's first line of defense—the mechanical, chemical, and biological barriers—the **innate immune system** provides the second line of defense (the first immunologic line of defense) against infection. Because its components are always in an activated or near-activated state, responses by the innate immune system occur much faster than those of the adaptive immune system that provides the third line of defense (the second immunologic line of defense). Once the adaptive system becomes involved, the innate and adaptive immune systems often interact with one another to coordinate their activities. To respond quickly, components of the innate immune system are genetically programmed to recognize molecules associated with broad classes of pathogens. Innate immune responses include the rapid destruction of an infectious organism, activation of phagocytic cells, and the localized protective response known as **inflammation.** In inflammation, innate (and sometimes adaptive) cells and molecules are stimulated to isolate and destroy infectious agents and trigger tissue repair.

II. RECOGNITION

The innate immune system uses a limited number of **pattern recognition receptors** (**PRRs**) to recognize **pathogen-associated molecular patterns** (**PAMPs**)—conserved, structural features expressed by microbes but not by the host (see Fig. 2.5). Unlike the epitope-specific somatically generated receptors of the adaptive immune system expressed by B and T lymphocytes, genes encoding PRRs are encoded within the genome and require no additional modification. Because the host does not produce PAMPs, the innate immune system is able to discriminate between self and nonself.

A. Pathogen-associated molecular patterns

The innate immune system distinguishes infectious microbes from noninfectious self cells by recognizing a limited number of widely expressed viral and bacterial molecular structures. PAMPs may be sugars, proteins, lipids, nucleic acids, or combinations of these types of molecules. PRRs on phagocytic cells recognize PAMPs either directly or indirectly by cell-surface PRRs or by soluble molecules that engage a microbe prior to cell-surface receptor contact (e.g., complement and complement receptors, discussed later in this chapter). PAMP binding immobilizes the infectious organism and may culminate in its ingestion by phagocytes. In addition, PRR engagement often leads to the activation of the host cell, causing it to alter its activity and increase its secretion of antimicrobial substances (Fig. 5.1).

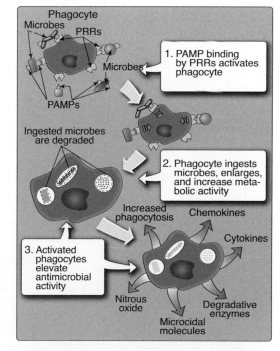

Figure 5.1
PAMP-PRR engagement activates phagocytes. Binding of PAMPs on microbial surfaces by PRRs on the surfaces of phagocytes activates the phagocytes to ingest and degrade the microbes.

Two common bacterial products that contain PAMPs are lipopolysaccharide and peptidoglycan. Bacterial **lipopolysaccharide (LPS)** is a major constituent of the outer cell membrane of Gram-negative bacteria. Cell-surface molecules on monocytes, macrophages, dendritic cells, mast cells, and intestinal epithelial cells bear toll-like receptor 4 (TLR4; see Table 2.2) and other cell-surface molecules that bind LPS. **Peptidoglycans** are major components of the cell walls of Gram-positive bacteria and are recognized by TLR2 receptors on host phagocytic cells (Fig. 5.2). Peptidoglycans are also expressed to a lesser degree and in a slightly different form on Gram-negative bacteria. As a result of receptor engagement, the microbes are ingested and degraded, the macrophage is activated, and cytokine production and inflammation result (see Section IV.A).

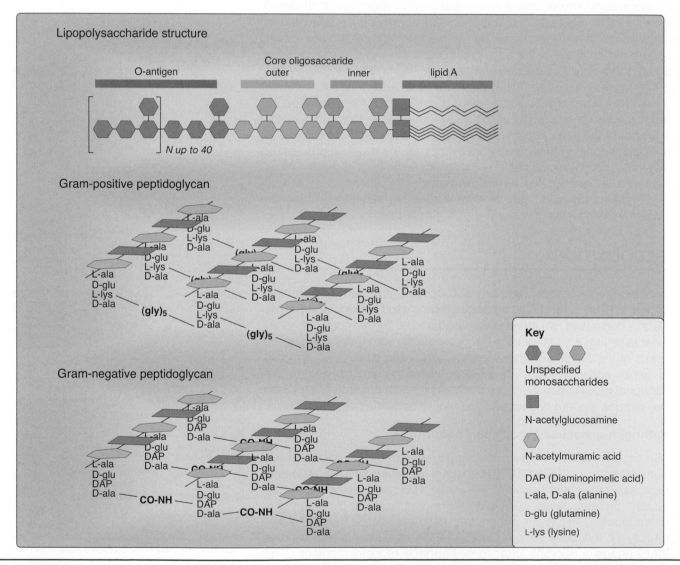

Figure 5.2

Lipopolysaccharide and peptidoglycan structures. Major bacterial PAMPs are found in lipopolysaccharides (carbohydrates + lipids) of Gram-negative bacteria and in peptidoglycans (carbohydrates + proteins) associated with both Gram-negative and Gram-positive bacteria.

B. Pattern recognition receptors

PRRs are divided into the categories described below and are present as extracellular proteins or as membrane-bound proteins on phagocytic cells in the bloodstream. During recognition of PAMPs, multiple receptors may be simultaneously engaged to mediate internalization, activate the killing of microbes, and induce the production of inflammatory cytokines and chemokines.

1. **Toll-like receptors** (**TLRs**) mediate recognition of diverse pathogens. After binding to PAMPs, signal transduction from a TLR to the nucleus leads to enhanced activation of genes encoding cytokines and other molecules involved in antimicrobial activity. The result is synthesis and secretion of the cytokines that promote inflammation and the recruitment of leukocytes to the site of infection.

2. **Scavenger receptors** are involved in binding of modified low-density lipoproteins, some polysaccharides, and some nucleic acids. They are involved in the internalization of bacteria and in the phagocytosis of host cells undergoing apoptosis. The mechanisms involved are currently being investigated.

3. **Opsonins** are molecules that, when attached to the surface of microbes, make them more attractive to phagocytic cells, thus facilitating microbe destruction. Opsonins bind to microbial surfaces. Receptors for opsonins are present on phagocytic cells, and the subsequent increased phagocytic destruction of microbes is termed **opsonization**.

C. Markers of abnormal self

An evasive maneuver that microorganisms sometimes employ to avoid recognition by the immune system is to subvert the host cells. Some viruses cause an infected host cell to reduce its expression of MHC class I molecules that are critical to the proper functioning of the adaptive immune system (discussed in Chapters 7 and 10). Similar changes sometimes occur in cells undergoing cancerous transformation. Host cells that become abnormal as a result of such events can alert the immune system to their situation by expressing molecules on their surfaces that act as stress signals. In humans, these include some heat shock proteins and two molecules known as MICA and MICB (Fig. 5.3). These stress signals are detected by various receptors, including some of the TLRs (e.g., TLR2 and TLR4; see Table 2-2) and the killer activation receptors (KARs) of natural killer (NK) cells (see Section IV.B).

III. SOLUBLE DEFENSE MECHANISMS

In addition to the actions of whole cells, the innate immune system employs soluble molecules as weaponry for protection from viral infection, for lytic destruction of microbes, or for increasing the susceptibility of microbes to ingestion by phagocytic cells.

A. Type I interferons

Type I **interferons** (IFNs) are produced by a subset of dendritic cells (**IFN-α**), by nonleukocytes such as fibroblasts (**IFN-β**), and by other

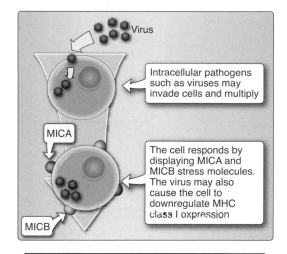

Figure 5.3
Infection of cells may lead to the surface expression of stress molecules. In response to viral infection, host cells may express stress molecules such as MICA and MICB on their surface and may also reduce their surface expression of MHC class I molecules. These surface changes can be detected by NK cells that seek to eliminate virally-infected cells.

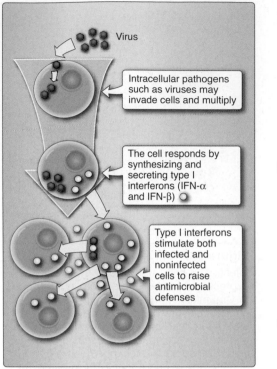

Figure 5.4
Type 1 interferon response to intracellular microbial invasion. Some cells respond to infection by producing and secreting type I interferons that signal adjacent cells to activate their antimicrobial defenses.

cells in response to viral infection (Fig. 5.4). IFN-α and -β are rapidly produced, within 5 minutes, by cells when viral PAMPs interact with certain PRRs. Very little is currently known about the signal transduction pathways responsible for expression and secretion of IFN-α and -β. Secreted type I IFNs induce both virally infected and non-infected cells to activate numerous antiviral defenses, including RNA-dependent protein kinase (PKR) and apoptotic (programmed cell death) pathways. In addition, IFN-α and -β influence the activities of macrophages and dendritic cells.

B. Microcidal molecules

A variety of cells, including epithelial cells, neutrophils, and macrophages, in the skin and mucous membranes secrete cysteine-rich peptides called **defensins.** These peptides form channels in the cell membranes of bacteria, which cause the influx of certain ions and eventually bacterial death. Other molecules with microcidal functions include cathelicidin, lysozyme, DNases and RNases, and others, as discussed in Chapter 3.

C. Complement

Complement is a collective term for a system of enzymes and proteins that function in both the innate and adaptive branches of the immune system as soluble means of protection against pathogens that evade cellular contact. A series of circulating and self-cell-surface regulatory proteins keep the complement system in check. In the innate immune system, complement can be activated in two ways: via the **alternative pathway**, in which antigen is recognized by particular characteristics of its surface, or via the **mannan-binding lectin** (**MBL**) **pathway**. Complement can also be activated in the adaptive immune system via the classical pathway that begins with antigen-antibody complexes (which is described in subsequent chapters) (Fig. 5.5). Regardless of the pathway of activation, functions of complement include lysis of bacteria, cells, and viruses; promotion of phagocytosis (opsonization); triggering of inflammation and secretion of immunoregulatory molecules; and clearance of immune complexes from circulation.

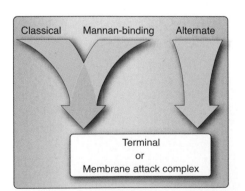

Figure 5.5
Three complement pathways lead to formation of the membrane attack complex.

> **Complement nomenclature**
> - Components C1 through C9, B, $\overline{D}$, and P are native complement (protein) components.
> - Fragments of native complement components are indicted by lowercase letter (e.g., C4a, C5b, Bb). Smaller cleavage fragments are assigned the letter "a," and major (larger) fragments are assigned the letter "b."
> - A horizontal bar above a component or complex indicates enzymatic activity, e.g., $\overline{C4bC2b}$.

1. **The alternative pathway** is initiated by cell-surface constituents that are recognized as foreign to the host, such as LPS (Fig. 5.6). A variety of enzymes (e.g., kallikrein, plasmin, elastase) cleave C3,

the most abundant (~1300 µg/ml) serum complement component, into several smaller fragments. One of these, the continuously present, short-lived, and unstable C3b fragment, is the major **opsonin** of the complement system and readily attaches to receptors on cell surfaces (Fig. 5.7).

1. C3b binds **Factor B**.

2. Factor B in the complex is cleaved by **Factor D̄** to produce $\overline{C3bBb}$, an unstable **C3 convertase**.

3. Two proteins, C3b inactivator (**I**) and β1H-globulin (**H**), function as important negative regulators, making an inactive form of C3b (C3b) to prevent the unchecked overamplification of the alternative pathway.

4. Alternatively, $\overline{C3bBb}$ binds **properdin** (**Factor P**) to produce **stabilized C3 convertase**, $\overline{C3bBbP}$.

5. Additional C3b fragments join the complex to make $\overline{C3bBbP3b}$, also known as **C5 convertase.** C5 convertase cleaves C5 into C5a and C5b.

6. C5b inserts into the cell membrane and is the necessary step leading to formation of the **membrane attack complex** (**MAC**) and cell lysis.

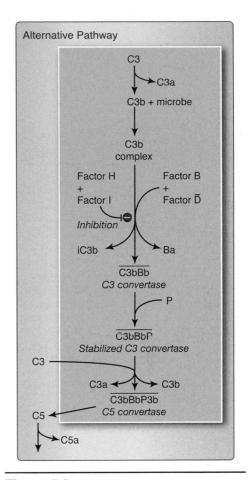

Figure 5.6
Alternative pathway of complement activation. Beginning with the binding of C3b to a microbial surface, this pathway results in an amplified production of C3b and formation of a C5 convertase.

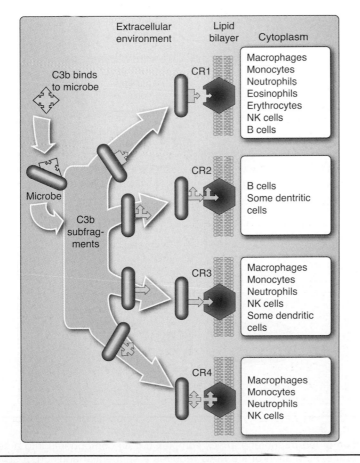

Figure 5.7
Multiple functional roles for complement fragment C3b.

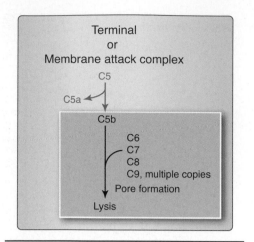

Figure 5.8
Terminal or membrane attack complex (MAC) of complement. The MAC forms a pore in the surfaces of microbes to which it is attached, causing lytic death of those microbes.

2. **The terminal or lytic pathway** can be entered from the alternative, mannan-binding lectin, or classical pathway of complement activation. Attachment of C5b to the bacterial membranes initiates formation of the **membrane attack complex** (**MAC**) and lysis of the cell (Fig. 5.8). The attachment of C5b leads to the addition of components C6, C7, and C8. C8 provides a strong anchor into the membrane and facilitates the subsequent addition of multiple C9 molecules to form a pore in the membrane. Loss of membrane integrity results in the unregulated flow of electrolytes and causes the lytic death of the cell (Fig. 5.9).

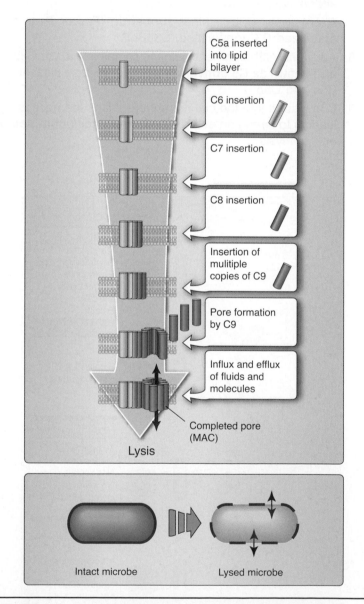

Figure 5.9
Insertion of the membrane attack complex (MAC) components into a cell membrane. Formation of the MAC requires a sequential addition of several complement components, beginning with C5a and terminating with multiple C9 components, to form the pore in the microbial membrane.

3. **Mannan-binding lectin pathway.** **Lectins** are proteins that bind to specific carbohydrates. This pathway is activated by binding of **mannan-binding lectin (MBL)** to mannose-containing residues of glycoproteins on certain microbes (e.g., *Listeria* spp., *Salmonella* spp., *Candida albicans*). MBL is an acute phase protein, one of a series of serum proteins whose levels can rise rapidly in response to infection, inflammation, or other forms of stress. MBL, once bound to appropriate mannose-containing residues, can interact with **MBL-activated serine protease (MASP)**. Activation of MASP leads to subsequent activation of components C2, C4, and C3 (Fig. 5.10).

4. **Anaphylotoxins.** The small fragments (C3a, C4a, C5a) generated by the cleavage of C3 and C5 in the alternative pathway and of C3, C4, and C5 in the MBL pathway act as anaphylotoxins. **Anaphylotoxins** attract and activate different types of leukocytes (Table 5.1). They draw additional cells to the site of infection to help eliminate the microbes. C5a has the most potent effect, followed by C3a and C4a.

D. Cytokines and chemokines

Cytokines are secreted by leukocytes and other cells and are involved in innate immunity, adaptive immunity, and inflammation (Table 5.2). Cytokines act in an antigen-nonspecific manner and are involved in a wide array of biologic activities ranging from chemotaxis to activation of specific cells to induction of broad physiologic changes. **Chemokines** are a subgroup of cytokines of low molecular weight and particular structural patterns that are involved in the **chemotaxis** (chemical-induced migration) of leukocytes. The roles of specific cytokines and chemokines are described in the contexts of the immune responses in which they participate (see Section IV.A of this chapter).

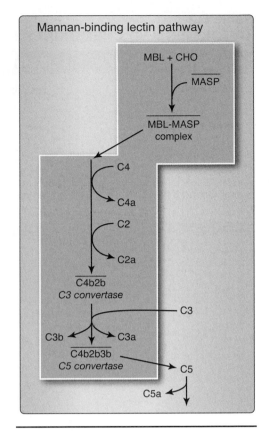

Figure 5.10
Mannan-binding lectin (MBL) pathway of complement activation. The lectin binding pathway is initiated by the binding of certain glycoproteins commonly found on microbial surfaces, and results in the formation of a C3 convertase (that acts to produce C3b) and a C5 convertase (that can lead to MAC formation).

Table 5.1
ANAPHYLOTOXINS IN DECREASING ORDER OF POTENCY

Fragment	Acts on	Actions
C5a	Phagocytic cells	Increased phagocytosis
	Endothelial cells	Phagocyte activation
	Neutrophils	Activation of vascular endothelium
	Mast cells	Attraction/activation of neutrophils
		Mast cell degranulation
C3a	Phagocytic cells	Increased phagocytosis
	Endothelial cells	Phagocyte activation
	Mast cells	Activation of vascular endothelium
		Mast cell degranulation (release of cytoplasmic granules)
C4a	Phagocytic cells	Increased phagocytosis
	Mast cells	Mast cell degranulation

Table 5.2
CYTOKINES AND CHEMOKINES PRODUCED BY ACTIVATED PHAGOCYTES

Cytokine/Chemokine	Acts on	Actions
Interleukin-1 (IL-1)	Vascular endothelium	Increased permeability of vascular endothelium
		Stimulates production of IL-6
Interleukin-6 (IL-6)	Liver	Production of acute phase proteins (e.g., C-reactive protein; elevated temperature (fever)
Interleukin-8 (IL-8)	Vascular endothelium	Activation of vascular endothelium
		Attraction/activation of neutrophils
Interleukin-12 (IL-12)	NK cells	Activates NK cells
		Influences lymphocyte differentiation
Tumor necrosis factor-α (TNF-α)	Vascular endothelium	Increased permeability of vascular endothelium
		Activation of vascular endothelium

IV. CELLULAR DEFENSE MECHANISMS

In addition to soluble means of defense, the innate immune system employs cellular mechanisms to combat infection. Receptors that recognize ligands from pathogens trigger inflammation and destruction of microbes by phagocytes. In addition, NK cells detect and destroy host cells that have been infected, injured, or transformed. We will discuss each of these cellular actions.

A. Phagocytosis

Phagocytosis is the engulfment and degradation of microbes and other particulate matter by cells such as macrophages, dendritic cells, neutrophils, and even B lymphocytes (prior to their activation). These cells are part of the body's "cleansing" mechanism. They not only defend the body by ingesting microbes, but also remove cellular debris and particulate matter that arise from normal physiologic functions.

Phagocytosis involves cell-surface receptors associated with specialized regions of the plasma membrane called **clathrin-coated pits**. Dendritic cells use an additional mechanism to sample large amounts of soluble molecules, a process known as **macropinocytosis**. This process does not involve clathrin. Instead, plasma membrane "ruffles" or projections fold back upon the membrane to engulf extracellular fluids in large intracellular vesicles.

1. **Recognition and attachment of microbes by phagocytes:** Phagocytosis is initiated when a phagocyte binds a cell or molecule that has penetrated the body's barriers. The binding occurs at various receptors on the phagocyte surface (Fig. 5.11). These include PRRs (including TLRs) that recognize microbe-related molecules, **complement receptors** (**CR**) that recognize certain fragments of complement (especially C3b) that adhere to microbial surfaces, Fc receptors that recognize immunoglobulins that have bound to microbial surfaces or other particles (discussed in Chapter 11), scavenger receptors, and others.

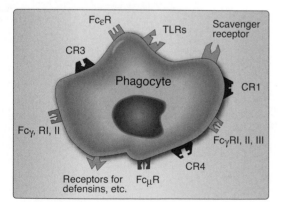

Figure 5.11
Phagocyte receptors. Phagocytosis is initiated when any of several types of receptors on the phagocyte surface recognize an appropriate molecule that indicates the presence of a foreign cell or molecule.

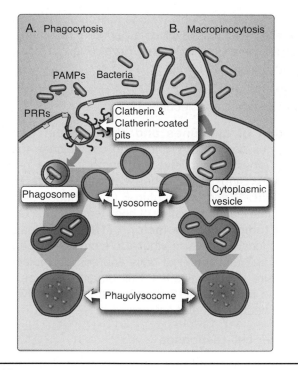

Figure 5.12
Phagocytosis, phagosome, and phagolysosome formation. **A.** In phagocytosis, molecules and particles are captured and ingested by receptors associated with membrane regions called clathrin-coated pits. **B.** In macropinocytosis, protrusions of the plasma membrane capture extracellular fluids whose contents are subsequently ingested. In both cases, the ingested material is degraded in phagolysosomes.

2. **Ingestion of microbes and other material:** Following attachment to the cell membrane, a microorganism or foreign particle is engulfed by extensions of the cytoplasm and cell membrane called **pseudopodia** and is drawn into the cell by internalization or **endocytosis** (Fig. 5.12). In addition to phagocytosis, dendritic cells can extend plasma membrane projections and encircle large amounts of extracellular fluids to form cytoplasmic vesicles independent of cell surface attachment. Once internalized, the bacteria are trapped within **phagocytic vacuoles (phagosomes)** or cytoplasmic vesicles within the cytoplasm. The attachment and ingestion of microbes trigger changes within the phagocyte. It increases in size, becomes more aggressive in seeking additional microbes to bind and ingest, and elevates production of certain molecules. Some of these molecules contribute to the destruction of the ingested microbes; others act as chemotactic agents and activators for other leukocytes.

3. **Destruction of ingested microbes and other materials:** Phagosomes, the membrane-bound organelles containing the ingested microbes/materials, fuse with **lysosomes** to form **phagolysosomes**. Lysosomes employ multiple mechanisms for killing and degrading ingested matter. These include

   • lysosomal acid hydrolases, including proteases and nucleases.
   • several oxygen radicals, including superoxide radicals (O_2^-), hypochlorite (HOCl$^-$), hydrogen peroxide (H_2O_2), and hydroxyl

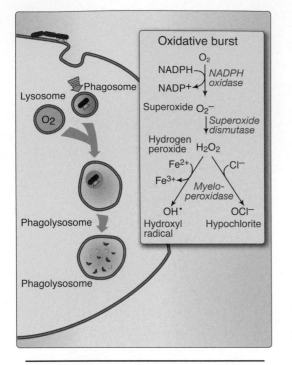

Figure 5.13
Oxidative burst. Phagolysosomes contain
enzymes capable of generating free radicals
that can efficiently kill microbes.

radicals, that are highly toxic to microbes. The combined action
of these molecules involves a period of heightened oxygen uptake known as the **oxidative burst** (Fig. 5.13).

*   nitrous oxide (NO).
*   decreased pH.
*   other microcidal molecules.

4. Secretion of cytokines and chemokines: Once activated,
phagocytes secrete cytokines and chemokines that attract and
activate other cells involved in innate immune responses (see
Table 5-2). Cytokines or chemical messengers such as **inter-
leukin-1 (IL-1)** and **interleukin-6 (IL-6)** induce the production of
proteins that lead to elevation of body temperature. Other cytokines,
such as **tumor necrosis factor-α (TNF-α)**, increase the permeability of local vascular epithelia to increase its permeability and
enhance the movement of cells and soluble molecules from the
vasculature into the tissues. Still others, such as **interleukin-8
(IL-8)** and **interleukin-12 (IL-12)**, attract and activate leukocytes
such as neutrophils and NK cells.

B. Natural killer cell responses

NK cells detect aberrant host cells and target them for destruction
(Fig. 5.14). NK cells possess **killer activation receptors (KAR)** that
recognize stress-associated molecules, including MICA and MICB in
humans, that appear on the surface of infected and transformed
host cells. Binding of KAR to MICA and MICB generates a kill signal.
Before proceeding to kill the targeted cells, however, NK cells use
killer inhibition receptors (KIR) to assess MHC I molecules on the
target cell surface. Expression of these molecules is often depressed
by some viruses and malignant events. If insufficient levels of KIR-MHC
I binding occurs, the NK cell will kill the target host cell. Sufficient
binding by the KIRs will override the KAR kill signal, and the host cell
will be allowed to survive.

V. INFLAMMATION

Components of both the innate and adaptive immune systems may respond to certain antigens to initiate a process known as inflammation.
The cardinal signs of inflammation are **pain** (*dolor*), **heat** (*calor*), **redness**
(*rubor*), **swelling** (*tumor*), and **loss of function** (*functio laesa*). Enlarged
capillaries that result from vasodilation cause redness (**erythema**) and
an increase in tissue temperature. Increased capillary permeability allows
for an influx of fluid and cells, contributing to swelling (**edema**). Phagocytic cells attracted to the site release lytic enzymes, damaging healthy
cells. An accumulation of dead cells and fluid forms pus, while mediators released by phagocytic cells stimulate nerves and cause pain. The
innate immune system contributes to inflammation by activating the
alternative and lectin-binding complement pathways, attracting and
activating phagocytic cells that secrete cytokines and chemokines, activating NK cells, altering vascular permeability and increasing body temperature (Fig. 5.15 and Table 5.2). The adaptive immune system also
plays a role in inflammation, which is discussed in Chapter 11.

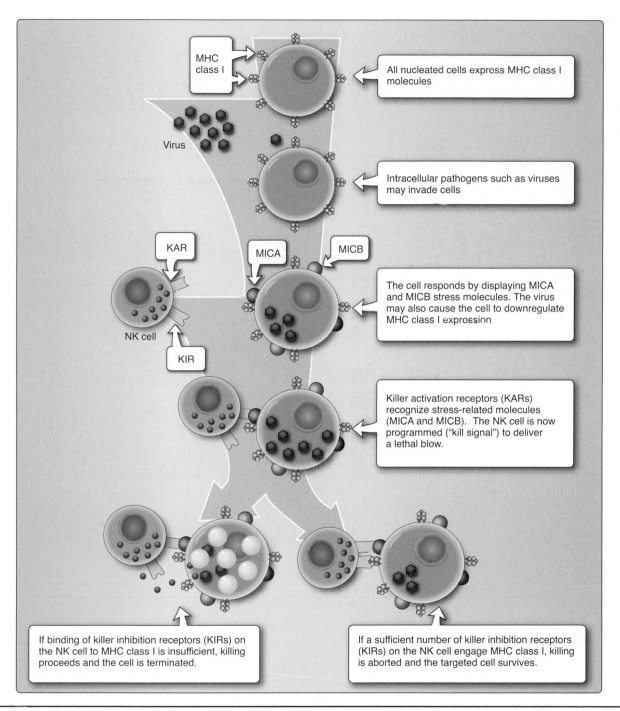

Figure 5.14

NK cell recognition by KIR and KAR. NK cells have killer activation receptors (KARs) that recognize stress-associated molecules (e.g., MICA and MICB in humans) on the surface of abnormal host cells. Binding of KAR to MICA and MICB provides a kill signal. NK cells also use killer inhibition receptors (KIRs) to assess MHC I molecules on the target cell surface. If insufficient KIR-MHC I binding occurs, the NK cell will proceed to kill the target host cell. But sufficient binding by KIRs will override the KAR kill signal, sparing the life of the host cell.

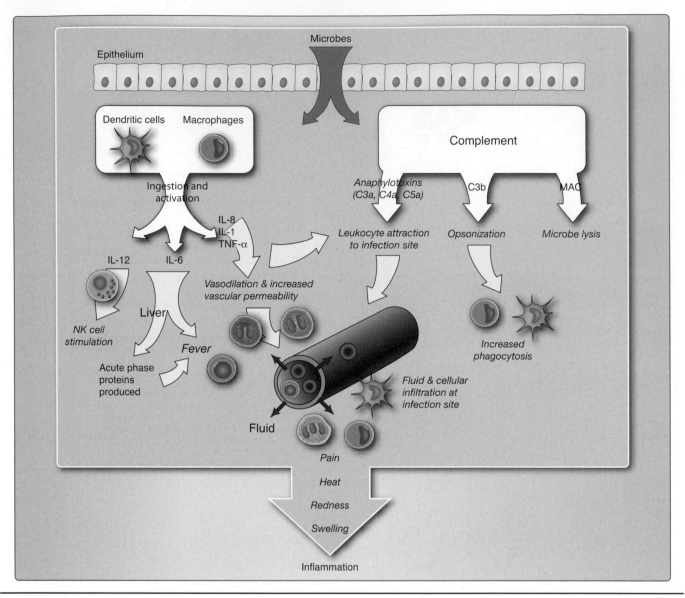

Figure 5.15
Inflammation. Inflammation results from the composite action of several immune responses to infection and injury, and results in pain, heat, redness, and swelling.

Chapter Summary

- The **innate immune system** provides a rapid, initial means of defense against infection using genetically programmed receptors that recognize structural features of microbes that are not found in the host.

- **Pattern recognition receptors** (**PRRs**) on or in **phagocytic cells** bind to **pathogen-associated molecular patterns** (**PAMPs**).

PAMPS are conserved, microbe-specific carbohydrates, proteins, lipids, and/or nucleic acids.

- Common bacterial structures that contain **PAMPs** include **lipopolysaccharides** and **peptidoglycans**.

- **PRR** binding to **PAMPs** results in **phagocytosis** and enzymatic degradation of the infectious organism. PRR engagement can lead to the activation of the host cell and its secretion of antimicrobial substances.

- **Toll-like receptors** are PRRs that bind specific PAMPs. This binding signals the synthesis and secretion of the cytokines to promote inflammation and recruit leukocytes to the site of infection.

- **Scavenger receptors** are PRRs that are involved in internalization of bacteria and in the phagocytosis of host cells undergoing apoptosis.

- **Opsonins** bind to microbes to facilitate their phagocytosis.

- Infected or transformed host cells display **stress molecules** on their surfaces and sometimes show **decreased MHC I expression**.

- Stress molecules are recognized by **killer activation receptors (KAR)** on NK cells. **Killer inhibition receptors (KIR)** on NK cells assess MHC I molecules on the target cell surface.

- Soluble defense molecules include the type I **interferons**, **defensins**, **complement**, and **cytokines**.

- **Complement** is a system of enzymes and proteins that functions in both the innate and adaptive branches of the immune system. In the innate immune system, complement can be activated through either the **alternative pathway** or the **mannan-binding lectin pathway**.

- **Phagocytosis,** a direct mechanism to combat infection, is the engulfment and degradation of microbes by phagocytic cells that secrete cytokines and chemokines to attract and activate other cells of the innate immune system. The oxidative burst, producing several highly reactive oxygen metabolites, and a series of degradation enzymes are important means by which ingested microbes are destroyed.

- The innate immune system contributes to **inflammation** by activating complement pathways, attracting and activating phagocytic cells that secrete cytokines and chemokines, activating NK cells, altering vascular permeability, and increasing body temperature.

- Cardinal signs of inflammation are **pain** (*dolor*), **heat** (*calor*), **redness** (*rubor*), **swelling** (*tumor*), and **loss of function** (*functio laesa*).

Study Questions

5.1 Pathogen-associated molecular patterns

    A. allow B and T lymphocytes to recognize bacteria and destroy them.

    B. are cysteine-rich peptides that form channels in bacterial membranes.

    C. are recognized by pattern recognition receptors of the innate immune system.

    D. closely resemble host cell surface proteins and sugars.

    E. induce secretion of interferons by virally infected host cells.

The answer is C. Pattern recognition receptors of the innate immune system bind structural patterns composed of proteins, sugars, and lipids that are found on microbes but are not found in the human host. This mechanism allows for a rapid and precise recognition of potential pathogens. In contrast, B and T lymphocytes are components of the adaptive immune system in which somatically generated receptors recognize precise molecular details of antigens as opposed to broad structural characteristics found in pathogen-associated molecular patterns.

5.2 A 76-year-old man is diagnosed with *E. coli* septicemia. The initial immune response to *E. coli* (Gram-negative bacteria) will include

A. binding by LPS-binding proteins and delivery to receptors on macrophages.

B. formation of specific somatically generated receptors to bind *E. coli*.

C. generation and secretion of specific antibodies to recognize *E. coli*.

D. production of *E. coli*–specific cytokines by lymphocytes.

E. stimulation of killer activation receptors on NK cells.

The answer is A. LPS of Gram-negative bacteria is recognized by LPS-binding protein in the bloodstream and tissue fluids. The LPS-LPS-binding protein complex is then delivered to the cell membrane of a macrophage, where resident LPS receptors, composed of a complex of proteins (TLR-CD14-MD-2) bind the bacterial LPS. As a result of receptor engagement, the microbes are ingested and degraded, the macrophage is activated, and cytokine production and inflammation result. Actions of somatically generated receptors of B and T cells and of antibodies are part of the adaptive immune response as opposed to the innate response. Cytokines do not have antigen-specific activities, and killer activation receptors on NK cells recognize stress-related molecules on the surfaces of abnormal host cells.

5.3 Double-stranded RNA-dependent protein kinase mediates the action of

A. chemokines.

B. complement.

C. defensins.

D. natural killer cells.

E. type I interferons.

The answer is E. The double-stranded RNA-dependent protein kinase (PKR), a serine/threonine kinase, is a component of host responses to infection and various situations of cellular stress. PKR is a key mediator of interferon (IFN) action, the first line of defense against viral infection. Chemokines are a subgroup of cytokines of low molecular weight that affect chemotaxis of leukocytes. Complement provides a soluble means of protection against pathogens that evade contact with cells of the immune system. Defensins are peptides that form channels in bacterial cell membranes, allowing for increased permeability to certain ions and resulting in death of a variety of bacteria. Natural killer cells detect aberrant host cells and target them for destruction.

5.4 Which of the following are examples of molecules that are expressed on the cell surfaces of human cells that are unhealthy or abnormal?

A. α and β defensins

B. C3 convertase and properdin

C. cytokines and chemokines

D. interferon-α and interferon-β

E. MICA and MICB

The answer is E. Defensins increase bacterial cell permeability to certain ions, resulting in death of the bacteria. C3 convertase and properdin are both components of the complement pathway, a soluble means of protection against pathogens that evade contact with cells of the immune system. Cytokines and chemokines are secreted by a variety of leukocytes and by endothelial cells, and are involved in innate immunity, adaptive immunity, and inflammation. Cytokines act in an antigen-nonspecific manner and are involved in a wide array of biologic activities, while chemokines are a subgroup of cytokines involved in chemotaxis. The type I interferons (interferon-α and interferon-β) are secreted by some virally infected cells in response to the infection.

5.5 The alternative complement pathway is initiated by

A. cell-surface constituents that are recognized as foreign to the host.

B. mannose-containing residues of glycoproteins on certain microbes.

C. stimulation of killer activation receptors on NK cells.

D. the formation of antibody-antigen complexes.

E. toll-like receptor binding to pathogen-associated molecular patterns.

The answer is A. Mannose-containing residues of glycoproteins on certain microbes activate the mannan-binding lectin pathway of complement. Killer activation receptors on NK cells recognize stress-related molecules on the surfaces of abnormal host cells. Antigen-antibody complexes are not required to initiate the alternative complement pathway. Toll-like receptor binding to pathogen-associated molecular patterns stimulates synthesis and secretion of the cytokines to promote inflammation and recruitment of leukocytes to the site of infection.

UNIT III
The Adaptive Immune System

"Those who cannot remember the past are condemned to repeat it."

George Santayana, 1863–1952

Eventually, some types of animals began to add even more items to their immunologic tool kits. These new tools enabled the body to supplement the innate immune system with a new set of protective mechanisms that make up the adaptive immune system. One of these new tools, appearing in organisms as ancient as corals, was the development of molecules that served as identification tags for all the cells of a given body. While these molecules could be variable within a population, each individual in the population (and each cell within that individual) expressed only one or a few forms. Thus the distinction of self from nonself could require not only the absence of nonself molecules, but also the presence of particular self molecules.

A second feature arose in some of the primitive fishes, perhaps around 500 million years ago, that provided a means to expand the number of receptors that could be generated for use in the detection of self and nonself molecules. Enzymes evolved that could delete and reanneal segments of DNA to create new sets of genes encoding receptors. This mechanism gave each individual the capacity to use a limited number of genes (a hundred or less) to generate many millions of different receptors and to enormously increase the scope of the immune system. However, this diversity is clonally distributed within the body. Rather than having specialized immune cells, each bearing the same set of millions of receptors, the adaptive immune system consists of millions of specialized cells, each bearing a single type of rearranged receptor. This ability remains restricted to fishes and the other vertebrates that eventually arose from them.

The clonal nature of the adaptive immune system permitted the emergence of a third feature that enabled the immune system to alter its responses to molecules (whether free or cell-bound) that it encountered on multiple occasions. This ability to modify its activity on the basis of previous exposure is the basis of immunologic memory.

The combination of "self markers," receptors generated by DNA rearrangement, and immunologic memory allows the adaptive immune system to function in ways that the innate system cannot. However, the innate and adaptive immune systems also interact constantly. The innate system is required to "ignite" the adaptive immune system. The adaptive immune system, in turn, can identify an extremely broad range of targets (e.g., a specific part of a specific molecule on a specific infectious organism) and then direct and focus the destructive activities of the innate system upon those targets.

Molecules of Adaptive Immunity

6

I. OVERVIEW

The adaptive immune system uses a broad range of molecules for its activities. Some of these molecules are also used by the innate immune system (see Chapter 5). Others, including antigen-specific B cell receptors (BCR) and T cell receptors (TCR) of B and T lymphocytes, are unique to the adaptive immune system. Immunoglobulins are synthesized by and reside within the cytoplasm and are present on the surfaces of B lymphocytes. Each B cell synthesizes immunoglobulins of a single specificity that bind to a specific molecular structure (epitope). The immunoglobulins on the B cell surface serve as the BCRs. Stimulated B cells may further differentiate into plasma cells that secrete soluble forms of these immunoglobulins. The immunoglobulins recognize and bind to the same epitopes that activate the classical complement pathway. T cells express a wide variety of membrane-bound TCRs. Each T cell produces single-specificity TCRs that recognize a specific peptide epitope contained within a major histocompatibility complex (MHC) molecule. Epitope engagement of BCRs or TCRs leads to the initiation of signal transduction pathways and the expression of both soluble (cytokines and chemokines) and cell-surface (receptors and adhesion) molecules.

II. IMMUNOGLOBULINS

Immunoglobulins are synthesized by **B lymphocytes (B cells)** and are both synthesized and secreted by **plasma cells.** Plasma cells are B cells that have terminally differentiated. The term **antibody** is applied to an immunoglobulin molecule with specificity for an epitope of the molecules that make up antigens (see Chapter 2). Antibodies noncovalently bind to antigens to immobilize them, render them harmless, or "tag" the antigen for destruction and removal by other components of the immune system. In doing so, antibodies facilitate the ability of other cells and molecules in the immune system to identify and interact with antigens. Because antibodies are often in soluble form, they are important components of humoral (soluble) immune responses (see Chapter 11).

A. Basic structure

Human **immunoglobulin** contains four polypeptides: two identical light chains and two identical heavy chains linked by **disulfide bonds** (Fig. 6.1) to form a monomeric unit. Heavy and light chains

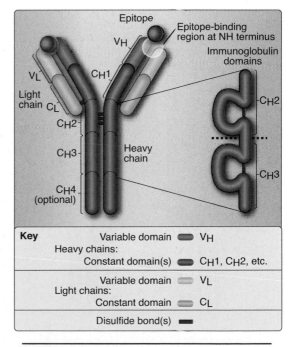

Figure 6.1
Immunoglobulin monomer. An immunoglobulin monomer contains 2 identical light (L) chains and two identical heavy (H) chains connected by disulfide bonds. Each chain contains a variable domain and one or more constant domains.

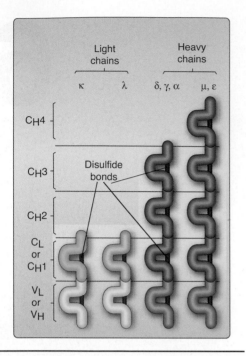

Figure 6.2
Immunoglobulin domains. Light chains are of two types (κ and λ) while there are five types of heavy chains (α, δ, ε, γ, μ). Immunoglobulin light and heavy changes are divisible into domains that consist of approximately 110 amino acids and contain an intrachange disulfide bond (V_L = light chain variable domain, V_H = heavy chain variable domain, C_L = light chain constant domain, C_H = heavy chain constant domain).

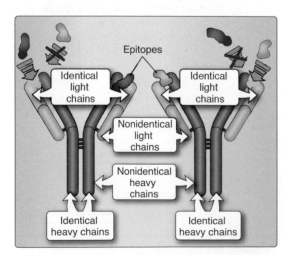

Figure 6.3
Immunoglobulin epitope-binding regions. Two identical epitope-binding regions are formed by pairing of a single V_L domain with a single V_H domain.

are aligned such that the amino portion (NH terminus) of a single heavy and a single light chain form an epitope-binding site (more about this later in the chapter). Each heavy and light chain may be subdivided into homologous regions termed **domains**. **Light chains,** termed κ (kappa) or λ (lambda), are encoded on chromosomes 2 and 22, respectively. There are five types of **heavy chains**, all encoded on chromosome 14, termed mu (μ), delta (δ), gamma (γ), epsilon (ε), and alpha (α). The genetically different forms of light chains (κ and λ) and of heavy chains (μ, δ, γ, ε, and α) are known as **isotypes**. Immunoglobulin class or subclass is determined by the heavy chain isotype.

1. **Light chains:** An immunoglobulin monomer contains two identical κ or two identical λ light chains but never one of each. Light or L chains contain a **variable (V_L) domain** and a **constant (C_L) domain** (Fig. 6.2). Each domain contains about 110 amino acids and an intrachain disulfide bond. Variable regions (in both heavy and light chains) are so named for their variation in amino acid sequences between immunoglobulins synthesized by different B cells.

2. **Heavy chains:** Heavy chains contain one variable (V_H) and three or four constant (C_H) domains (Fig. 6.2). Heavy (H) chain variable domains (V_H) are extremely diverse, and constant domains (C_H) display a relatively limited variability for members of an isotype. The δ, γ, and α heavy chains contain three constant domains (C_H1, C_H2, C_H3), and μ and ε heavy chains contain a fourth constant domain (C_H4), making them both longer and heavier than δ, γ, or α heavy chains.

3. **Antigen-binding sites:** A light chain variable domain and a heavy chain variable domain together form a pocket that constitutes the **antigen (epitope)-binding region** of the immunoglobulin molecule. Because an immunoglobulin monomer contains two identical light chains and two identical heavy chains, the two binding sites found in each monomeric immunoglobulin are also identical (Fig. 6.3). The variability in the amino acid sequences of the V_L and V_H domains, together with the random pairing of light and heavy chain that occurs from one B cell to another, creates a pool of binding sites capable of recognizing a very large number of different epitopes.

4. **Immunoglobulin landmarks:** Immunoglobulin molecules can be enzymatically cleaved into discrete fragments by either pepsin or papain (Fig. 6.4). Disulfide bonds join the heavy chains at or near a proline-rich **hinge region**, which confers flexibility on the immunoglobulin molecule.

The fragments of immunoglobulin are as follows:

- **Fab** or antigen (epitope)-binding fragment, produced by **papain** cleavage of the immunoglobulin molecule, contains V_H, C_H1, V_L, and C_L. Two Fab fragments are produced by papain cleavage of an immunoglobulin monomer; each fragment has an epitope-binding site.

- **Fc** or constant (crystallizable) fragment is produced by cleavage of the immunoglobulin molecule with **papain**. The Fc portion contains the C_H2, C_H3, and (sometimes) C_H4 regions of the immunoglobulin molecule. It is responsible for many biologic activities that occur following engagement of an epitope.

- **Fd** is the heavy chain (V_H, C_H1) portion of Fab.

- **Fd′** is a heavy chain (V_H, C_H1) portion of Fab. The prime (′) mark denotes extra amino acids due to a **pepsin** cleavage site.

- **F(ab′)₂** is a dimeric molecule produced by pepsin cleavage. An immunoglobulin monomer will produce a single F(ab′)₂ fragment containing two (V_H,C_H1′) segments joined by disulfide bonds. An F(ab′)₂ contains two epitope-binding sites.

B. Isotypes

Heavy chain isotypes (μ, δ, γ, α, and ε) also determine immunoglobulin isotype or class (IgM, IgD, IgG, IgA, and IgE, respectively) (Table 6.1). Normally, humans produce all five immunoglobulin isotypes. Of the two light chain isotypes, an individual B cell will produce only κ or λ chains, never both. B cells express surface-bound immunoglobulin monomers as epitope-specific receptors; B cells produce and display only one isotype, with the exception that unstimulated B cells express both IgM and IgD. When secreted into the body fluids, soluble IgG and IgE remain monomeric, soluble IgM forms a pentamer, and soluble IgA can be found in either a monomeric or dimeric form.

- **IgM** is found either as a cell-surface-bound monomer ($2\mu + 2\kappa$ or 2λ) or as a secreted pentamer with 10 H and L chains linked by disulfide bonds and a J ("joining") chain [five monomers + J, i.e., $5 \times (2\mu + 2\kappa$ or $2\lambda) + J$]. Most B cells display IgM on their cell surfaces. In general, IgM is the first immunoglobulin to be formed following antigenic stimulation. IgM is effective both at immobilizing antigen (**agglutination**; see Chapter 20, Fig. 20.2) and in activating the classical pathway of complement.

- **IgD** has a monomeric structure ($2\delta + 2\kappa$ or 2λ) and is almost exclusively displayed on B cell surfaces. Little is known of its function.

- **IgG** exists as both surface and secreted monomeric ($2\gamma + 2\kappa$ or 2λ) molecules. Four **subclasses** (γ_1, γ_2, γ_3, and γ_4) of γ heavy chains account for the four human IgG subclasses, **IgG1**, **IgG2**, **IgG3**, and **IgG4**. Collectively, IgG subclasses make up the greatest amount of immunoglobulin in the serum. Many IgG antibodies are effective in activating complement (see below), opsonizing and neutralizing microorganisms and viruses, and initiating antibody-dependent cell-mediated cytotoxicity, and they function in a wide variety of hypersensitivity functions.

- **IgA** is present in both monomeric and dimeric forms. Monomeric IgA ($2\alpha + 2\kappa$ or 2λ) is found in the serum. The addition of a J or joining chain to two IgA monomers forms a dimer. Epithelial cells use a specialized receptor to transport the IgA dimer to mucosal surfaces. This specialized receptor becomes an accessory molecule

(text continues on page 62)

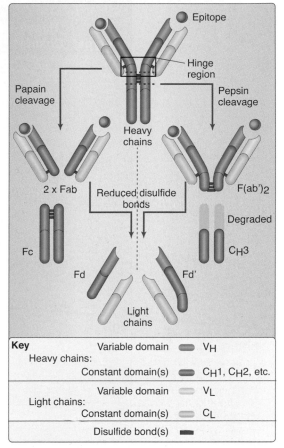

Figure 6.4
Enzyme cleavage of immunoglobulin determines landmarks. Papain cleaves heavy chains to form two identical Fab fragments (each containing one binding site) and one Fc fragment. Pepsin cleaves heavy chains at a point that produces an F(ab′)₂ fragment containing two linked binding sites and remaining heavy chain material that is degraded and eliminated.

Table 6.1
IMMUNOGLOBULIN ISOTYPES

Isotype	Heavy Chains[a]	Heavy Chain Subclass	Additional Chains	Formula[a]	Number of Monomers[b]	Subclass
IgM	μ			$2\mu^d + 2\kappa$ or 2λ	1	
	μ		J chain	$5[2\mu + 2\kappa$ or $2\lambda] + J$	5	IgM
IgD	δ			$2\delta + 2\kappa$ or 2λ	1	
IgG	γ			$2\gamma + 2\kappa$ or 2λ	1	
		γ_1		$2\gamma_1 + 2\kappa$ or 2λ	1	IgG1
		γ_2		$2\gamma_2 + 2\kappa$ or 2λ	1	IgG2
		γ_3		$2\gamma_3 + 2\kappa$ or 2λ	1	IgG3
		γ_4		$2\gamma_4 + 2\kappa$ or 2λ	1	IgG4
IgA	α			$2\alpha + 2\kappa$ or 2λ	1	
		α_1		$2\alpha_1 + 2\kappa$ or 2λ	1 — serum	IgA1
			J chain & SC[f]	$2[2\alpha_1 + 2\kappa$ or $2\lambda] + J + SC^f$	2 — external[g] upper body and GI	sIgA1
		α_2		$2\alpha_2 + 2\kappa$ or 2λ	1 — serum	IgA2
			J chain & SC[f]	$2[2\alpha_2 + 2\kappa$ or $2\lambda] + J + SC^f$	2 — external[g] GI	sIgA2
IgE	ε			$2\varepsilon + 2\kappa$ or 2λ	1	

[a]All monomers contain two identical heavy (μ, δ, γ, α, or ε) and two light (κ or λ) chains.

[b]Number of monomeric subunits expressed on the surface of the B cell (always 1) or in the form secreted by a plasma cell.

[c]Molecular weight.

[d]The carboxyl-terminal cytoplasmic tail portion of the μ chain of the surface-bound IgM monomer differs significantly from the μ chain present in the pentameric secreted form of IgM.

Table 6.1
(CONTINUED)

Valence	MW[c]	Half Life (days)	Serum Level (mg/dl)	Percent	Stick Figure
2	180,000				
10	900,000	1	45–150[e]	5–8	
2	180,000	2.8	3	<1	
2	150,000	23	720–1500[e]	75–85	
2	150,000	23	430–1050		
2	150,000	23	100–300		
2	150,000	8	30–90		
2	150,000	23	15–60		
	170,000	5.8	90–325	10–16	
2	170,000	5.8	80–290		
4	390,000	na	na		
2	170,000	5.8	10–35		
4	390,000	n.a.	n.a.		
2	190,000	2.5	0.03	<1	

[e]Serum level for all members of this class.

[f]Secretory component.

[g]The dimeric form is transported across specialized epithelial cells to the external environment. sIgA1 is found in tears, nasal secretions, saliva and milk. sIgA2 is found in the gastrointestinal system.

that binds to the IgA dimers is known as **secretory component** (SC) [2 × (2α + 2κ or 2λ) + J + SC]. Secretory IgA dimers are found in mucus, saliva, tears, breast milk, and gastrointestinal secretions. The SC provides increased resistance to enzymatic degradation. Two isoforms of IgA (α_1 and α_2) show slightly different functions. IgA1 predominates in the serum and in secretions above the diaphragm. Secretory IgA2 accounts for the majority of IgA found in the lumen of the lower portion of the gastrointestinal tract. Large amounts of IgA are synthesized and secreted daily at the mucosal surfaces of the GI tract, respiratory tracts, and other secretory epithelia. More IgA is produced daily than all the other isotypes combined.

- **IgE** is present in relatively low serum concentration; most is adsorbed onto the surfaces of mast cells, monocytes, and eosinophils. Its basic structural formula is (2ε + 2κ or 2λ). Mast cells and basophils have isotype-specific receptors (FcRε, CD23) for the Fc portion of free IgE molecules. Cross-linking of IgE on mast cell surfaces by antigen triggers the release of histamine and other inflammatory mediators, leading to immediate hypersensitivity (allergic) responses.

III. CLASSICAL PATHWAY OF COMPLEMENT ACTIVATION

Interaction of antibody with antigen initiates the **classical pathway** of complement activation. (Fig. 6.5). This biochemical cascade of enzymes and protein fragments facilitates destruction of microbes by the **membrane attack complex,** by increased opsonization through C3b binding of microbial surfaces, and by the production of **anaphylotoxins** C3a, C5a, and C4a. The cascade begins with the activation of component C1.

A. Activation of C1

Binding of IgM or IgG antibody to antigen causes a conformational change in the Fc region of the immunoglobulin molecule. This conformational change enables binding of the first component of the classic pathway, C1q. Each head of C1q may bind to a C_H2 domain (within the Fc portion) of an antibody molecule. Upon binding to antibody, C1q undergoes a conformational change that leads to the sequential binding and activation of the serine proteases C1r and C1s. The C1qrs complex has enzymatic activity for both C4 and C2, indicated by a horizontal bar as either C1$\overline{qrs}$ or C1$\overline{s}$.

B. Production of C3 convertase

Activation of C1$\overline{qrs}$ leads to the rapid cleavage and activation of components C4, C2, and C3. In fact, both the classical and mannan-binding lectin (MBL) pathways of complement activation are identical in the cleavage and activation of C4, C2, and C3 (Fig. 6.6).

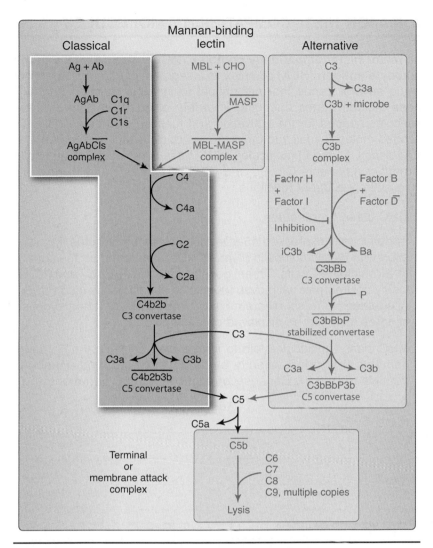

Figure 6.5
Classical pathway of complement activation. The classical pathway is initiated by the binding of antibody (usually IgG or IgM) to an antigen and then to the C1 complement component. The pathway produces a C3 convertase (responsible for production of C3b) and a C5 convertase (that can lead to MAC formation).

C. Production of C5 convertase

The binding of $\overline{\text{C4b2b}}$ to C3b leads to the formation of the $\overline{\text{C4b2b3b}}$ complex. This complex, a C5 convertase initiates the construction of the **membrane attack complex** on the microbial surface (see Figs. 5.8, 5.9, and 6.5). Thus, as in the case of the alternative (see Fig. 5.7) and MBL pathways (see Fig. 5.10), production of C5 convertase by the classical pathway leads to the development and insertion of a structure that is capable of damaging the cell surfaces.

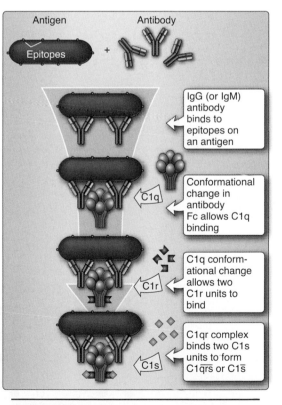

Figure 6.6
Activation of complement component C1. Activation of C1 involves serial binding and activation of its three subunits (C1q, C1r, C1s).

IV. MAJOR HISTOCOMPATIBILITY MOLECULES

The **major histocompatibility complex** (**MHC**), also called the **human leukocyte antigen** (**HLA**) complex, is a segment of chromosome 6 containing several genes that are critical to immune function (Fig. 6.7). These include genes encoding a variety of enzymes and structural molecules needed for the activation and function of B and T cells. The encoded molecules fall into three groups or classes known as MHC (or HLA) class I, II, and III molecules. MHC class III molecules include complement components C4, Bf, and C2. MHC class I and II molecules serve entirely different functions.

A. MHC class I molecules

Codominantly expressed 45-kDa **MHC class I** molecules, in association with β_2 microglobulin (β_2**m**, 12 kDa), are found on the surfaces of all nucleated cells. Three genetic loci, *HLA-A*, *-B*, and *-C*, are highly polymorphic, with over 100 alleles at each locus (see Fig. 6.7). Altogether, up to six different class I molecules (if heterozygous at all three loci) can be displayed on each cell.

MHC class I molecules fold to form a cleft between the α_1 and α_2 domains that noncovalently binds an eight- to nine-amino-acid peptide (Fig. 6.8). Because of slight structural variations in the

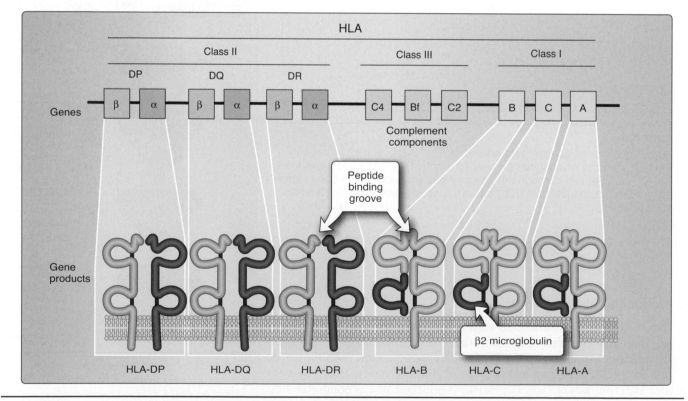

Figure 6.7
Genetic and protein organization of MHC class I, II, and III. Located on chromosome 6, HLA (human leukocyte antigen) genes are arranged as shown. They are grouped into Class I, Class II, and Class III based on structural and functional characteristics.

binding cleft (or binding groove) among the different allelic forms, different peptides may preferentially fit into clefts of some MHC class I molecules better than others. Additional ("nonclassical") class I molecules (e.g., those encoded by the *HLA-E, -F, -G, -H* loci) show limited variability and tissue distribution and may function to present carbohydrate and peptide fragments to $\gamma\delta$ T cells.

B. MHC class II molecules

MHC class II molecules are normally only expressed on dendritic-, macrophage-, and B cell surfaces; on some activated T cells; and on some specialized epithelial cells in the thymus and intestine. Codominantly expressed as noncovalent heterodimers, a 32- to 38-kDa α chain and a 29- to 32-kDa β chain form a binding groove (α_1 and β_1 domains) that can accommodate peptides of 18- to 20-amino-acid length (see Fig. 6.8). Encoded within the *HLA-DP, -DQ,* and *-DR* regions (see Fig. 6.7) are both α and β loci (DPα, DPβ, DQα, DQβ, etc.). After synthesis, MHC class II α and β chains combine only with others encoded within the same region (e.g., DPα associates only with DPβ but never with DQβ or DRβ). However, within each of these regions, α chains can combine with β chains encoded on the same chromosome (*cis*) or on the other member of the chromosome pair (*trans*). Termed ***cis-trans* complementation**, this allows individuals that are heterozygous at one or more of the class II loci to produce a greater variety of class II dimers than would be possible if they were homozygous. The range of different MHC class I and II molecules expressed can affect the overall immune capacity of an individual.

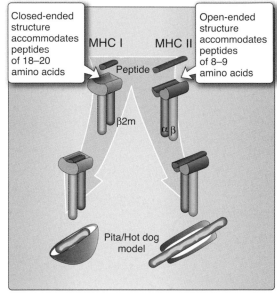

Figure 6.8
Peptide-binding clefts of MHC class I and class II molecules. MHC class I molecules (HLA-A, HLA-B, or HLA-C), in association with β_2 microglobulin (β_2m), form peptide binding clefts that are closed at the ends and bind peptides of 8-9 amino acids in length. MHC class II molecules (HLA-DP, HLA-DQ, or HLA-DR) are α chain - β chain heterodimers that form open-ended peptide binding clefts that bind peptides of 18-20 amino acids in length.

V. T CELL RECEPTORS

The antigen-specific T cell receptor (TCR) is an $\alpha\beta$ or a $\gamma\delta$ heterodimer polypeptide pair. (*Note: Despite the similarity in terminology, $\alpha\beta$ TCR loci/molecules and MHC class II $\alpha\beta$ loci/molecules are genetically and molecularly distinct.*) Each polypeptide of the TCR contains variable and constant domains that are genetically and molecularly distinct from immunoglobulins. The choice of whether to express an $\alpha\beta$ or $\gamma\delta$ heterodimer is made early in T cell development, and clonal descendants retain the same type of TCR.

A. Basic structure

The TCR is bound to the membrane of the T cell. The short cytoplasmic tails of $\alpha\beta$ or $\gamma\delta$ polypeptide chains lack signaling sequences or **immunoreceptor tyrosine activation motifs (ITAMs)** to initiate activation signals to the nucleus (see Chapter 8). These signals are provided by the CD3 complex molecules [(CD3δ, CD3γ, CD3ε, and CD247 (ζ chain)] that noncovalently associate with the TCR. Unlike antibodies, TCRs cannot bind soluble epitopes. They bind only to fragments of larger molecules that fit within the binding grooves of MHC class I or class II molecules as peptide-MHC (**pMHC**) complexes. Interaction of the TCR with pMHC is stabilized by the associated interaction of CD4 or CD8 with constant

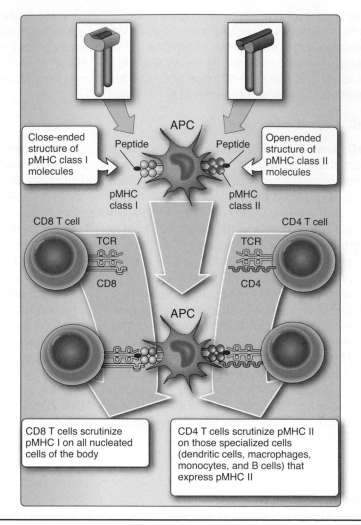

Figure 6.9
CD4$^+$ and CD8$^+$ T cells only interact with peptides bound to MHC class II or class I molecules.

domains of MHC class II or MHC class I molecules, respectively (Fig. 6.9).

B. Variable and constant regions

Each polypeptide chain of the TCR pair contains a variable (V_α or V_β, V_γ or V_δ) and a constant (C_α or C_β, C_γ or C_δ) region domain. Together, variable regions of α and β (or γ and δ) chains form hypervariable or **complementarity-determining regions** (**CDRs**) that interact with pMHC. Similar to immunoglobulins, each T cell expresses a unique TCR. Unlike immunoglobulins, T cells must "see" pMHC and do not recognize soluble peptides.

VI. MOLECULES OF CELLULAR INTERACTION

Many adaptive and innate immune responses require leukocyte-to-leukocyte interaction. These interactions take place by direct cell-to-cell contact or by the sending and receiving of signals via soluble molecules. Leukocytes respond to these signals by upregulating or downregulating their functions, by migrating to specific anatomic sites, or by making life-or-death decisions about the fate of a cell within the body.

A. Cytokines

Cytokines are low-molecular-weight soluble protein messengers that are involved in all aspects of the innate and adaptive immune response, including cellular growth and differentiation, inflammation, and repair. Originally called *lymphokines* and *monokines* to reflect lymphocytic or monocytic origin, we now recognize that these substances are produced by a wide variety of leukocytes and nonleukocytes. A large number of cytokines have been identified, although the roles of many of them are not yet fully understood (Table 6.2). Many cytokines are crucial in regulating lymphocyte development and in determining the types of immune responses evoked by specific responses.

B. Chemokines

Low-molecular-weight cytokines known as **chemokines** (chemoattractant cytokines) stimulate leukocyte movement. Leukocytes are guided by chemokine concentration gradients to the site of an infection or inflammation (a process called *homing*). They are divided into four types based on the presence of certain structural motifs involving the numbers and intervals between cystine residues: C, CC, CXC, and CX_3C (Table 6.3).

C. Adhesion molecules

Often, leukocytes must interact directly to contact other cells under somewhat adverse conditions, such as during rapid fluid flow within the circulatory system or under weak ligand-receptor binding. **Adhesion molecules** provide stable cell-to-cell contact necessary for both innate and adaptive immune responses as well as for many other intercellular activities. While a seemingly simple activity, the ability of cells to examine the surface of other cells and to establish stable contact with them is vital. For cells to communicate and for cell-surface receptors and ligands to interact, the cells must be able to establish and maintain relatively prolonged surface-to-surface contact.

Types of adhesion molecules include integrins, selectins, and addressins.

1. **Integrins** are found on the surfaces of many types of leukocytes. Integrins are heterodimers consisting of various combinations of α and β chains (e.g., $\alpha_5\beta_1$ on monocytes and macrophages). They interact with other molecules that are based on the Ig superfamily motif (found on a wide variety of cells and has the generalized intrachain disulfide bond domain, e.g., Fig. 6.2) and with extracellular matrix. Their main function is to strengthen contact between leukocytes and many types of cells (e.g., vascular endothelium) so that more extensive interactions can then take place. Individual integrins and their activities are discussed in upcoming chapters in the more detailed descriptions of various immune responses

Table 6.2
CYTOKINES

Cytokine	Cellular Source[†]	Targets[†]	Function	Receptor
IL-1α				
IL-1β	M, B	T, B, M, End, other	Leukocyte activation, increase endothelium adhesion.	CD121a or CD121b
IL-2	T	T, B, NK, M, oligo	T cell proliferation, regulation	CD122/CD25
IL-3	T*, Mas, Eos, NK, End	Ery, G	Proliferation and differentiation of hematopoietic precursors	CD123/CDw131
IL-4	Mas, T, M	B, T, End	Differentiation of Th2 and B cells	CD124/CD132
IL-5	Mas, T, Eos	Eos, B	Growth differentiation of B cells and eosinophils	CD125/CDw131
IL-6	T, B, M, Astrocytes, End	T, B, others	Hematopoiesis, differentiation, inflammation	CD126/CD130
IL-7	Bone marrow and thymic stroma	pB, pT	Pre/pro-B cell proliferation, T cell, upregulation of pro-inflammatory cytokines	CD127/CD132
IL-8	M, L, others	PMN, Bas, L	Chemoattractant	CD128
IL-9	Th2*	T, B	Potentiates production of IgM, IgG, IgE	
IL-10	CD8⁺ T, Th2, (B) M	T, B, Mas, M	Inhibits IFN-γ, TNF-β, IL-2 by TH1 cells, DTH, stimulates Th2	CD210
IL-11		Bone marrow stroma	Osteoclast formation	
IL-12	DC, B, T	T, NK	Potentiates IFN-γ and TNF-α production by T and NK, down-regulates IL-10	CD212
IL-13	Th2*, Mas, NK	Th2, B, M	Th2 modulator, down-regulated IL-1, IL-6, IL-8, IL-10, IL-12	
IL-14	T	B*	Stimulates proliferation, inhibits Ig secretion	
IL-15	M, Epi	T, B*	Proliferation	
IL-16	Eos, CD8⁺ T	CD4⁺ T	CD4⁺ chemoattractant	
IL-17	(T)	Epi, End, others	Osteoclastogenesis, angiogenesis	
IL-18	M	Th1, NK	Induces IFN-γ production, enhances NK activity	
TGF-β	Eos, others?	Many cell types	Anti-inflammatory, promotes wound healing	
TNF-α	M*, PMN, T, B, NK	M, PMN, T, End, others	Mediator of inflammatory reactions	CD120a and CD120b
TNF-β	L	Wide variety	Mediator of inflammatory reactions	CD120a and CD120b
IFN-α	L, Epi, fibroblasts	Wide variety	Upregulates MHC class I, inhibits viral proliferation	
IFN-β	Epi, fibroblasts	Wide variety	Upregulates MHC class I, inhibits viral proliferation	
IFN-γ	CD8⁺*, (CD4⁺*), NK	T, B, M, NK, End	Antiviral, antiparasite, inhibits proliferation, enhances MHC class I and II expression	CD119
M-CSF	L, M, G, End, Epi, others	M	Growth and differentiation of macrophages	CD115
G-CSF	T*, M, End	G	Growth and differentiation of granulocytes	
GM-CSF	T, M, End, Mas	PG, pMye	Stimulates growth and differentiation of granulocytes and myeloid lineage cells	CD116
MIF	M	M	Antiapoptotic activity for macrophages, promotes macrophage survival	

[†]Abbreviation key: Activated cells (*), B cells (B), basophils (Bas), dendritic cells (DC), endothelium (End), eosinophil (Eos), epithelium (Epi), erythrocytes (Ery), granulocytes (G), lymphocytes (L), macrophage (M), mast cells (Mas), myeloid (Mye), natural killer cells (NK), neutrophils (PMN), oligodendrocytes (oligo), parenthesis (cellular subset), and T cell (T). Within the table, parentheses are used to indicate when only a subset of the designated cell types produce the cytokine.

Table 6.3
CHEMOKINES AND THEIR RECEPTORS

Chemokine family	Chemokine receptors	Ligand	Chemokines
C	XCR1	XCL1, XCL2	ATAC, Lymphotactin, SCM-1
CC	CCR1	CCL3, CCL5, CCL14, CCL15, CCL16, CCL23	HCC-1, HCC-2, HCC-4, LD78α, Lkn-1, MCP-4, LEC, MIP-1α, MPIR-1, RANTES
	CCR2	CCL2, CCL7, CCL8	MCP-1, MCP-2, MCP-3, MCP-4, MCAF
	CCR3	CCL5, CCL7, CCL16, CCL24, CCL26	Eotaxin, Eotaxin-3, HCC-2, HCC-4, LEC, Lkn-1, MIP-1α, MCP-3, RANTES, MPIF-2
	CCR4	CCL17, CCL22	MDC, STCP-1, TARC
	CCR5	CCL3, CCL4, CCL5, CCL8	LD78α, MCP-2, MIP-1α, MIP-1β, RANTES
	CCR6	CCL20	exodus-1, LARC, MIP-3α,
	CCR7	CCL19, CCL21	6Ckine, ELC, exodus-3, exodus-2, MIP-3β, SLC
	CCR8	CCL1	I-309
	CCR9	CCL25	TECK
	CCR10	CCL27	TACK, ILC
CXC	CXCR1	CXCL1, CXCL2, CXCL3, CXCL6, CXCL7, CXCL8	GCP-2, GROα, GROβ, IL-8, MCSA-α, MGSA-β, MGSA-γ, NAP-2
	CXCR2	CXCL5, CXCL6, CXCL7, CXCL8	ENA-78, GCP-2, IL-8, NAP-2
	CXCR3A	CXCL9, CXCL10, CXCL11	I-TAC, Mig
	CXCR3B	CXCL4, CXCL9, CXCL10, CXCL11	IP-10, Mig , PF4
	CXCR4	CXCL12	SDF-1α, SDF-1β
	CXCR5	CXCL13	BCA-1, BLC
CX₃C	CX3CR1	CX3CL1	Fractalkine

Source: http://www.nchi.nlm.nih.gov/

2. **Selectins and addressins** are limited in their tissue distribution and are designed to identify particular tissues and to facilitate the interactions of particular cell combinations. For example, newly differentiated lymphocytes need to migrate to lymph nodes to undergo their next stage of development. This migration is accomplished by interactions between selectin molecules found on the lymphocytes (e.g., **CD62L,** also known as L-selectin) and addressin molecules (e.g., GlyCAM-1) located on the high vascular endothelium of blood vessels passing through lymph nodes. Other selectins and addressins assist in the movement of lymphocytes and other cells to the gut, epithelium, and sites of tissue inflammation. Individual selectins and adhesions and their activities are discussed in upcoming chapters in the more detailed descriptions of various immune responses.

D. Cluster of differentiation molecules

Cluster of differentiation (**CD**) molecules populate the surfaces of many cell types and often serve as indicators of the functional capacities of leukocytes and other cells. It is beyond the scope of this book to describe more than just a few of the over 250 CD molecules that have been identified so far. Fortunately, for a basic understanding of the underlying mechanisms of the adaptive immune response, you need to know only a few of these. Among those that you will frequently encounter are the following:

- *CD3 complex* contains several molecules associated with the TCR. It is composed of six polypeptides (2 CD3ε + 1 CD3γ + 1 CD3δ + 1 CD247 ζ–ζ homodimer). Its functions are to support the TCR and to transduce transmembrane signaling when the TCR is engaged.

- *CD4* is a single-chain member of the immunoglobulin supergene family and is expressed on the surfaces of approximately two thirds of mature T cells. CD4 molecules recognize a nonpeptide-binding portion of MHC class II molecules. As a result, $CD4^+$ T cells, also known as helper T (Th) cells, are "restricted" to the recognition of pMHC class II complexes.

- *CD8* is a two-chain cell-surface molecule expressed as a homodimer ($\alpha\alpha$) or heterodimer ($\alpha\beta$) by about one third of mature T cells. CD8 molecules recognize the nonpeptide-binding portion of MHC class I molecules. $CD8^+$ T cells, "restricted" to the recognition of pMHC I complexes, are also known as cytotoxic T (Tc) and suppressor T (Ts) cells.

E. Signal transduction molecules

Leukocytes use their cell-surface receptors to sense their extracellular environment. Binding of certain ligands causes a conformational change in the receptor or its accessory molecules. This change is then communicated inside the cell via the receptor's cytoplasmic tail (the part that is inside the cell), initiating a signal transduction cascade within the cell. Such cascades usually involve the binding of one or more specific intracellular signal transduction proteins. Receptor engagement often initiates a series of chemical signals that regulate gene transcription in the nucleus and alteration of cellular activity. Two stylized, tyrosine-kinase pathways cascades are described.

1. **JAK-STAT pathway:** Many extracellular stimuli activate a JAK (an acronym that stands for "Janus kinase" or sometimes "just another kinase") –STAT (signal transducers and activators of transcription) signal transduction pathway. Ligand (e.g., cytokines, growth factors) -binding induces receptor polypeptides to dimerize and bind cytosolic JAK (Fig. 6.10). Activated JAKs are tyrosine kinases that phosphorylate tyrosine residues within the intracellular portion of the receptor chains. The phosphorylated tyrosine residues provide docking sites for SRC homology 2 (SH2) domains of inactive, cytosolic STAT molecules. Receptor-bound STAT molecules are phosphorylated by the receptor-associated JAKs, allowing the STATs to disassociate from the cytoplasmic tail and dimerize with another phosphorylated STAT. The STAT dimer translocates to the nucleus, where it binds to specific DNA response element(s) to regulate gene transcription.

2. **Ras-MAP kinase pathway:** This pathway is named for guanosine triphosphate (GTP)-binding protein and MAP or mitogen-activated protein. Receptor dimerization promotes the phosphorylation of intracellular tyrosine kinase domains on the cytoplasmic

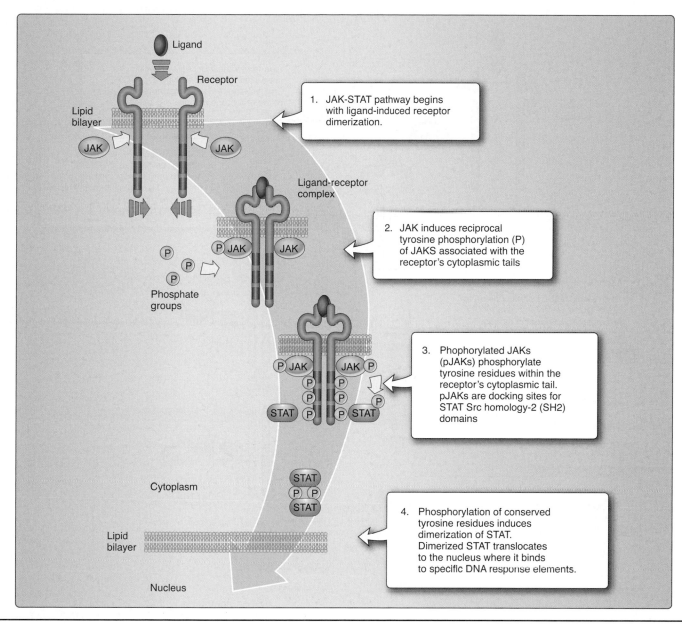

Figure 6.10

A stylized JAK-STAT signal transduction pathway. Ligand (e.g., a cytokine) engagement induces receptor dimerization and the binding and activation of cytosolic JAKs (Janus kinases). Phosphorylation of STATs induces their dimerization, translocation to the nucleus, and binding to specific DNA response elements.

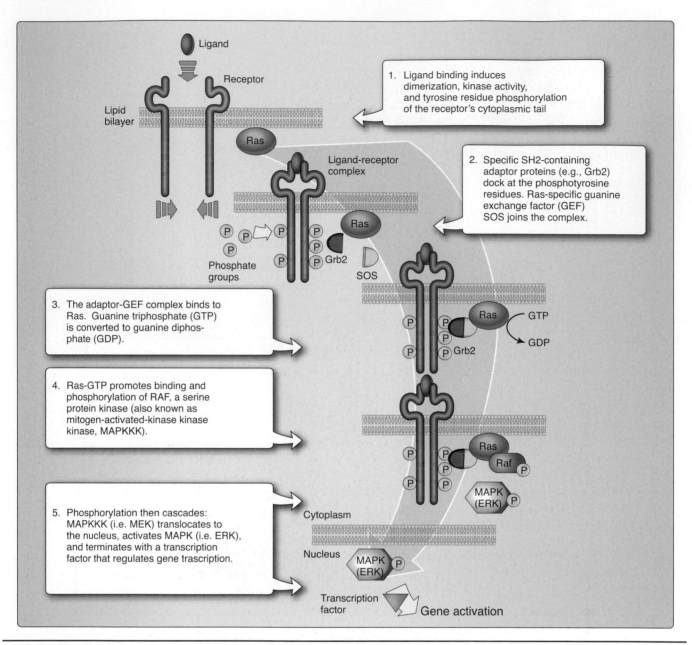

Figure 6.11

A stylized Ras-MAPK signal transduction pathway. Ligand engagement induces receptor dimerization and intrinsic tyrosine kinase activity by the cytoplasmic tail of the receptor and its phosphorylation. A sequential phosphorylation cascade, involving several intermediates, results in the phosphorylation of MAPK and its movement into the nucleus, terminating in the binding of transcription elements to specific DNA response elements.

tail of a catalytic receptor with intrinsic tyrosine kinase activity or allows activation of receptor-associated tyrosine kinases such as JAKs (Fig. 6.11). The receptor's phosphotyrosine provides a "docking" or binding site for a specific intracellular SH2-containing (e.g., SHC and Grb2) adaptor protein. Upon docking, SHC activates its SH3 domain and binds the SOS protein. SOS is a guanine nucleotide exchange factor (GEF) for Ras, a monomeric plasma membrane protein. The SHC-SOS-Ras complex exchanges GTP for guanosine diphosphate (GDP) on Ras. Ras-GTP promotes binding of the Raf serine protein kinase (also known as MAPKKK, which stands for mitogen-activated protein kinase kinase kinase). Raf initiates a sequential phosphorylation cascade involving MAPKK (also known as MEK, which translocates to the nucleus) and MAPK (also known as ERK, or extracellular-signal regulated kinases). The cascade terminates with a gene transcription factor (such as ELK) that leads to gene transcription.

Chapter Summary

- The **immunoglobulin monomer** contains two identical light and two identical heavy polypeptide chains linked by disulfide bonds. **Light chains** contain one **variable** and one **constant domain. Heavy chains** contain one variable and three or four constant domains. The combination of one light and one heavy chain variable domains form an **epitope-binding site**.

- Normal individuals express five immunoglobulin **classes** or **isotypes**: **IgM,** the heaviest, is present as either a cell-surface-bound monomer or as a secreted pentamer. **IgD,** a monomer, is almost exclusively displayed on B cell surfaces. Human **IgG** is a monomer present in four subclasses; **IgG1, IgG2, IgG3,** and **IgG4.** Monomeric **IgA** is present in the serum and in its dimeric form is found in association with mucosal surfaces and secretions. **IgE** is present in relatively low serum concentration; most is adsorbed onto the surfaces of mast cells, basophils, and eosinophils.

- Binding of IgM or IgG antibody to antigen causes a conformational change in the Fc region of the immunoglobulin molecule, initiating the **classical pathway** of complement activation.

- The **major histocompatibility complex** (**MHC**), also called the **human leukocyte antigen** (**HLA**) complex, is a segment of chromosome 6 containing several genes critical to immune function. Codominantly expressed **MHC class I** molecules, in association with β_2 microglobulin (β_2**m),** are found on the surfaces of all nucleated cells. **MHC class II molecules** are normally expressed only on dendritic-, macrophage-, and B-cell surfaces, on some activated T cells, and on some specialized epithelial cells in the thymus and intestine.

- The epitope-specific T cell receptor contains $\alpha\beta$ or $\gamma\delta$ heterodimer polypeptide pairs. Each polypeptide contains one variable and one constant region domain. TCRs recognize and bind peptides that lie within the binding grooves of MHC class I or class II molecules as peptide-MHC (**pMHC**) complexes.

- **Cytokines** are low-molecular-weight soluble protein messengers that are involved in all aspects of the innate and adaptive immune response, including cellular growth and differentiation, inflammation, and repair.

- Low-molecular-weight cytokines known as **chemokines** (chemo-attractant cytokines) stimulate leukocyte movement.

- Adhesion molecules provide stable cell-to-cell contact. **Integrins** are found on the surfaces of a wide variety of leukocytes. **Selectins and addressins** are limited in their tissue distribution and designed to identify particular tissues and to facilitate the interactions of particular cell combinations.

- **Cluster of differentiation** molecules populate the surfaces of a wide variety of cell types and serve as indication of the functional capacities leukocytes and a number of other cells.

- Leukocytes use receptors to sense their extracellular environment. Ligand binding by a receptor leads to a signal transduction from the receptor-bound ligand to the nucleus involving phosphorylation of serine/tyrosine residues. Two stylized, prototypic signal transduction cascades are JAK-STAT and Ras-MAP pathways.

Study Questions

6.1   Epitope-specific receptors of T lymphocytes are found

     A. as either cytosolic or membrane-bound proteins.
     B. in blood plasma, lymph, and other secretory fluids.
     C. on the surface of plasma cells.
     D. as transmembrane polypeptides.
     E. in the nuclear lipid bilayer.

> The answer is D. The epitope specific receptors of T cells (TCRs) are displayed as membrane-bound molecules on their cell surfaces. TCRs are not found as soluble molecules. Epitope-specific molecules produced by plasma cells are genetically distinct from T cell receptor molecules.

6.2   Antibodies (immunoglobulins)

     A. are synthesized and secreted by both B and T cells.
     B. bind to several different epitopes simultaneously.
     C. contain four different light chain polypeptides.
     D. recognize specific epitopes together with self molecules.
     E. tag antigens for destruction and removal.

> The answer is E. Antibodies bind to epitopes on antigens to identify them or tag them for destruction by other elements of the immune system. They are synthesized only by B cells and plasma cells. An antibody molecule contains two (IgD, IgG, IgE, and serum IgA), four (secretory IgA), or ten (secreted IgM) *identical* epitope-binding sites. An antibody monomer contains two identical light chains and two identical heavy chains. Self-recognition is not required for antibody molecules.

6.3 The constant regions of the five major types of heavy chains of immunoglobulin molecules dictate the molecule's

A. epitope.
B. Fab fragment.
C. isotype.
D. tyrosine activation motif.
E. variable domain.

The answer is C. The heavy chain constant regions determine immunoglobulin isotypes: mu (μ, IgM), delta (δ, IgD), gamma (γ, IgG), epsilon (ε, IgE), and alpha (α, IgA). Fab fragments are enzymatic cleavage products of immunoglobulin monomers. (Immunoreceptor) tyrosine activation motifs are not present on immunoglobulin molecules. Variable domains show extensive amino acid sequence variability among immunoglobulins, even within the same isotype.

6.4 When an immunoglobulin molecule is subjected to cleavage by pepsin, the product(s)

A. are Individual heavy and light chains.
B. can no longer bind to antigen.
C. consist of two separated antigen-binding fragments.
D. crystallize during storage in the cold.
E. is a dimeric antigen-binding molecule.

The answer is E. Enzymatic cleavage of the immunoglobulin monomer by pepsin occurs distal to the variable domain and distal to heavy-heavy chain disulfide bonds, which remain intact, resulting in a molecule with two epitope-binding sites. Interchain disulfide bonds are unaffected by pepsin cleavage. The epitope-binding site remains intact upon pepsin cleavage of the heavy chain. Papain cleavage of the immunoglobulin monomer occurs distal to the variable domain but proximal to the heavy-heavy chain disulfide bond, resulting in two separate epitope-binding Fab fragments. Pepsin enzymatically degrades the $C_H 2$ portion of the immunoglobulin molecule resulting in fragments that rarely, if ever, form crystals.

6.5 In an individual with an immediate hypersensitivity response (allergy) to dust mites, cross-linking of which of the following dust-mite-specific molecules will trigger inflammatory mediator release?

A. IgA
B. IgE
C. IgG
D. histamine
E. mast cells

The answer is B. Cross-linking of IgE bound to the surfaces of basophils and mast cells causes cellular degranulation and release of vasoactive amine responsible for inflammation. In humans, neither IgA nor IgG is associated with allergic responses. Histamine is released from mast cells are a result of cross-linking of surface-bound IgE.

6.6 The classical pathway of complement begins with

A. activation of C1.
B. cleavage and activation of C4, C2, and C3.
C. IgA binding to a specific epitope.
D. initiation of membrane attack complex formation.
E. production of C3 convertase.

The answer is A. The classical pathway of complement begins with the recognition of antigen-antibody complexes by the first component of complement, C1q. Subsequent steps in the classical pathway involve activation of components C4, C2, C3, and the production of C3 convertase leading to the production of C5 convertase and entry into the membrane attack complex. Antigen binding by IgA does not activate the classical pathway.

6.7 The classical pathway of complement functions to

A. cleave immunoglobulins into Fc fragments.
B. facilitate destruction of microbes.
C. recognize specific epitopes on microbes.
D. regulate lymphocyte development.
E. trigger histamine release.

The answer is B. Complement functions to facilitate the lysis of microbes by recognition of microbes tagged by antibody, by the opsonization of microbes by the attachment of C3 fragments, and by the release of anaphylotoxins C3a, C5a, and C4a. Immunoglobulin molecules are not cleaved by complement. The classical pathway is activated only by antigen-antibody complexes and by itself does not recognize microbial epitopes. Complement is not involved in lymphocyte development and does not trigger the release of histamine.

6.8   In humans, MHC class II molecules are expressed by

    A. all nucleated cells.
    B. B cells, dendritic cells, and macrophages.
    C. erythrocytes.
    D. mast cells.
    E. naïve T cells.

> The answer is B. B cells, dendritic cells, monocytes, and macrophages constitutively express MHC class II molecules. Only a subset of nucleated cells expresses MHC class II molecules, and it does not include mast cells or naïve T cells. Erythrocytes do not express MHC class II molecules.

6.9   The basic structure of a T cell receptor consists of

    A. a membrane-bound $\alpha\beta$ or $\gamma\delta$ heterodimer.
    B. a complex of disulfide-linked heavy and light chains.
    C. covalently linked CD3 and CD247 molecules.
    D. peptide-MHC complexes.
    E. soluble antigen-binding homodimers.

> The answer is A. The T cell receptor (TCR) is a heterodimer composed of $\alpha\beta$ or $\gamma\delta$ polypeptide chains. Neither the $\alpha\beta$ or $\gamma\delta$ heterodimers nor their associated molecules (CD3 and CD247) are linked by disulfide bonds. TCR recognize pMHC complexes on antigen-presenting cells. TCRs are found only on the surfaces of T cells and are not soluble.

6.10   Migration of a B lymphocyte to specific sites (such as a lymph node) is dependent in part on the utilization of

    A. antibodies.
    B. CD8.
    C. CD3.
    D. complement.
    E. selectins.

> The answer is E. Selectins are adhesion molecules that participate in the recognition that occurs between different types of cells and tissues. Antibodies do not serve as guides for such homing. CD8 and CD3 are expressed on T cells, not on B cells, and are responsible for lymphocyte homing. Complement fragments may be chemoattractants for leukocytes, but they attract those cells to the site of immune responses rather than to specific organs.

6.11   Which of the following molecules is expressed by a mature T cell that functions as a helper T cell?

    A. CD4
    B. CD8
    C. GlyCAM-1
    D. IgA
    E. IgG

> The answer is A. $CD4^+$ T cells are also called T helper cells. $CD8^+$ T cells have cytotoxic or suppressive functions. GlyCAM-1 is an adhesion molecule found on certain vascular epithelial cells within lymph nodes. IgA and IgG are not expressed on T cells.

6.12   Following cytokine binding to a specific cell-surface receptor, a lymphocyte is stimulated to undergo signaling via the JAK-STAT pathway. In this pathway, which of the following will be induced to translocate to the cell's nucleus to regulate transcription?

    A. a JAK
    B. Ras
    C. SH2-containing adapter proteins
    D. STAT dimers
    E. tyrosine kinase

> The answer is D. STAT dimers translocate into the nucleus. JAKs are cytosolic tyrosine kinases that bind to the intracellular domain of the tyrosine-phosphorylated receptor and never enter the nucleus. Ras is a membrane-bound GTP binding protein that is bound by cytosolic proteins with SH2 domains that also bind to phosphotyrosine residues within the intracellular portion of the receptor. Catalytic receptors signal by stimulating tyrosine kinase, either of the receptor itself (intrinsic activity) or by associating with nonreceptor tyrosine kinases (e.g. JAK), neither of which enters the nucleus.

Cells and Organs

7

I. OVERVIEW

In contrast to the morphologically distinct cells of the innate immune system, lymphocytes of the adaptive immune system generally look alike except for size, ranging from small (4 to 7 μm) to medium (7 to 11 μm) to large (11 to 15 μm). Lymphocytes may be broadly categorized by the antigen-specific receptors they generate through gene rearrangement and by the organs in which they develop. These cells may be likened to the soldiers of the adaptive immune system. Like soldiers, they often display combinations of additional surface molecules that serve essentially as molecular "badges" of rank and function. Also, cells of the adaptive immune response undergo "basic training" in specialized training centers (thymus or bone marrow), "bivouac" in specialized areas (spleen, lymph nodes, and lymphocyte accumulations), may be "promoted" (differentiation), and are transported from one anatomic site to another via the bloodstream or in their own lymphatic circulatory system.

II. LYMPHOCYTES

The immune system must be able to distinguish its own molecules, cells, and organs (**self**) from those of foreign origin (**nonself**). The innate immune system does this by expressing germline-encoded pattern recognition receptors (PRRs) on the surfaces of its cells, receptors that recognize structures on potentially invasive organisms (see Chapter 5). The adaptive immune system, on the other hand, utilizes somatically generated epitope-specific T cell and B cell receptors (TCRs and BCRs). These receptors are created anew and randomly within each individual T and B lymphocyte by gene recombination prior to antigen encounter (more about this in Chapter 8). No two individuals, even identical twins, have identical adaptive immune systems. Lymphocytes are usually defined by where they undergo "basic training": in the thymus (**thymus-derived lymphocytes** or **T cells**, and **natural killer T** or **NKT cells**) or in the bone marrow (**B lymphocytes** or **B cells**). They are also defined by the type of receptors they display on their cell surfaces: TCR (T cells and NKT cells), BCR or immunoglobulins (B cells), or neither (natural killer or NK cells).

A. Thymus-derived cells

T cells are the key players in most adaptive immune responses. They participate directly in immune responses as well as orchestrating and regulating the activities of other cells. T cells arise from hematopoietic stems cells in the bone marrow. Immature T cells called prothymocytes migrate to the thymus, where, as thymocytes, they develop TCRs and are screened for their ability to distinguish self from nonself. Although most thymocytes fail the screening process and are eliminated, those that pass scrutiny and survive are able to further differentiate and mature to become thymus-derived lymphocytes or T cells and enter the circulation. The developmental pathways for T cells are discussed in greater detail in Chapter 9. Although T cells show a wide diversity in adaptive immune function (see Chapters 8–19), all can be identified by the presence of the CD3 (cluster of differentiation–3) molecule that is associated with the TCR on the T cell surface. Two other CD molecules are also used to identify CD3$^+$ T cell subsets, CD4$^+$ and CD8$^+$, and to readily distinguish their potential immune function.

1. **CD4$^+$ T cells:** These cells account for approximately two thirds of mature CD3$^+$ T cells. CD4 molecules displayed on the surfaces of these T cells recognize a nonpeptide-binding portion of MHC class II molecules (Fig. 7.1). As a result, CD4$^+$ T cells, also known

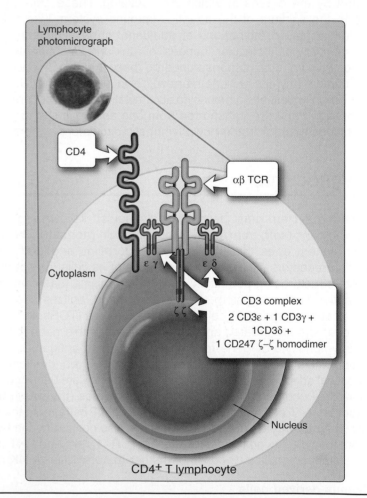

Figure 7.1

Comprising approximately two thirds of all T lymphocytes, CD4$^+$ T cells are the workhorses of the adaptive immune system. They display T cell receptors (TCRs), associated CD3 signalling complex molecules, and CD4 molecules on their cell surfaces.

as helper T (Th) cells, are "restricted" to the recognition of pMHC class II complexes.

2. **CD8⁺ T cells** account for approximately one third of all mature CD3⁺ T cells. CD8 molecules displayed on the surfaces of these T cells recognize the nonpeptide-binding portion of MHC class I molecules. As a result, CD8⁺ T cells are "restricted" to the recognition of pMHC I complexes (Fig. 7.2). Functionally, CD8⁺ T cells are also known as **cytotoxic T (Tc)** and **suppressor T (Ts) cells**. Tc cells identify body cells that are infected with intracellular organisms, such as viruses and intracellular bacteria, and eliminate the cells harboring these organisms. Ts cells function to downregulate and thus control adaptive immune responses.

B. Bone marrow-derived cells

Not all lymphocytes of bone marrow origin are destined for thymic education. Certain cells of lymphoid lineage remain and develop within the bone marrow and are the precursors of immunoglobulin-producing

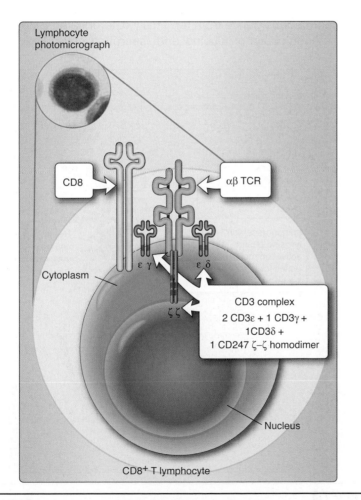

Figure 7.2
Approximately one third of the T cells found in peripheral blood, CD8⁺ T cells display T cell receptors (TCRs), associated CD3 molecules, and CD8 dimers on their cell surfaces.

lymphocytes. These bone marrow–derived lymphocytes, also known as B lymphocytes or B cells, synthesize immunoglobulin and display it on their surfaces, where it functions as their BCR. Plasma cells are derived from differentiated, mature B cells and both synthesize and secrete immunoglobulin.

1. **B cells** arise from pluripotent hematopoietic stem cells in the bone marrow. They do not migrate to the thymus but develop within the bone marrow. B cells arise from two distinct lineages: B-1 and B-2 cells. So named because they are the first to develop embryologically, B-1 cells are a self-renewing population that dominate the plural and peritoneal cavities. In contrast, conventional or B-2 cells arise during and after the neonatal period, are continuously replaced from the bone marrow, and are widely distributed throughout the lymphoid organs and tissues. Each B cell is specific, that is, it produces immunoglobulin of only one antibody specificity that recognizes only one epitope. Like T cells, it is the extreme diversity among B cells, each producing a single form of immunoglobulin, that generates the overall diversity of the immunoglobulin (or antibody) response (Fig. 7.3).

2. **Plasma cells** derive from terminally differentiated B cells and are immunoglobulin-producing and -secreting cells. They cease to

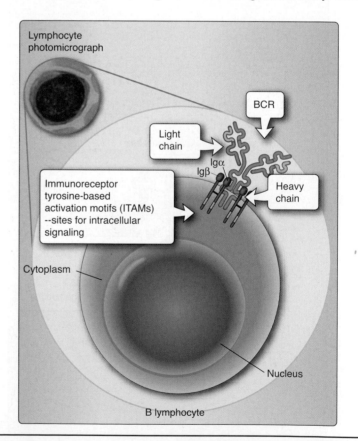

Figure 7.3

Bone-marrow derived lymphocytes or B cells synthesize immunoglobulin molecules that are found both within and displayed on their cell surface. On the surface they function as the B cell epitope-specific receptor (BCR). BCR-associated Igα and Igβ molecules signal the cell when an epitope is bound by the BCR.

use immunoglobulin as a membrane receptor and instead secrete it into the fluids around the cells. Plasma cells, with increased size and metabolic activity, are factories that produce large quantities of immunoglobulin during their short lifespan of less than 30 days. They are characterized by basophilic cytoplasm, a nucleus that has a stellate (starlike) pattern within it, and nonstaining Golgi (Fig. 7.4).

C. Natural killer cells

Approximately 5% to 10% of peripheral blood lymphocytes lack both T cell (CD3) and B cell (surface immunoglobulin) markers. These cells are known as **natural killer (NK) cells** to reflect their ability to kill certain virally infected cells and tumor cells without prior sensitization (see Chapters 4 and 5). Their granular appearance is due to the presence of cytoplasmic granules that can be released to damage the membranes of the cells they attack. NK cells develop within the bone marrow and lack TCR produced by rearrangement of TCR genes (see Chapter 8). However, they do bear another set of receptors called killer activation receptors (KARs) and killer inhibition receptors (KIRs) that allow them to recognize host cells that might need to be destroyed (Fig. 7.5, left). In addition, a unique subset of T cells, designated NKT because they share some functional characteristics

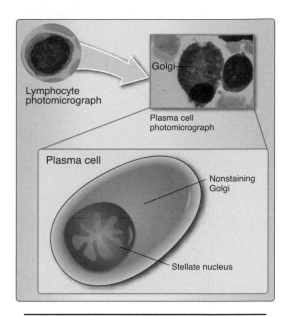

Figure 7.4
Plasma cells are terminally differentiated B cells that both synthesize and secrete immunoglobulin. Anatomically distinguishable from lymphocytes, their cytoplasm reflects increased ribosomes and endoplasmic reticulum. Immunoglobulin molecules are assembled within their (nonstaining) Golgi prior to export to the fluids surrounding the cell.

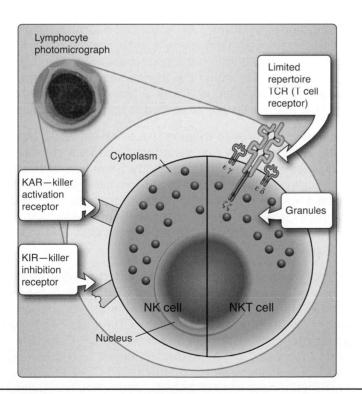

Figure 7.5
Natural killer (NK) and natural killer T (NKT) cells bridge both adaptive and innate immune systems. NK cells are characteristically large granular lymphocytes that express neither TCRs nor BCRs and bear receptors for stress molecules (killer activation receptors or KARs) and for MHC class I molecules (killer inhibition receptors or KIRs). Unlike NK cells, NKT cells express low levels of TCRs with extremely limited repertoires.

with NK cells, develop within the thymus and express a rearranged TCR of extremely limited repertoire (Fig. 7.5, right). Unlike conventional T cells, NKT cells respond to lipids, glycolipids, or hydrophobic peptides presented by a specialized, nonclassical MHC class I molecule, CD1d, and secrete large amounts of cytokines, especially interleukin-4 (IL-4).

III. LYMPHOID TISSUES AND ORGANS

Leukocytes may be found in the body distributed as single cells in the tissues and circulation, as lymphoid accumulations (e.g., Peyer's patches), or within lymphoid organs (e.g., thymus, spleen, lymph nodes) (Fig. 7.6). Lymphoid organs are classified as **primary** or **secondary.** Lymphocytes develop within the primary organs: thymus and bone marrow. The secondary lymphoid organs (e.g., spleen, lymph nodes, lymphoid accumulations) trap and concentrate immunogens and provide sites where large numbers of circulating immune cells can make contact with each another. Specific immune reactions are initiated with the interactions that occur in secondary lymphoid organs.

A. Primary organs

The primary lymphoid organs, the thymus and bone marrow, serve as lymphocyte educational centers. While all lymphocytes originate within the bone marrow, those destined to become T cells are sent at an early age to the thymus for "advanced education" in distinguishing self from nonself. Other lymphocytic lineage cells are "home schooled" and remain within the bone marrow, destined to become B cells. Stromal cells within the thymus and bone marrow closely regulate the development of T and B lymphocytes. Developmental details of B and T cells are described in upcoming chapters.

1. **Thymus:** The bilobed **thymus** is the first lymphoid organ to develop. It increases in size during fetal and neonatal life and progressively involutes following puberty. Stem cells of bone marrow origin called prothymocytes that are committed to the T cell lineage migrate via the circulation to the thymic cortex. In this new environment, they are called **cortical thymocytes** (see Fig. 8.4) and acquire a nascent TCR, as well as CD4 and CD8 surface molecules.

One of the first tests that these so-called **double positive** (DP, because they express both CD4 and CD8 molecules) thymocytes encounter, called **positive selection,** is the recognition of MHC class I (by CD8) or MHC class II (by CD4) (Fig. 7.7). Failure to do so appropriately means the demise of the DP thymocyte. Thymocytes that "pass" positive selection cease to express both CD4 and CD8 to become **single positive** (SP) CD4$^+$ or CD8$^+$ cells. SP thymocytes move into the medulla, where they encounter antigen-presenting cells. At this stage, termed **negative selection**, those that show strong interaction with MHC or pMHC are fated to die by programmed cell death (**apoptosis**). Tremendous numbers of thymocytes are processed by the thymus, but fewer than 5% of the thymocytes successfully complete this process. We will revisit

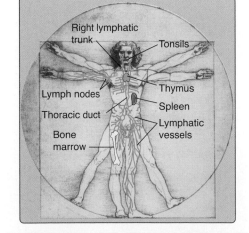

Figure 7.6
Lymphatics, lymphoid organs, and tissues. The lymphatics serve as a drainage system to remove cellular debris and microbes from the body's tissues to the lymph nodes. Lymphatic trunk vessels join to form the thoracic duct, which returns fluid (lymph) to the cardiovascular circulation.

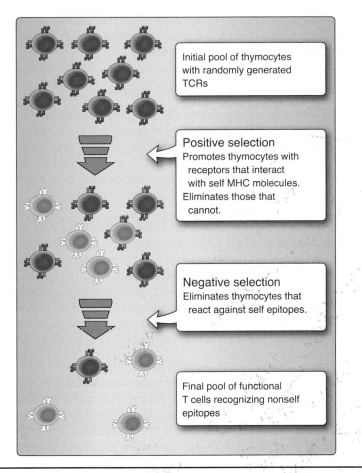

Figure 7.7

Thymic education: Many are "admitted," but few "graduate." "Freshman" thymocytes are called double positive (DP) because they express both CD4 and CD8 molecules in addition to T cell receptors (TCRs). *Positive selection*: Thymocytes that recognize MHC class I (using CD8) or MHC class II (CD4) pass their first exam are promoted; those that don't do this die. *Negative selection*: Thymocytes that show strong interaction with MHC or peptide-MHC combinations fail and meet an apoptotic death. Those few cells that pass the negative selection are destined to "graduate" from the thymus as T cells.

the processes of positive and negative selection in greater detail in Chapter 9.

2. **Bone marrow:** Lymphocytic lineage cells fated to become immunoglobulin-producing lymphocytes undergo their early stages of differentiation within the **bone marrow**. They develop their BCRs by DNA rearrangement, express auxiliary molecules such as Igα and Igβ, and begin to display IgM on their surfaces prior to leaving the bone marrow. As with T cells in the thymus, interactions with stromal cells of the bone marrow serve to carefully regulate the development of B cells. While still within the bone marrow, the randomly generated BCRs of some B cells may recognize and bind molecules in their local environment. By definition, these B cells would be self-reactive. At this early stage of development, the binding of BCRs triggers the cells bearing

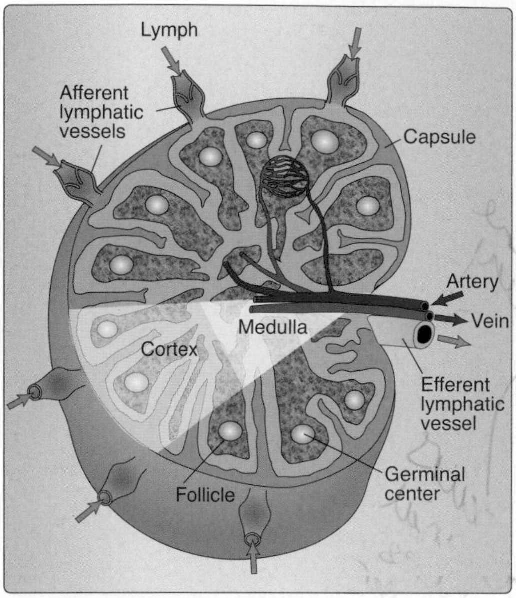

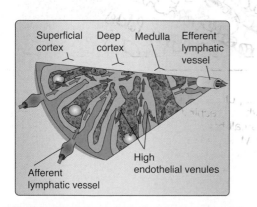

Figure 7.8

Circulation of lymph through a lymph node. Afferent lymphatic vessels enter the cortical portion of the lymph node. Leukocyte- and debris-rich lymph percolates through the body of the lymph node where it encounters phagocytic cells (macrophages and dendritic cells) that remove dead and dying cells, cellular debris, and microorganisms from the lymph. The "scrubbed" lymph exits the lymph node via an efferent lymphatic vessel. The vessels of the cardiovascular system transport leukocytes to and from the lymph node.

Figure 7.9

Section from lymph node in Figure 7.8 (see white triangle). Specialized high endothelium vessels provide a portal for leukocyte entry into the lymph node from the cardiovascular system. B cell–rich areas (superficial cortex and germinal centers) are anatomic sites of immunoglobulin production. The deep cortex and medullary regions are sites for T cell homing and activation.

them to undergo apoptotic death. This mechanism removes self-reactive cells. The developmental pathways of B cells are discussed in greater detail in Chapter 9.

B. Secondary lymphoid tissues and organs

Cellular interactions are critical for the development of adaptive immune responses. The secondary lymphoid tissues function as filtration devices removing foreign matter, dead cells, and protein aggregates from the circulation. Blood vessels and lymphatic vessels that facilitate movement of lymphocytes, monocytes, and dendritic cells into and out of these organs richly supply secondary lymphoid tissues. Specialized regions of the vasculature, called high endothelial venules, permit the movement of cells between the blood and the tissues or organs through which they are passing. The leukocyte-rich nature of the secondary lymphoid tissues facilitates cellular interaction, providing leukocytes an environment in which they can "compare notes," exchange regulatory signals, undergo further development, and proliferate before reentering the circulation. The major secondary lymphoid organs are the spleen and lymph nodes. The tonsils and Peyer's patches also act as secondary lymphoid accumulations.

1. **Spleen:** The largest lymphoid organ, the **spleen** clears particulate matter from the blood and concentrates blood-borne antigens and microbes. In addition to B and T lymphocytes and other leukocytes, the spleen contains large numbers of plasma cells secreting immunoglobulins into the circulation. It is histologically divided into the lymphocyte-rich **white pulp** and erythrocyte-rich **red pulp**. The white pulp surrounds small arterioles.

2. **Lymph nodes:** Small round or oval-shaped peripheral or secondary lymphoid organs, **lymph nodes** are leukocyte accumulations occurring periodically throughout the lymphatic circulatory system (see Fig. 7.6). They function as filters to purify **lymph**, the fluid and cellular content of the lymphatic circulatory system, and provide sites for mingling of lymphocytes, monocytes, and dendritic cells for initiation of immune responses. Anatomically, a lymph node is divided into the **cortex** and **medulla** (Fig. 7.8). The **reticulum** or framework of the organ is composed of phagocytes and specialized kinds of reticular or dendritic cells. Lymphocytes are distributed mainly in two areas of the cortex (Fig.7.9). **The superficial cortex** is closely packed with clusters of lymphocytes forming **nodules** or **follicles**. It is sometimes called the thymus-independent area and contains mostly B cells. When an immune response takes place, the follicles develop a central area, with large proliferating cells, termed a **germinal center**. The **deep cortex** is the T cell–rich area. Circulating cells enter the outer cortical area through blood or lymphatic vessels and then filter down through the deep cortex and into the medulla before leaving the lymph node and moving on.

3. **Mucosa-associated lymphoid tissues:** In addition to the spleen and lymph nodes, other sites that facilitate interaction among circulating leukocytes include tonsils in the nasopharynx and Peyer's patches in the submucosal surfaces of the small intestine (Fig. 7.10). These secondary lymphoid tissues defend the mucosa

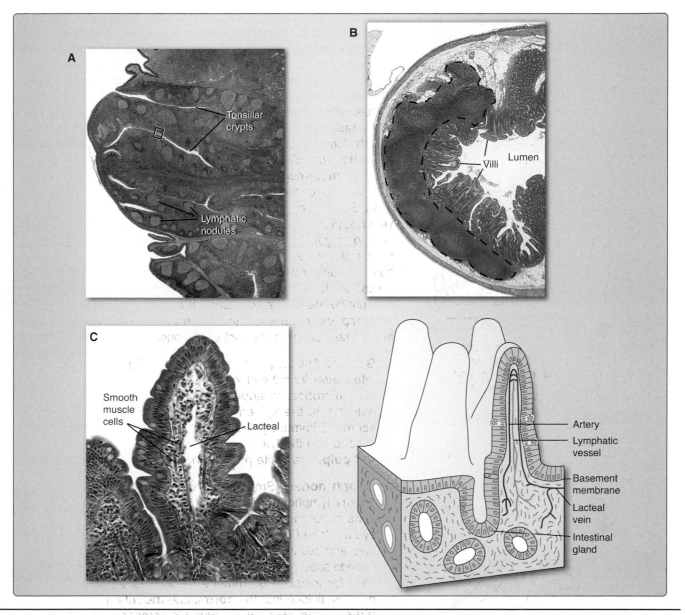

Figure 7.10
Mucosa-associated lymphoid tissues are anatomically placed at strategic areas of potential microbial entry. **A.** Tonsils are located as a defensive ring around the nasopharynx at the portal of entry for both the respiratory and gastrointestinal systems. **B.** Peyer's patches are lymphoid accumulations lying underneath the villi of the small bowel (within the area delineated by the dotted line). **C.** Intestinal villi contain intraepithelial lymphocytes, interstitial leukocytes, and draining lymphatics (lacteals) that serve to both sample the intestinal environment and defend the bowel from microbial invasion.

surfaces and are located at potential portals of microbial entry. Peyer's patches function similarly to lymph nodes and the spleen, with cells entering at the cortical end, promoting the intermingling of antigen-presenting cells, B cells, and T cells and the exit of cells at the medullary end.

C. Lymphatic circulatory system

Leukocytes and their products use two circulatory systems. One, the cardiovascular system, is responsible for the circulation of blood (both its soluble and cellular components) throughout the body. The other system, the lymphatic circulatory system (see Fig. 7.6), is an extensive capillary network that collects **lymph**, a watery clear fluid containing leukocytes and cellular debris, from various organs and tissues. Lymphatic vessels within small intestine villi, designated **lacteals**, contain a milk-white fluid, **chyle**, produced by digestion. The lymphatic capillaries drain into large lymphatic vessels that drain into lymph nodes for filtration. Ultimately, the lymphatic trunk vessels join to form the thoracic duct that conveys lymph into the subclavian artery.

Chapter Summary

- CD4$^+$ T cells account for approximately two thirds of mature CD3$^+$ T cells. CD4 molecules displayed on the surfaces of these T cells recognize a nonpeptide-binding portion of MHC class II molecules.

- **CD8$^+$ T cells** account for approximately one third of all mature CD3$^+$ T cells. CD8 molecules displayed on the cell surfaces of these T cells recognize the nonpeptide-binding portion of MHC class I molecules.

- **B cells** form two distinct lineages: B-1 and B-2 cells. B-1 cells develop before B-2 cells. Each B cell is specific; that is, it produces immunoglobulin of only one antibody specificity that recognizes only one epitope.

- **Plasma cells** derive from terminally differentiated B cells and are immunoglobulin-producing and secreting cells.

- Approximately 5% to 10% of peripheral blood lymphocytes lack T cell (CD3) and B cell (surface immunoglobulin) markers. These cells are known as **natural killer (NK) cells** to reflect their ability to kill certain tumor cells without prior sensitization.

- Lymphoid organs are classified as primary or secondary. Lymphocytes develop within the primary organs: the **thymus** and **bone marrow**. The secondary lymphoid organs (e.g., **spleen, lymph nodes**, lymphoid accumulations) trap and concentrate immunogens and provide sites where large numbers of circulating immune cells can make contact with each another. The largest lymphoid organ, the spleen, clears particulate matter from the blood and concentrates blood-borne antigens and microbes

- In addition to the spleen and lymph nodes, other sites that facilitate interaction among circulating leukocytes include tonsils in the nasopharynx and Peyer's patches in the submucosal surfaces of the small intestine

- Lymph nodes are located along lymphatic vessels that contain **lymph**, a watery mixture containing cellular debris and leukocytes. The lymph nodes act as filters to remove cellular debris and microorganisms from the lymph prior to its return to the cardiovascular circulatory system.

Study Questions

7.1 T cell receptors, when coexpressed with CD8 molecules, are restricted to recognizing and binding peptide fragments associated with

A. CD3 molecules.
B. CD4 molecules.
C. MHC class I molecules.
D. MHC class II molecules.
E. MHC class III molecules.

The correct answer is C. CD8$^+$ T cells are restricted to the recognition of pMHC I complexes. CD3 molecules are associated with the TCR on the T cell surface and are found on both mature CD4$^+$ and CD8$^+$ T cells. CD4$^+$ T cells are restricted to the recognition of pMHC class II complexes. MHC class III molecules include complement components C4, Bf, and C2 and are not involved in T cell recognition.

7.2 B lymphocytes synthesize and express immunoglobulin

A. containing multiple epitope specificities.
B. in cytoplasmic phagosomes.
C. in membrane complexes also containing CD3.
D. on their cell membrane surface.
E. only after leaving the bone marrow.

The correct answer is D. B cells synthesize and express immunoglobulin on their cell surfaces. Immunoglobulins within an individual B cell contain specificity for one epitope, not several. Cytoplasmic phagosomes are involved in degradation of unwanted materials. Membrane complexes also containing CD3 are T cell receptors (TCR) on the surfaces of T cells. B cells express surface IgM before leaving the bone marrow.

7.3 The primary lymphoid organs are those in which

A. adaptive immune responses are usually initiated.
B. filtration devices remove foreign matter.
C. large numbers of circulating leukocytes make contact with one another.
D. lymphocytes undergo their initial differentiation.
E. pattern recognition receptors bind antigens.

The correct answer is D. Primary lymphoid organs are sites where lymphocytes undergo their initial differentiation. Adaptive immune responses are initiated by mature lymphocytes that have migrated out of primary lymphoid organs. Secondary lymphoid organs contain filtration devices to remove foreign materials. Circulating leukocytes are found within blood and lymph and secondary lymphoid organs but not within primary lymphoid organs. Pattern recognition receptors (PRRs) are expressed by cells of the innate immune system (see Chapter 5).

7.4 The thymus is the site of initial differentiation for

A. B cells.
B. erythrocytes.
C. hematopoietic stem cells.
D. NK cells.
E. T cells.

The correct answer is E. The thymus is the site of initial differentiation of T cells. Erythrocytes develop from erythroid precursors in the bone marrow. Hematopoietic stem cells differentiate along any one of several lineages within the bone marrow. Natural killer (NK) cells develop within the bone marrow and lack rearranged TCR.

7.5 Lymph nodes have two main regions: the

A. cortex and medulla.
B. lymph and cortex.
C. reticulum and cortex.
D. lymph and medulla.
E. reticulum and medulla.

The correct answer is A. Lymph nodes are divided into the cortex and the medulla. Lymph is the watery fluid of the lymphatic circulatory system that contains leukocytes and cellular debris from various organs and tissues. Reticulum refers to the framework of a lymph node that is composed of phagocytes and specialized kinds of reticular or dendritic cells.

7.6 Which of the following molecules is expressed on the surface of mature CD4$^+$ cells?

A. B cell receptor
B. CD1d
C. CD3
D. CD8
E. CD19

The correct answer is C. Mature T cells (both CD4$^+$ and CD8$^+$) express CD3, a molecular complex associated with the TCR. CD4$^+$ cells are T cells with T helper function and do not express B cell receptors. CD1d is a specialized, nonclassical MHC class I molecule on NKT cells. CD8 is a molecule expressed by T cytotoxic and suppressor cells. CD19 is expressed on B cells.

7.7 Positive selection refers to

A. the ability of single positive cells to bind both MHC class I and II.
B. cortical thymocytes' acquisition of TCR.
C. migration of stem cells to the thymus to become T cells.
D. programmed cell death of single positive T cells.
E. recognition of MHC by CD4$^+$CD8$^+$ thymocytes.

The correct answer is E. Positive selection refers to recognition of MHC class I (by CD8) or MHC class II (by CD4) by double-positive (CD4$^+$CD8$^+$) thymocytes. Single positive thymocytes (and T cells) are either CD4$^+$ or CD8$^+$ and recognize either MHC class II (CD4) or MHC class I (CD8), but not both. Cortical thymocytes acquire a nascent TCR as well as CD4 and CD8 surface molecules, resulting in formation of double-positive (CD4$^+$CD8$^+$) thymocytes. Precursor T cells migrate or traffic from the bone marrow to the thymus before acquiring CD4 and CD8, which they will do as cortical thymocytes. Programmed cell death, or apoptosis, is the fate of cells that undergo negative selection after failure to undergo positive selection.

7.8 Which of the following is a primary lymphoid organ?

A. bone marrow
B. lymph node
C. Peyer's patch
D. spleen
E. tonsil

The correct answer is A. The bone marrow is a primary lymphoid organ. Lymph nodes, Peyer's patches, spleen, and tonsils are all secondary lymphoid organs.

7.9 The white pulp of the spleen is enriched in

A. erythrocytes carrying hemoglobin.
B. CD4$^+$CD8$^+$ T cells binding to MHC.
C. natural killer cells recognizing targets.
D. plasma cells secreting immunoglobin.
E. precursor cells developing into mature B cells.

The correct answer is D. The white pulp of the spleen is enriched in plasma cells secreting immunoglobulin, in addition to B and T lymphocytes. Erythrocytes are found within the red pulp of the spleen. CD4$^+$CD8$^+$ T cells are found in the thymus. Natural killer cells function within peripheral blood. Precursors of B cells are located in the bone marrow.

Generation of Immune Diversity: Lymphocyte Antigen Receptors

8

I. OVERVIEW

Epitope specificity of immunoglobulin molecules produced by B cells and of T cell receptors is determined before they encounter antigen. Moreover, the number of possible epitope-binding specificities greatly exceeds the number of genes within the human genome. This presents a paradox: How does the immune system generate a diverse array of antigen-specific molecules from a limited number of genes? The immune system's genetic solution is both fascinating and elegant.

II. PROPERTIES OF LYMPHOCYTE ANTIGEN RECEPTORS

Domains located at the amino (NH) terminus of immunoglobulin heavy and light chains (variable or V_H and V_L regions) produced by different B cells are highly variable in amino acid sequence. In contrast, other regions, termed C or constant regions, are limited in variability for immunoglobulins of the same isotype produced by different B cells. Light chains have a single constant domain (C_L, also designated as C_κ for kappa chains or C_λ for lambda chains), and heavy chains contain multiple constant regions C_H1, C_H2, C_H3, and for some C_H4 domains. Heavy or light chain DNA gene segments for both variable and constant regions are rearranged, transcribed into RNA, and translated into a single heavy or light chain polypeptide. Individuals codominantly inherit maternal and paternal sets of alleles for light chain and heavy chain loci. A single B cell or plasma cell may express only the kappa ($V_\kappa C_\kappa$) or the lambda ($V_\lambda C_\lambda$) light chain alleles, either maternal or paternal, to the exclusion of all others (Fig. 8.1). Likewise, a single B cell may express only the maternal or paternal $V_H C_H$ heavy chain alleles but not both. The restriction of $V_L C_L$ and $V_H C_H$ expression to a single member of each of the involved chromosome pairs is termed **allelic exclusion**. However, the combined contributions of all of the B cells mean that the both maternal and paternal **allotypes** (allelic forms) are expressed within any particular individual.

The same principles apply to the genes encoding the $\alpha\beta$ and $\gamma\delta$ T cell receptors, which also include light chains (α or γ) and heavy chains (β

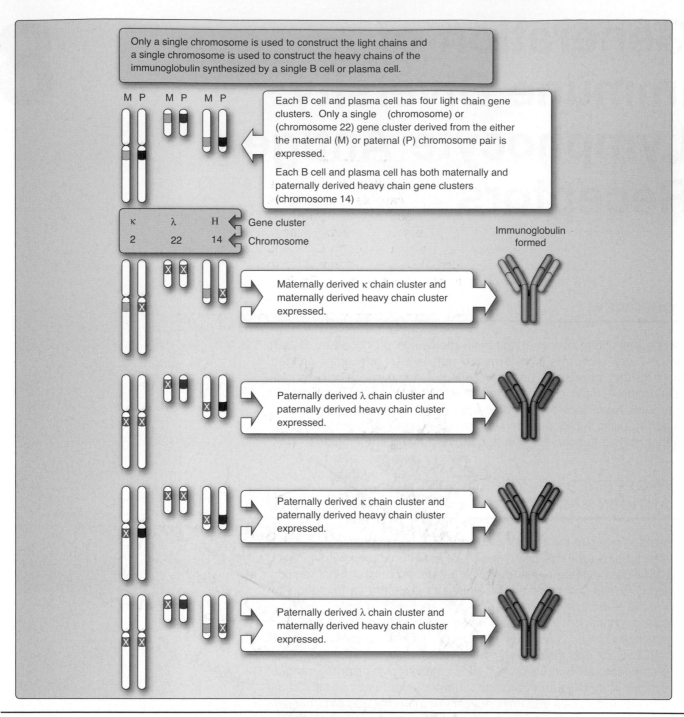

Figure 8.1

Allelic exclusion. Immunoglobulin light and heavy gene clusters are located on different chromosome pairs, each pair having a maternally derived and a paternally derived chromosome. Each B cell and its progeny use only one parental chromosome to encode its light (#2 or #22) and heavy (#14) chains. A given B cell uses these same variable region gene clusters throughout its lifetime for the immunoglobulins it produces to the exclusion of all others.

or δ). Each chain consists of a variable region at its amino terminus and a constant region at its carboxy terminus. The variable regions of the chains are determined by rearrangement of the DNA encoding them and the production of an mRNA transcript, including both the variable and constant regions. Splicing of the mRNA that is then translated into the polypeptide chains unites the variable and constant regions.

III. DNA REARRANGEMENT

Immunologists estimate that each person has the ability to produce a range of individual antigen-specific receptors capable of binding as many as 10^{15} different epitopes. DNA chromosomal rearrangement is responsible for a significant portion of epitope-specific diversity among T and B cell receptors. Rearrangement occurs at both the DNA and RNA levels by the **deletion** of nucleotides, followed by reannealing, to bring together gene segments that were previously separated (Fig. 8.2).

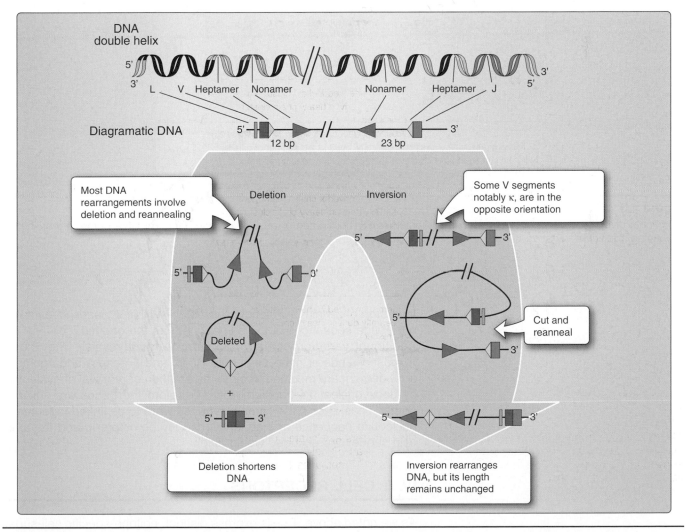

Figure 8.2

Chromosome rearrangement. Segments of DNA encoding a series of genes are rearranged by the deletion of intervening DNA. Joining of the remaining segments (a process called *annealing*) then brings together genes that were originally separated on the chromosome. In addition, DNA rearrangement is sometimes accomplished by the inversion of DNA segments, changing the linear sequence of genes without the removal of intervening DNA.

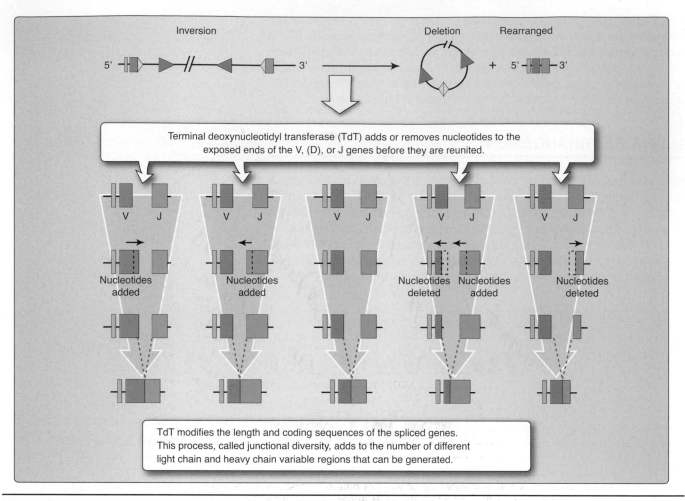

Figure 8.3

Junctional diversity. Terminal deoxynucleotidyl transferase (TdT) can add or remove exposed ends of DNA before annealing, producing additional variation in nucleotide sequence.

Inversion of certain DNA sequences, notably within V_κ, leads to rearranged nucleotide sequences of the same length as the original (see Fig. 8.2). Additional variation comes from **junctional diversity** (Fig. 8.3) as "exposed" ends of gene segments (V, D, and J genes) undergoing rearrangement are modified through the addition or removal of nucleotides by deoxynucleotidyl transferase (TdT) before the genes are linked together. Thus, even if the same two genes were to be linked together, the nucleotide sequence at their junctions may be different, and the amino acid sequences encoded would differ.

IV. T CELL RECEPTORS

As we noted above, T cells express distinct, epitope-specific cell-surface receptors (TCRs) that are heterodimers composed of either $\alpha\beta$ or $\gamma\delta$ light-heavy chain pairs. Each polypeptide contains a single variable region domain and a single constant region domain. T cells express and

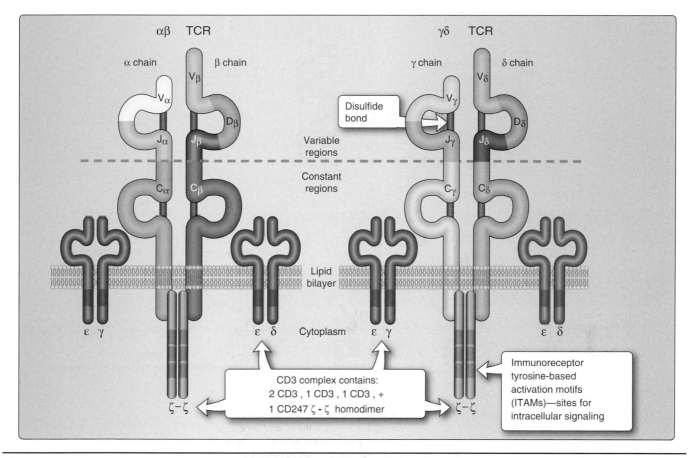

Figure 8.4
T cell receptors (TcRs). T cells express either αβ or γδ TCR heterodimers. The CD3 complex associates with the TCR to transduce a signal to the interior of the cell when the TCR engages a peptide-MHC complex.

display T cell receptor (TCR) complexes composed of an αβ or a γδ TCR (but never both) heterodimer pair, associated CD3 (γ, δ, and ε and a CD247 ζ-chain homodimer), and CD4 or CD8 molecules. Associated transmembrane molecules, such as CD4 or CD8, stabilize the interaction of the TCR with a specific peptide-MHC (pMHC) combination. Others, such as those in the CD3 complex, participate in signal transduction events after TCR-ligand engagement (Fig. 8.4). The short cytoplasmic tail of the TCR lacks signaling sequence or immunoreceptor tyrosine activation motifs (ITAMs). The CD3 and CD247 molecules supply these. Unlike antibodies, TCRs cannot bind free epitopes. They can bind only enzymatically cleaved fragments of larger polypeptides that are presented as pMHC complexes.

A. Gene clusters encoding T cell receptors

Gene clusters encoding α and δ chains of the TCR on chromosome 14 are arranged such that the entire δ chain gene cluster (D_δ, J_δ, and C_δ) lies within the α gene cluster between the D_α and J_α chain genes (Fig. 8.5). Genes encoding β and δ chains are located in separate clusters on chromosome 7.

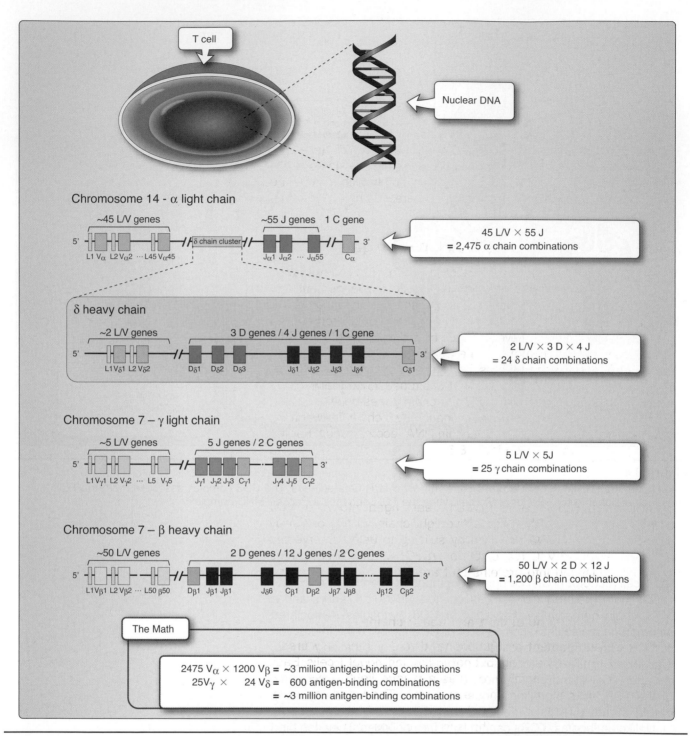

Figure 8.5

Gene clusters encoding TCR chains. Gene clusters encoding TCR light chains are located on chromosomes 14 (α chain) and 7 (γ chain) and heavy chains on chromosomes 7 (β chain) and 14 (δ chain).

The first level of TCR diversity comes from DNA recombination to produce the variable regions. The selection of V, D, and J genes for rearrangement appears to be random from cell to cell: 2475 α chain sequences (45 $V_\alpha \times$ 55 J_α) $\times$ 1200 β chain sequences (50 V_β $\times$ 2 $D_\beta \times$ 12 J_β). Random association of α and β chains yields nearly 3 million different epitope-binding sites for $\alpha\beta$ chains. For $\gamma\delta$ TCRs, 25 γ chain sequences (5 $V_\gamma \times$ 5 J_γ) $\times$ 24 δ chain sequences (2 $V_\delta \times$ 3 $D_\delta \times$ 4 J_δ) yields 600 $\gamma\delta$ TCR epitope-binding site possibilities. Junctional diversity, a process mediated by TdT (see Fig. 8.3), contributes a second level of diversity by the insertion or deletion of up to 20 nucleotides at the time of recombination. Thus, the total number of possible TCR specificities increases by many orders of magnitude.

B. Variable regions: Rearrangement of V, D, and J genes

TCRs are generated by recombination enzymes or **recombinases** (e.g., Rag-1 and Rag-2) that mediate genetic rearrangement and recombination, processes similar to those seen for immunoglobulin (see sections 8.V.B and 8.V.C, on page 98). Each T cell produces $\alpha\beta$ or $\gamma\delta$ TCR heterodimers, never both. Gene rearrangement begins by the excision and deletion of DNA between V_α and J_α (light, Fig. 8.5) or V_δ and D_δ (heavy) chain genes. Because the entirety of the δ chain genetic material lies within the α light chain sequence (between V_α and J_α), initiation of recombination by α chain genes deletes δ chain DNA. Conversely, initiation of recombination by δ chain (between V_δ, D_δ, and D_δ) DNA precludes α light chain DNA recombination. For the details of this process, see Figure 8.6.

C. Uniting variable and constant regions

TCR constant region genes (already rearranged into VJ or VDJ units) are united with their respective light chain VJ (C_α or C_γ) by transcription into mRNA, followed by splicing to delete intervening mRNA. The united VJC (C_α or C_γ) or VDJC (C_β or C_δ) transcripts are then translated into proteins that are the joint product of the rearranged genes.

D. Random combinations of light and heavy chains

Genetic rearrangement and junctional diversity randomly create TCR chains that vary among, but not within, individual T cells. Each developing T cell randomly produces a unique light-heavy chain ($\alpha\beta$ or $\gamma\delta$) combination with unique specificity. The theoretical number of possible combinations produced within the body may be estimated to be the product of the number of possible light chains and the number of possible heavy chains (Fig. 8.7). Immunologists estimate that 1 million to 5 million epitope-binding combinations are possible for TCRs. However, unlike immunoglobulin genes, TCRs do not undergo subsequent changes equivalent to the isotype switching and somatic hypermutation that occur in immunoglobulins to further increase their diversity (see Sections 8.V.E and 8.V.G, on page 102).

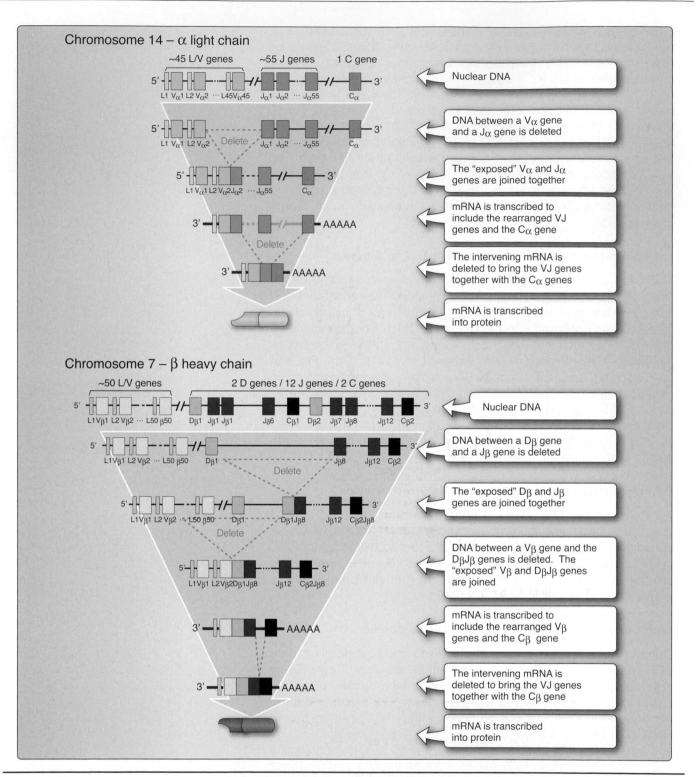

Figure 8.6

Rearrangement to form an αβ TCR. For the α chain, DNA is deleted to join randomly selected V and J genes. An mRNA transcript is then produced containing united VJ genes and a constant gene. This transcript is then spliced to unite the VJ and C genes to form mRNA that can be directly translated to a polypeptide containing conjoined VJC segments. A similar process occurs for the β chain with the addition of D genes toe form a VDJ variable region. γδ TCRs are synthesized in a similar manner.

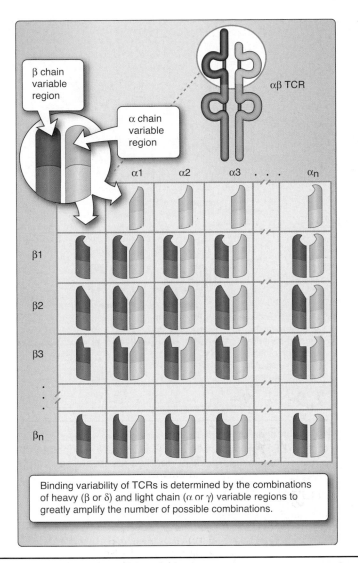

Figure 8.7
Formation of TCR peptide-MHC binding regions.

V. B CELL RECEPTORS

Immunoglobulin gene rearrangements occur in the early stages of B cell precursor differentiation and prior to antigen exposure. These gene rearrangements, along with allelic exclusion, allow for the construction of variable regions that recognize a great portion of the antigenic universe. A single B cell produces immunoglobulins of one epitope specificity (and one isotype), formed from the association of light and heavy chains and inserted within the plasma membrane (Fig. 8.8). The rearranged DNA encoding immunoglobulins within B cells is transcribed into primary RNA, intervening sequences are edited out of mRNA, and polypeptides

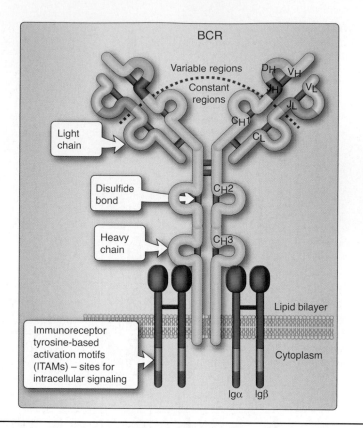

Figure 8.8
B cell receptors (BCR or immunoglobulin). BCRs are composed of two identical immunoglobulin light (κ or λ) and two identical heavy chains. Cell-surface associated Igα and Igβ chains transmit signals to the interior of the cell when ligands are bound by the BCR.

are assembled in the Golgi apparatus and targeted to either the membrane in B cells or for secretion by plasma cells.

A. Gene clusters encoding B cell receptors

Gene clusters encoding κ light chains are found on chromosome 2, while those encoding λ light chains are on chromosome 22. The heavy chain gene cluster is located on chromosome 14. Potential antigen-binding combinations are greater than 26 million. Details of this process are shown in Figure 8.9.

B. Light chains

As we have seen, immunoglobulin light chains contain two regions or domains, a **variable** (V_L) domain and a **constant** (C_L) domain. Any given B lymphocyte will generate only identical light chain proteins of either the κ or λ type ($V_κC_κ$ or $V_λC_λ$), never of both types or a combination of the two.

1. **Variable regions: Rearrangement of V and J genes:** To generate a light chain variable region of the κ or λ type, one of about 100 variable (V_k or $V_λ$) gene segments recombines with one of

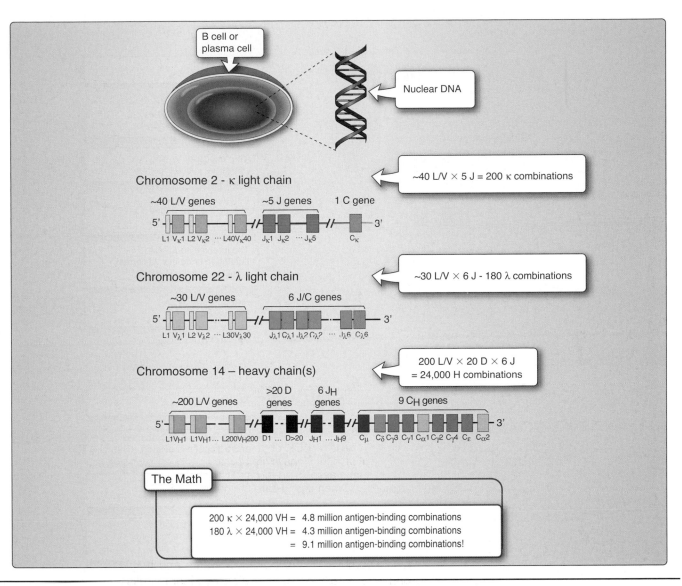

Figure 8.9
Gene clusters encoding the BCR chains. Clusters of genes encoding the BCR light chains (κ and λ) are located on chromosomes 2 and 22, respectively. Each cluster includes a series of V genes, a series of J genes, and one or more constant (C) genes. The single BCR heavy chain cluster is located on chromosome 14. It includes a series of V genes, a series of D genes, a series of J genes, and a series of constant (C) genes.

four to five joining (J_λ) segments at the DNA levels to create a conjoined VJ pair. The intervening DNA is then removed and degraded. The choice of which V and which J gene to include occurs randomly for each cell. Thus, across a large number of B cells, several hundred different VJ units can be generated.

2. **Uniting variable and constant regions:** This occurs at the mRNA level, where a transcript including both the variable (now a VJ unit) region and a constant region is generated. The transcript is then spliced to unite the two regions to produce an mRNA transcript that can be translated directly into a single polypeptide. Details of this process are shown in Fig 8.10.

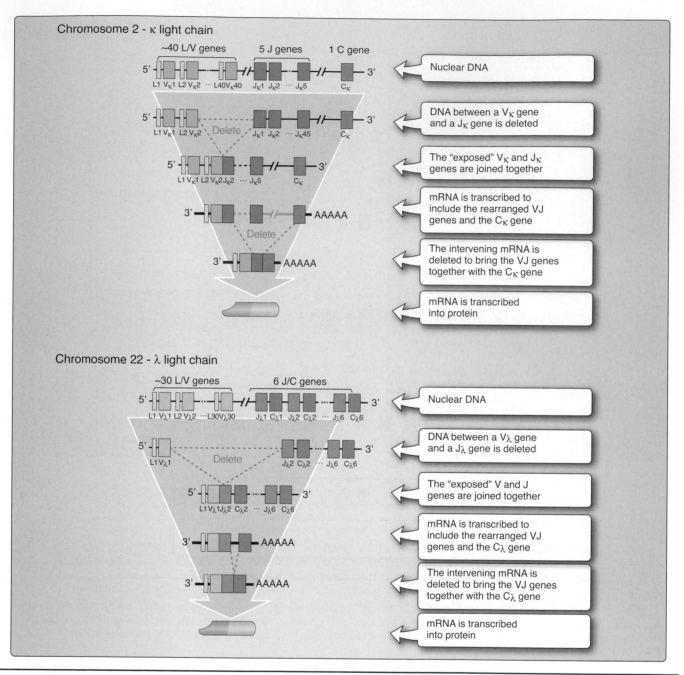

Figure 8.10

Rearrangement to form BCR light chains. The rearrangements to form κ and λ chains are illustrated. DNA is deleted to join a randomly selected V gene with a randomly selected J gene. An mRNA transcript is then produced that contains the united VJ genes and a constant gene. This transcript is subsequently spliced to unite the VJ and C genes to form an mRNA that can be translated directly to a polypeptide with conjoined VJC segments.

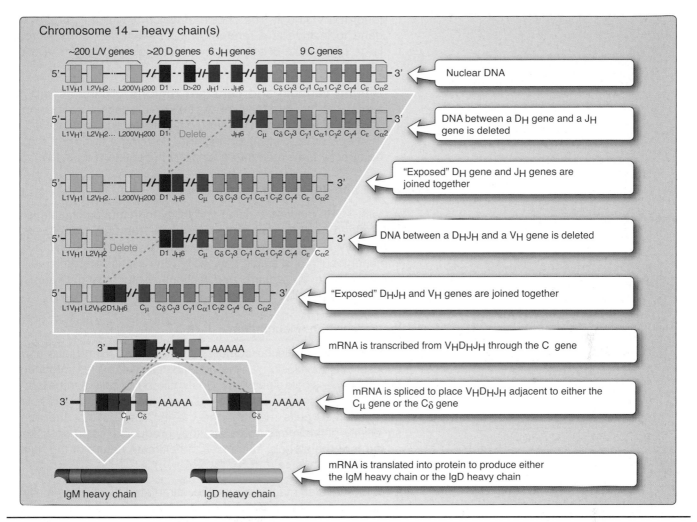

Figure 8.11
Rearrangement to form BCR heavy chains. Intervening DNA is deleted between randomly selected D and J genes to form as DJ sequence followed by a second random deletion to form a VDJ unit. An mRNA transcript is produced and spliced to unite the VDJ genes together with the μ or δ genes (the remaining constant region genes are utilized at a later stage in B cell development) that can be directly translated into IgM or IgD heavy chains. Naïve B cells simultaneously express both IgM and IgD with identical epitope specificity on their cell surfaces.

C. Heavy chains

A single cluster of genes encode the immunoglobulin heavy chain. Heavy chains contain a single variable (V_H) and three or four constant (C_H1, C_H2, C_H3, and sometimes C_H4) region domains.

1. **Variable regions: Rearrangement of V, D and J genes:** To generate a heavy chain variable region, one of about 200 heavy chain variable (V_H) genes is combined with one of several diversity (D_H) genes and one of numerous joining (J_H) genes. The intervening DNA is removed and degraded (see details in Fig. 8.11). A DNA deletion unites randomly selected D and J to form DJ, and second deletion unites a randomly selected V gene with the DJ

to form a VDJ unit. The choice of which V, which D, and which J gene to include is a random one for each cell. Thus, across a large number of B cells, many thousands of different VDJ units can be generated.

2. **Uniting variable and constant regions** occurs, as with light chains, at the mRNA level. An mRNA transcript containing the separated variable (VDJ) and constant regions is produced and then spliced to bring them together, forming a transcript that can be directly translated into a single polypeptide (Fig. 8.11).

D. Heavy and light chain combinations

As with TCRs, antigen-binding variability in immunoglobulins is also determined by the combination (random from cell to cell) of light and heavy chain variable regions. An individual B cell synthesizes immunoglobulin of a single specificity (one particular combination of V_L region and V_H region), and millions of such combinations are theoretically possible (Fig. 8.12).

E. Isotype switch: Mechanism

Because of its particular combination of V_L and V_H regions and the effect of allelic exclusion, an individual B cell synthesizes immunoglobulin of only a single specificity. Unstimulated B cells synthesize and display monomeric IgM (and IgD) on their cell surfaces. Upon stimulation, B cells may change the isotype, but not the epitope specificity, of the immunoglobulins they produce. This process, known as the **isotype switch,** influences the ultimate nature of the humoral immune response.

The intracellular machinery of the stimulated B cell produces immunoglobulins of only a single isotype at a time. Immunoglobulins may be considered the "ballistic missiles" of the adaptive immune system, their V regions forming a specific "warhead" and their constant regions constituting the "rocket" portion of the molecule. Although a single B cell can manufacture a single type of "warhead," it can be placed on different "rockets" or constant regions. The isotype ultimately determines whether an antibody activates complement or is secreted into a lumen, secreted onto a mucous membrane, or immobilized by certain tissues of the body. Isotype switching permits the adaptive immune system to produce antibodies with identical specificity that are capable of initiating a variety of different immune responses. As will be discussed in later chapters, T cells are usually required to activate and stimulate B cells to proliferate, switch isotype, and differentiate into immunoglobulin-secreting plasma cells.

F. Isotype switch: Consequence

The initial or primary antibody response to an epitope is dominated by production of the IgM isotype. Not all B cells initially stimulated by antigen (primary response) become plasma cells, synthesizing and secreting immunoglobulins for the remainder of their lifespan. Some stimulated B cells, **memory B cells**, are held in reserve

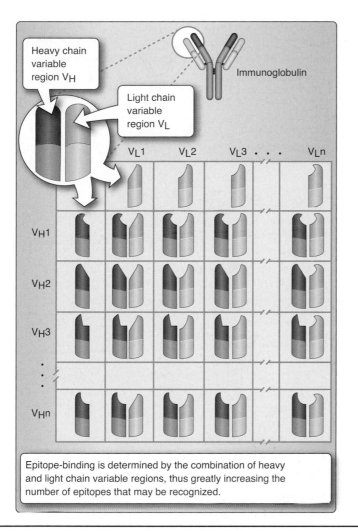

Epitope-binding is determined by the combination of heavy and light chain variable regions, thus greatly increasing the number of epitopes that may be recognized.

Figure 8.12
Formation of TCR epitope-binding regions by the combination of light and heavy chain variable regions. Each B cell produces a single light chain variable region and a single heavy chain variable region. However, among a population of B cells, the number of possible combinations of light and heavy chains creates a large number of different epitope-binding sites.

against future exposures to antigen. In response to restimulation by the appropriate epitopes, T cell cytokines (e.g., IL-4, IFN-γ, IL-5), and other signals, memory B cells synthesizing IgM can undergo further DNA rearrangement to change the class or isotype of the immunoglobulin through isotype switching. These memory B cells undergo further DNA rearrangement to juxtapose their rearranged VDJ gene regions to different heavy chain C region genes (Fig. 8.13A) and thereby alter the mRNA transcript and ultimately the immunoglobulin isotype (e.g. IgG, IgA, or IgE) that is produced.

Rearrangements to produce particular isotypes may occur through excision of large DNA segments or through deletion of smaller DNA segments (Fig. 8.13B). As a result, if you were to follow the B cell

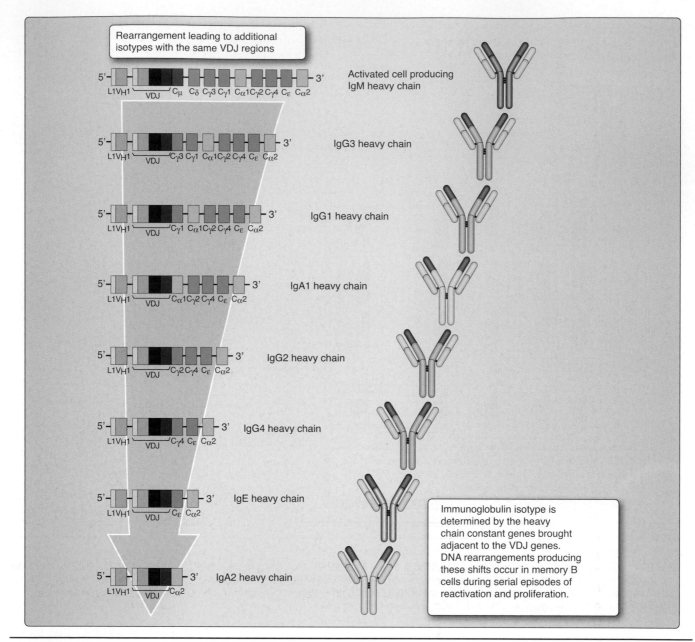

Figure 8.13

The isotype switch **A.** Following initial activation after contact with its specific epitope (plus other interactions), B cells cease production of IgD, and most of them differentiate into plasma cells that concentrate on secretion of IgM. However, some B cells become memory B cells and remain quiescent for future use. At this point, they express only IgM on their surface. However, if reactivated by a new contact with their specific epitope and appropriate interactions with T cells, they can begin to undergo additional rearrangements of their heavy chain genes at the DNA level to juxtapose their VDJ units with other constant genes. The VDJ units are not altered by these rearrangements. Whatever constant gene is brought adjacent to the VDJ determines what heavy chain gene will be produced. Again, most of these cells will differentiate into plasma cells secreting immunoglobulins of the newly generated isotype, but some will again be reserved as memory cells for subsequent use.

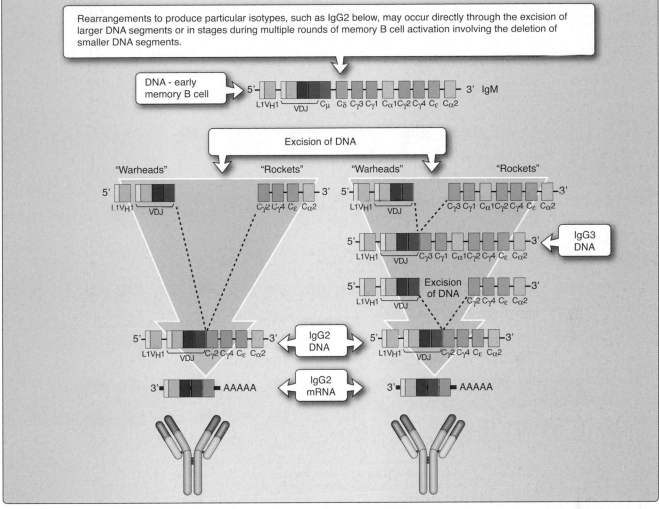

Figure 8.13
B. Isotype switches can occur in multiple ways. Some isotype switches may involve the deletion of large tracts of DNA to bring VDJ segments together with distant constant genes. In other cases, serial reactivations of memory B cells may result in a series of shorter deletions as IgM memory B cells may switch and become IgG memory B cells, then be reactivated again and switch to yet another isotype.

response to a given epitope over time and repeated stimulation, you would observe that it is typically dominated initially by IgM-producing cells, then by IgG-producing cells, with the eventual appearance of IgA- and IgE-producing B cells as well (Fig. 8.14). The isotype switch is restricted to B cells; there is no equivalent process in T cells.

G. Somatic hypermutation

Upon subsequent epitope exposure, memory B cells may switch their expressed isotype, and they may also accumulate small point mutations in the DNA encoding their V_L or H_L regions during the

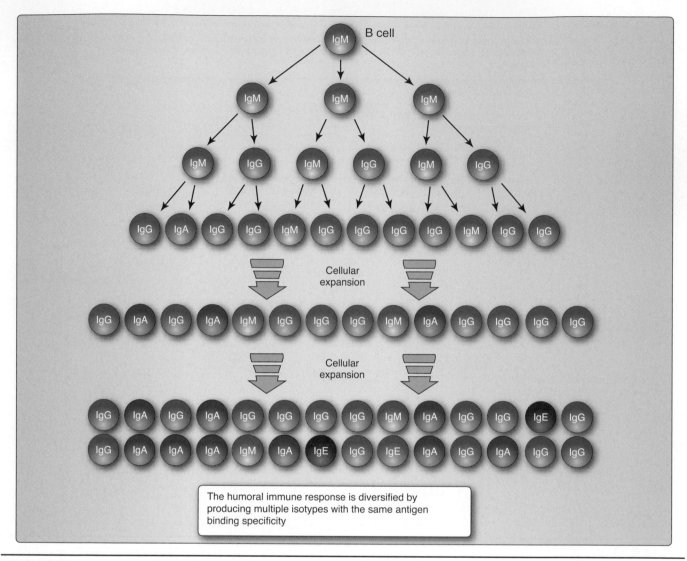

Figure 8.14

Consequences of the isotype switch. Repeated or constant stimulation by the same epitope drives B cells from IgM expression to other isotype. The cells epitope specificity is not alters by isotype switching.

rapid proliferation that follows restimulation (Fig 8.15). This process, **somatic hypermutation**, provides additional variation that "fine-tunes" the antibody responses to antigens that are frequently or chronically present. Some mutations may increase the binding affinity of the antibody for its epitope, and this increase in affinity causes those cells to proliferate more rapidly after binding to antigen. As a result, the interaction of antibody with a given epitope becomes tighter and more effective over time, a process called **affinity maturation**. Like the isotype switch, somatic hypermutation occurs only in B cells, not in T cells.

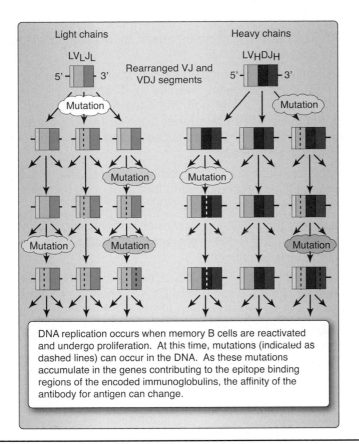

Figure 8.15
Somatic hypermutation. B cells undergo multiple round of rapid proliferation upon antigenic stimulation. Cells carrying mutations that result in tighter binding are stimulated to proliferated come to dominate the response. Thus antibodies with ever-increase affinity for that epitope are produced, a process called *affinity* maturation.

Chapter Summary

• Both heavy and light chain chains of immunoglobulins and T cell receptors contain variable regions that are extremely diverse and constant regions that are relatively consistent.

• The restriction of V_LC_L and V_HC_H expression to a single member of the chromosome pair in any given B cell or T cell is termed **allelic exclusion**. The presence of both maternal and paternal **allotypes** (allelic forms) is observed within a particular individual.

• The variable regions of immunoglobulins and T cell receptors are formed by the rearrangement (at the DNA level) of multiple genes that are then transcribed into a single mRNA transcript that includes both the variable and constant regions. The variable and constant regions are then brought together by splicing of the mRNA to produce a transcript that can be directly translated into a single polypeptide.

- DNA chromosomal rearrangement is responsible for a significant portion of epitope-specific diversity for T and B cell receptors. Rearrangement occurs at both the DNA and RNA levels by the removal of nucleotides (**deletions)** followed by reannealing or by **inversion** of certain DNA sequences. Additional variation comes from **junctional diversity.**

- Recombination enzymes or recombinases mediate the genetic rearrangement and recombination that generates the variable regions of TCR and immunoglobulin chains.

- TCR and immunoglobulin gene rearrangements occur in the early stages of T cell and B cell precursor differentiation, prior to exposure of the cells to antigen.

- Gene clusters encoding α and δ chains of the TCR are arranged such that all of the δ chain genes (D_δ, J_δ, and C_δ) lie between the D_α and $J_\alpha + C_\alpha$ α chain gene

- Gene clusters encoding immunoglobulin κ light, λ light, and heavy chains are found on different chromosomes.

- The initial or primary antibody response to epitopes is dominated by production of the IgM isotype.

- Memory B cells, in response to subsequent restimulation by antigen and interaction with T cells, undergo further DNA rearrangement to juxtapose their rearranged VDJ genes next to different heavy chain C region genes, thereby altering the immunoglobulin isotype (e.g. IgG, IgA, or IgE) produced. This is known as the **isotype switch**.

- **Somatic hypermutation** is the process whereby memory B cells are stimulated by subsequent exposures to the same epitope. Small point mutations occur in the DNA encoding their V_L or H_L regions during the rapid proliferation that follows restimulation.

- **Affinity maturation** is the process whereby the binding of antibodies to a given antigen becomes better over multiple exposures. It is caused by the accumulations of small mutations that may affect the antigen-binding sites and the positive selection of those cells carrying mutations that result in tighter binding.

Study Questions

8.1 In a patient who later developed an allergy to a certain antigen, the initial response to the antigen consisted of immunoglobulin of the IgM class. However, over time, antigen-specific IgE came to be predominant. This change from an IgM to an IgE response is caused by:

A. affinity maturation.
B. allelic exclusion.
C. isotype switching.
D. junctional diversity.
E. somatic hypermutation.

The answer is C. Isotype switching is a process in which rearranged VDJ genes within a memory B cell become juxtaposed through DNA excision from an upstream (5') C region gene with a different C region gene farther downstream (3'). Affinity maturation of antibody for its epitope is independent of isotype. For B cells that have "selected" their maternal or paternal immunoglobulin variable region genes, there are no "do-overs." Both junctional diversity and somatic hypermutation involve the antigen-binding site for immunoglobulin and do not appear to influence a switch from one isotype to another.

8.2 A 2-year-old child exposed to an antigen for the first time already possesses a B cell with immunoglobulin specific for that antigen. This finding is best explained by:

A. antigen-independent immunoglobulin gene rearrangements.
B. antigen stimulation of T cell cytokine production.
C. maternally derived antibodies to that antigen.
D. memory B cells that recognize the antigen.
E. somatic hypermutation of immunoglobulins.

The answer is A. Determination of antibody specificity occurs prior to and independent from an individual's first encounter with antigen. This process begins developmentally during prenatal and neonatal life. This process is independent of soluble factors (cytokines) produced by T cells and occurs independently of maternal immune function. By definition, memory B cells have previously encountered antigen. Somatic hypermutation occurs only after previous exposure to antigen.

8.3 Serum immunoglobulins containing both maternally and paternally derived V_κ light chains are found within an individual. A given B cell, however, expresses only maternally-derived or paternally-derived V_κ chains, but never both. This finding is the result of

A. allelic exclusion.
B. antibody diversity.
C. isotype switching.
D. junctional diversity.
E. random VD and VDJ joining.

The answer is A. A given B cell or plasma cell expresses a single maternal or paternal allele of a chromosome pair. This process, known as allelic exclusion, applies to both heavy and light chain genes. An additional exclusion allows for the expression of only a κ (chromosome 2) or λ (chromosome 22) gene, never both within the same cell. Allelic exclusion has a slight impact upon genetic diversity, a process like isotype switching, junctional diversity, and random V(D)J joining that occurs after alleles are selected/excluded.

8.4 The role of terminal deoxynucleotidyl transferase (TdT) in development of antibody diversity is to

A. add/remove nucleotides of V, D, and J genes.
B. fuse VD and J segments together in heavy chains.
C. increase binding affinity of antibody for antigen.
D. join C_L to C_H1, C_H2, C_H3 or C_H4 domains.
E. transfer V_L alleles from maternal to paternal chromosomes.

The answer is A. TdT adds or removes nucleotides when the ends of V, (D), and/or J gene segments are exposed. This process, known as junctional diversity, occurs during DNA rearrangement. This process occurs in addition to the fusion of VDJ segments of the heavy chain and occurs prior to a B cell's exposure to antigen. The light chain constant region (C_L) never joins with constant region (C_H) domains of the heavy chain to make a polypeptide. A crossover between maternal and paternal V_L alleles is an exceedingly rare event, and TdT is not involved.

8.5 When a memory B cell is restimulated by its specific antigen, small point mutations that accumulate in the DNA encoding variable regions of both light and heavy chains may result in

A. antigen-stimulated VDJ joining and new antigen specificity.
B. change from production of IgM to IgG.
C. DNA chromosomal rearrangement and altered antigen specificity.
D. inactivation of either the maternal or paternal VL and VH allele.
E. generation of antibody with increased binding affinity for its epitope.

The answer is E. Accumulation of point mutations that affect light and heavy chain variable regions may increase binding affinity for antigen, by "fine-tuning" the antigen-binding site of the resulting immunoglobulin molecule. These point mutations occur after allelic exclusion and VDJ joining, they do not affect DNA rearrangement, and they do not appear to affect isotype switching.

Lymphocyte Development

9

I. OVERVIEW

Epitope-specific T cell and B cell receptors (TCRs and BCRs) are randomly generated within individual thymus- and bone marrow-derived lymphocytes by gene rearrangement. Not surprisingly, some lymphocytes develop receptors that react with self epitopes. However, a selection mechanism is in place that removes these cells before they become fully functional and attack the body's own and tissues. The adaptive immune system carefully regulates the development and differentiation of lymphocytes to prevent the maturation of self-reactive T and B cells.

Arising from **hematopoietic stem cells** in the bone marrow, a common lymphoid precursor (CLP) of lymphocytic lineage cells either differentiates within the thymus (T cells) or remains in the bone marrow (B cells). In addition, B and T cell lineages have major subdivisions (Table 9.1; also see Fig. 4.2). T lineage cells differentiate within the thymus along one of three developmental pathways: those that express $\alpha\beta$ TCRs, those that express $\gamma\delta$ TCRs, and those that share functional properties of natural killer (NK) cells. Thymic "graduates" in each of these groups can be differentiated from one another in several ways: the extent of their thymic "education," their arrival and departure from the thymus, the diversity or "repertoire" of their TCRs, their geographic distribution within the body, and the nature of their responses to different categories of epitopes. B cell lineages, designated B-1 and B-2 cells, can be distinguished

Table 9.1
PARALLELS AND DIFFERENCES OF TRANSITIONAL AND ADAPTIVE B CELL AND T CELL LINEAGES

	Transitional		Adaptive	
Cell type	$\gamma\delta$ T cell	B-1 cell	$\alpha\beta$ T cell	B-2 cell
Ontogeny	Develop earlier		Develop later	
Repertoire	Limited		Vast	
Receptor selection	None or very limited		Within the thymus	Within the bone marrow
Education	None		Thymus	None
Location of mature cells	Integument	Peritoneum and lungs	Throughout body	Throughout body
Response time to initial antigen encounter	Quick		Takes time to develop	Takes time to develop
Cell-to-cell cooperation required	None	Perhaps	Yes	
Memory	None		Yes	

from one another by many of the same characteristics used for categorizing the T cell subgroups.

II. T CELL LINEAGE

T cell precursors, known as **prothymocytes**, migrate from the bone marrow to the thymus attracted by thymic molecules (e.g., lymphotactin). Prothymocytes entering at the cortical region, now properly called **thymocytes**, lack TCRs, CD3, CD4, and CD8 surface molecules. The newly arrived thymocytes rapidly acquire TCRs, CD3, and both CD4 and CD8 molecules. They must then "run a gauntlet" of selective tests as they migrate from the thymic cortex to the medulla. The selection processes are so demanding that only an estimated 1% to 5% of all thymocytes "graduate" as T cells. The other 95% to 99% either leave the thymus before undergoing selection (e.g., γδ T cells) or die an apoptotic death after failing one of the selective tests.

A. Thymus structure

By the end of the third gestational month, the bilobed thymus is increasingly populated by lymphocytes, organized into a denser outer region or **cortex** and looser inner region or **medulla** (Fig. 9.1). A connective tissue **capsule** with inward-extending **trabeculae**

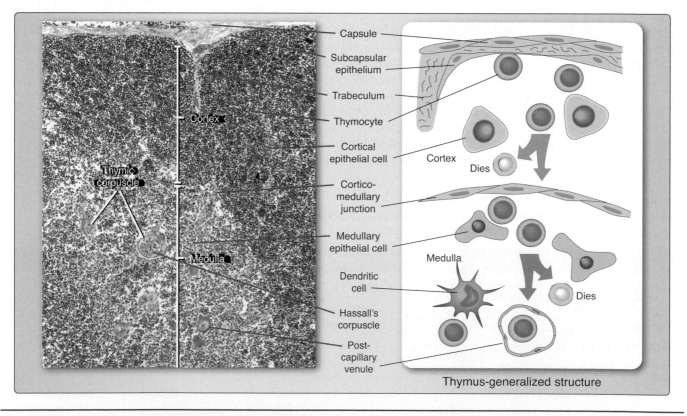

Figure 9.1

Thymocyte development: positive and negative selection. **A.** The thymus is organized into outer or cortical and inner or medullary regions. Prothymocytes enter the thymus to both increase in number and under several maturational steps. Thymocytes that "pass" exit from the thymus via postcapillary venules in the medulla. Thymic graduates are known as thymus-derived lymphocytes or T cells. Those thymocytes that fail their "tests" die. *(figure continues on following page.)*

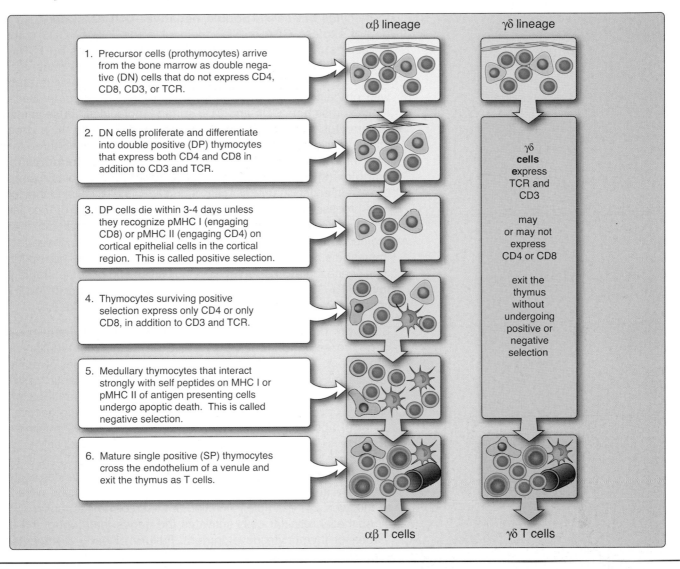

αβ lineage   γδ lineage

1. Precursor cells (prothymocytes) arrive from the bone marrow as double negative (DN) cells that do not express CD4, CD8, CD3, or TCR.

2. DN cells proliferate and differentiate into double positive (DP) thymocytes that express both CD4 and CD8 in addition to CD3 and TCR.

3. DP cells die within 3-4 days unless they recognize pMHC I (engaging CD8) or pMHC II (engaging CD4) on cortical epithelial cells in the cortical region. This is called positive selection.

4. Thymocytes surviving positive selection express only CD4 or only CD8, in addition to CD3 and TCR.

5. Medullary thymocytes that interact strongly with self peptides on MHC I or pMHC II of antigen presenting cells undergo apoptotic death. This is called negative selection.

6. Mature single positive (SP) thymocytes cross the endothelium of a venule and exit the thymus as T cells.

γδ **cells** **express** TCR and CD3

may or may not express CD4 or CD8

exit the thymus without undergoing positive or negative selection

αβ T cells   γδ T cells

Figure 9.1

B. Prothymocytes migrating from the bone marrow enter the cortical region of the thymus. As they migrate from the cortical to the medullary regions, they begin to express T cell receptors and other necessary accessory molecules. The γδ thymocytes exit quickly from the thymus, while the αβ thymocytes remain. Within the cortex, αβ thymocytes undergo positive selection. The survivors of positive selection then undergo a negative selection to remove cells that are potentially autoreactive.

surrounds the thymus. Additional cell types within the thymus are **epithelial reticular** cells, an inclusive term that includes several cells types such as dendritic cells, macrophages, and epithelial cells that serve as "instructors" for the thymocytes as they complete their education. The epithelial reticular cells, as well as those organized to form concentric rings called **Hassall's** corpuscles, express major histocompatibility molecules and secrete hormones associated with thymocyte differentiation. Medullary **postcapillary venules** are important for the egress of thymic graduates or T cells from the thymus.

B. αβ T cell development

Prothymocytes enter the subcapsular region of the thymus from the circulation, where they proliferate. These newly arrived cortical thymocytes are called **double negative (DN)** cells, because they do not express CD4 or CD8 molecules (or TCR or CD3 complex molecules). They soon begin to generate and express $\alpha\beta$ TCRs, associated CD3 complex, and both CD4 and CD8 molecules, as well receptors and adhesion molecules important for their interaction with other cells and their migration through the thymus. Because they express both CD4 and CD8 surface molecules, these immature thymocytes are called **double positive (DP)** cells. In a process known as **positive selection**, DP thymocytes die within three to four days unless they recognize and bind to **major histocompatibility complex (MHC)** or to **peptide + MHC (pMHC)** molecules expressed by certain epithelial reticular cells (cortical epithelial cells) in the cortex. This process eliminates thymocytes that are incapable of recognizing self MHC. Cells that pass the positive selection test, located at the corticomedullary junction, are allowed to enter the medulla; those that fail the test die. DP cells whose CD8 molecules have engaged (p)MHC I then cease the expression of CD4 molecules and become **single positive (SP)** $CD8^+$ cells. Likewise, those that are bound to (p)MHC II cease expression of CD8, becoming SP $CD4^+$ cells (Fig. 9.2).

Survivors of positive selection then run a second gauntlet called **negative selection** when they arrive at the corticomedullary junction. There, they meet and interact with a second set of epithelial reticular cells (antigen presenting cells such as dendritic cells and macrophages). Those that efficiently bind to self peptides of the pMHC I or pMHC II on these APCs are potentially autoreactive and undergo apoptotic death. Thymocytes that pass both positive and negative selection tests "graduate" from the thymus, entering the circulation through the medullary postcapillary venules as **T cells**. Each developmental stage is closely controlled by substances secreted by epithelial reticular cells that regulate gene expression within the thymocytes. For example, secretion of the cytokine interleukin-7 (IL-7) by epithelial reticular cells activates the genes that control the early stages of thymocyte development. Failure of early thymocytes to express IL-7 receptors terminates their development.

C. $\gamma\delta$ T cell development

The thymus is also the differentiation site for thymocytes that express $\gamma\delta$ TCRs and CD3 complex molecules. Many of these cells fail to express CD4 and/or CD8. Consequently, they do not undergo the same positive and negative selective processes as $\alpha\beta$ TCR-bearing thymocytes and depart from the thymus shortly after developing their TCR complexes (Tables 9.1 and 9.2, Fig. 9.1). $\gamma\delta$ cells are thought to be a transitional cell type that may represent a bridge between the innate and adaptive immune systems. $\gamma\delta$ T cells develop early in embryogenesis before many $\alpha\beta$ T cells and migrate preferentially to the respiratory organs, the skin, and the peritoneal cavity. They use a very limited set of V, D, and J genes in the generation of the variable regions of the γ and δ chains and thus are much more limited in their recognition repertoire than are $\alpha\beta$ T cells. They respond more quickly than do $\alpha\beta$ T cells, but they do so without generating memory.

D. NKT cell origin

Natural killer T (NKT) cells are a distinctive subset of T cells that share some characteristics with NK cells. They express several surface

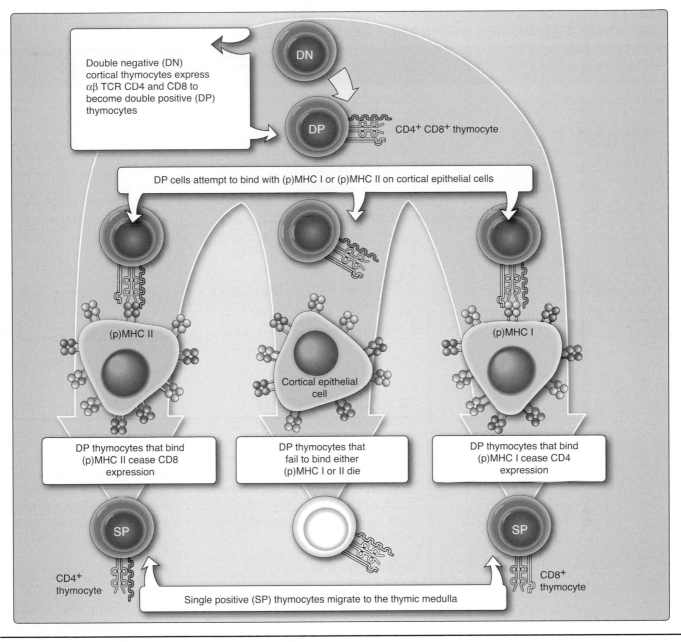

Figure 9.2

Development of CD4⁺ and CD8⁺ αβ T cells. The type of MHC molecule or peptide + MHC (pMHC) molecule to which a double-positive CD4⁺CD8⁺ (DP) binds determines its adult phenotype. Thymocytes that fail to bind to (p)MHC I or (p) MHC II die.

markers and receptors found on NK cells, but unlike NK cells, they undergo some development in the thymus and express TCRs generated by DNA rearrangement and junctional diversity. NKT cells express TCRs that are extremely limited in repertoire and are predominantly specific for lipids, glycolipids, and a few specialized types of peptides. Their TCRs have an unusual restriction pattern. Although they may be either CD4⁺ or CD4⁺CD8⁺, they specifically recognize epitopes presented by a "nonclassical" MHC class I molecule called CD1D. The nonclassical class I molecules, encoded by genes located in a chromosomal segment adjacent to the HLA complex, appear to present epitopes (often nonpeptide in nature) to T cells other than the most abundant αβ type.

Table 9.2
FUNCTIONAL CATEGORIES WITHIN THE T-CELL LINEAGE

Developmental Stage	Synonym	"Mature" Surface Markers			
Hematopoietic stem cell (HSC)		None			
Common lymphoid precursor (CLP)		None			
Prothymocyte		None			
Thymocyte	Double negative (DN)	None			
	Double positive (DP)	αβ TCR, CD3+, CD4+, CD8+		γδ TCR, CD3+	αβ TCR, CD3+
	Single positive (SP)	αβ TCR, CD3+CD4+ *or* CD8+		May not occur	May not occur
Mature T cell		αβ TCR, CD3+, CD4+	αβ TCR, CD3+, CD8+	γδ TCR, CD3+ sometimes CD4+ and/or CD8+	αβ TCR, CD3+, CD4+ or CD4+CD8+
Restriction element		MHC class II	MHC class I	unknown	CD1d
Common name	T lymphocyte or T cell	CD4+ T cell	CD8+ T cell	γδ T cell	Natural killer T (NKT) cell

III. B CELL LINEAGE

In humans, progenitors of immunoglobulin-producing cells are found in the yolk sac by the third week, in the fetal liver by the eighth week, and in the bone marrow by approximately the twelfth week of gestation. These cells are called bone marrow-derived lymphocytes or B cells, because this is where the majority of these cells differentiate. B cells are defined as cells that synthesize immunoglobulin and display it on their cell surfaces as their BCRs.

A. Bone marrow

The bone marrow contains connective tissue, blood vessels, fat, and cells. Among these structures are the hematopoietic stem cells capable of giving rise to the stem cells of the myeloid, granuloid, erythroid, and lymphoid cells (see Chapter 4). The vasculature provides an efficient route for cells originating in the bone marrow to move into the periphery and for the reentry of activated, matured immune cells (e.g., plasma cells) from the periphery. Unlike lymphoid cells that are destined to differentiate into T cells, those committed to the B cell lineage remain within the bone marrow for development.

B. B cell development

B cell development reflects the stages (also called bone marrow fractions) of immunoglobulin heavy and light chain rearrangement (see also Chapter 8) and surface expression (Fig. 9.3).

- Arising from a **common lymphoid progenitor** (CLP), the earliest identifiable cell committed to the B cell lineage is the **pre-pro-B cell** (Fraction A), within which the cell begins to express Igα and Igβ BCR accessory molecules.

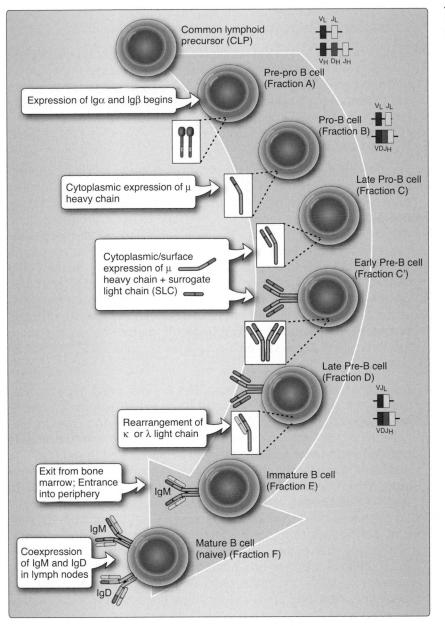

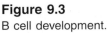

Figure 9.3
B cell development.

- Immunoglobulin DJ gene joining and cytoplasmic expression of **surrogate light chain (SLC)** occurs at the early **pro-B cell** (Fraction B) stage followed by VDJ gene joining and cytoplasmic SLC expression at the late pro-B cell (Fraction C) stage.

- The **early pre-B cell** (Fraction C-prime or C') stage is characterized by the surface expression of pseudo-IgM (rearranged μ heavy chains plus SLC) and is accompanied by a burst of cellular proliferation.

- In the **late pre-B cell** (Fraction D) stage, immunoglobulin light chain kappa (κ) or lambda (λ) genes rearrange, and their products (κ or λ light chains) replace the SLCs.

- **Immature B cells** (Fraction E) express μ heavy chains plus κ or λ light chains on their cell surfaces.

- **Mature B cells** (Fraction F) coexpress IgM and IgD on their cell surfaces. As they pass through the developmental stage, B cell

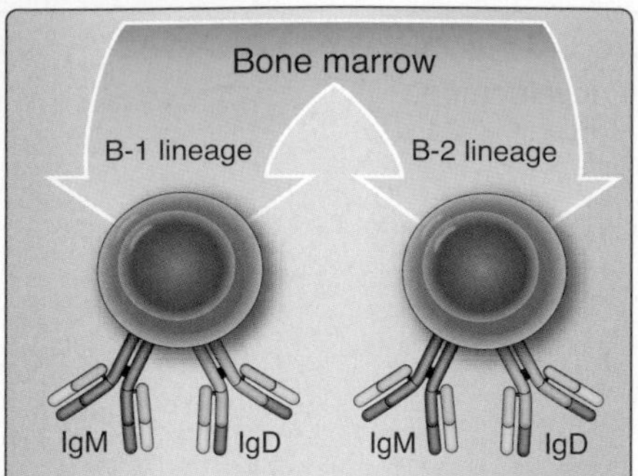

	B-1	B-2
Arise	Fetal	Perinatal/ Postnatal
Location	Respiratory & GI systems	Widespread
Diversity	Low	High
Memory	Little/none	Yes
Usual target	Carbohydrates	Proteins
Dominant isotype on surface of naive B cell	IgM>IgD = B1	IgD>IgM = B2
Isotype switch	Limited	Typical
Require T cell help	Almost never	Almost always
Replace-ment	Self-renewing in periphery	Continuously replaced from bone marrow

Figure 9.4
Characteristics of B-1 and B-2 B cells.

progenitors, like thymocytes, express molecules and receptors necessary for migration and interaction with other cells.

Some attributes (e.g., DNA recombinase expression) are lost by the time cells reach the immature B cell (Fraction E) stage. If the IgM on the developing cells should bind to epitopes they encounter in the bone marrow, such cells undergo apoptotic death to prevent production of autoreactive B cells.

C. B-1 and B-2 B cells

Two developmentally distinct B cell pathways are currently recognized (Fig. 9.4). Conventional B cells (**B-2 B cells**) are widely distributed throughout the body, require interaction with T cells for their activation and proliferation, and are continually replaced from the bone marrow throughout adult life. The range of epitopes that can be recognized by B-2 B cells is vast. Upon repeated antigen exposure, B-2 B cells respond quickly with increased antibody quantity and quality, often by "fine-tuning" the affinity of the antibody produced (affinity maturation; see Chapter 8). B-2 B cell responses are often accompanied by a change in immunoglobulin isotype. All of these properties are hallmarks of **immunologic memory**. Typically, more IgD than IgM is expressed on the surfaces of mature B-2 (Fraction F) B cells.

Appearing early in embryogenesis, **B-1 B cells**, arise from the fetal liver by the eighth gestational week. They might represent a transitional type of lymphocyte that bridges the innate and adaptive immune systems. First described about two decades ago, B-1 B cells have an importance in innate-related immunity and in autoimmune disorders that has become increasingly recognized. The B-1 B cell repertoire is quite limited in comparison to that of B-2 cells. B-1 BCRs and B-1 B antibodies are often directed against conserved microbial antigens (e.g., carbohydrates). It is thought that most, if not all, **natural antibodies** (e.g., IgMs directed against the A and B blood groups that exist in the absence of known immunization) are of B-1 B cell origin. B-1 B cells are found predominantly in tissues that are potential portals of microbial entry (e.g., the peritoneal cavity and respiratory tract) and are a self-renewing population within these tissues. Although they show little if any immunologic memory, limited isotype switching, and limited repertoires, they contribute greatly to protective immunity. It is estimated that over half the IgA secreted into the mucosa is of B-1 origin.

Chapter Summary

- Arising from **hematopoietic stem cells** in the bone marrow, lymphocytic lineage cells differentiate either within the thymus (T cells) or remain in the bone marrow (B cells).
- T cell precursors, known as **prothymocytes**, migrate from the bone marrow to the thymus attracted by thymic molecules (e.g., lymphotactin). The bilobed thymus is increasingly populated with lymphocytes, organized into a denser outer region or **cortex** and a looser inner region or **medulla**.

- In the thymus cortex, T cells begin to generate and express T cell receptors (TCRs), CD3 molecules, and sets of receptors and adhesion molecules. At this time, they begin to simultaneously express both CD4 and CD8 molecules and are known as "double positive" (DP). Those thymocytes that generate and express $\gamma\delta$ TCRs also express CD3, but many of them fail to express CD4 and/or CD8. The DP $\alpha\beta$ thymocytes undergo a set of selective processes referred to collectively as "education," in which the immune system begins to screen them on the basis of their ability to recognize self.

- The thymocyte population that moves from the cortex into the medulla consists of a mix of $CD4^+$ and $CD8^+$ cells. Fewer than 5% of thymocytes originally entering the thymus survive both **positive** and **negative selection** and leave the thymus to enter the body, where they may become activated and participate in a variety of immune responses.

- NKT cells are a distinctive subset of T cells that share some characteristics with natural killer (NK) cells.

- B cells undergo their entire developmental process within the bone marrow. Arising from a common lymphoid progenitor (CLP), the earliest identifiable cell committed to the B cell lineage is the **pre-pro-B cell.** Immunoglobulin DJ gene joining and cytoplasmic expression of **surrogate light chain** (**SLC**) occurs at the early **pro-B cell** (Fraction B) stage. The **early pre-B cell** (Fraction C-prime or C′) stage is characterized by the surface expression of pseudo-IgM. **Immature B cells** (Fraction E) express μ heavy chains plus κ or λ light chains on their cell surfaces. **Mature B cells** (Fraction F) coexpress IgM and IgD on their cell surfaces.

- Two developmentally distinct B cell pathways are currently recognized. Conventional B cells (**B-2 B cells**) are widely distributed throughout the body. **B-1 B cells** represent a transitional type of lymphocyte that bridges the innate and adaptive immune systems. The importance of B-1 B cells in innate-related immunity and autoimmune disorders is increasingly recognized.

Study Questions

9.1 DiGeorge syndrome is an immune deficiency disease due to impaired thymic development. Which of the following is/are affected in patients with DiGeorge syndrome?

   A. B cell development only
   B. complement only
   C. NK cell function
   D. T cell development only
   E. T cell development and B cell responses

The correct answer is E. The defective thymic environment inhibits T cell development and function. Because so much B cell activity depends upon interaction with T cells, B cell responses will also be impaired. Complement would not be impaired while sparing T and B cell activity. NK cell function should not be affected.

9.2 Negative selection of T cells occurs in the

   A. blood vessels.
   B. bone marrow.
   C. lymph node.
   D. spleen.
   E. thymus.

The correct answer is E. Negative selection of T cells occurs as they move from the thymic cortex into the thymic medulla. It does not occur at sites outside of the thymus.

9.3 T cell precursors, known as prothymocytes, migrate from the bone marrow to the thymus in response to

   A. eotactin.
   B. IL-4.
   C. IL-5.
   D. IL-10.
   E. lymphotactin.

The correct answer is E. Lymphotactin is one of the thymic products that help to guide prothymocytes from the bone marrow to the thymus. IL-4, IL-5, and IL-10 are cytokines produced by mature, activated T cells as well as by other cell types. Eotactin guides the movement of eosinophils.

9.4 What will be the fate of an early thymocyte that fails to express IL-7 receptors?

   A. apoptotic cell death
   B. development as a γδ T cell
   C. development as an NKT cell
   D. failure to traffic to the thymus
   E. maturation along the B cell lineage

The correct answer is A. Failure to bind IL-7 dooms the developing thymocyte. It will be unable to develop into either an αβ or a γδ thymocyte. This interaction occurs after migration of the thymocytes into the thymus. Thymocytes cannot switch to the B cell developmental pathway.

9.5 γδ T cells

   A. contain very extensive antigen recognition repertoires.
   B. express surface markers that are also characteristic of NK cells.
   C. generate memory when recognizing antigen on multiple occasions.
   D. migrate preferentially to respiratory organs, skin, and the peritoneal cavity.
   E. respond more slowly to antigen than do αβ T cells.

The correct answer is D. γδ T cells are found predominantly in the respiratory organs, skin, and peritoneal cavity. Their recognition repertoire is far less extensive that found in αβ T cells. They do not express significant immunologic memory but do react to antigenic stimuli more rapidly than do αβ T cells.

9.6 NKT cells

   A. are usually CD8 single positive cells.
   B. bind epitopes presented by MHC Class II molecules.
   C. express TCRs generated by DNA rearrangement and junctional diversity.
   D. recognize carbohydrates and complex proteins.
   E. synthesize immunoglobulin and display it on their cell surfaces.

The correct answer is C. NKT cells do express TCRs generated (like those of other T cells) by DNA re-arrangement and junctional diversity. They are either CD4$^+$ or CD4$^+$CD8$^+$. Despite this, their TCRs recognize lipid-related molecular fragments presented by the nonclassical class I molecule CD1D. They do not synthesize or express immunoglobulins.

9.7 Pre-pro B cells

   A. contain either κ or λ light chains.
   B. demonstrate surface expression of pseudo-IgM.
   C. express Igα and Igβ BCR accessory molecules.
   D. have VDJ joining of genes.
   E. show cytoplasmic expression of surrogate light chains.

The correct answer is C. Pre-pro B cells initially express Igα and Igβ molecules. The synthesis of heavy and light chains (including surrogate light chains) occurs at later stages of development.

9.8 In contrast to B-2 B cells, B-1 B cells

   A. appear later in development.
   B. are more important in innate-related immune responses.
   C. express more IgD than IgM on their cell surfaces.
   D. have a more extensive antigen recognition repertoire.
   E. require interaction with T cells for their activation.

The correct answer is B. B-1 B cells appear to be transitional types of lymphocytes whose functions are reminiscent of the innate immune system. B-1 B cells express more surface IgM than IgD and B-2 B cells express more surface IgD than IgM. The B-1 B cell repertoire is more limited, and their need for interaction with T cells is more limited than is seen for B-2 B cells. B-1 B cells appear developmentally earlier than B-2 B cells.

Lymphocyte Activation

10

I. OVERVIEW

Compared with innate immune responses, adaptive immune responses against newly encountered antigens initially develop slowly. Although many self-reactive cells are eliminated during development, lymphocytes undergo a further set of time-consuming checks and balances to minimize the potential for adverse immune responses. Different cell types for recognition, regulation, and effector function impose this system of checks and balances. T cells play a central role as arbiters of adaptive immune function, and because of this role, the manner in which T cells recognize and are activated by epitopes is stringently regulated. It is useful to think of the innate immune system as the gatekeeper for adaptive immune responses (Fig. 10.1). Adaptive immune system effector responses often activate and focus cells and/ or molecules of the innate system upon targets selected by the lymphocytes.

II. ANTIGEN PRESENTATION

Phagocytes sample their environment by phagocytosis and macropinocytosis. Ingested proteins are enzymatically degraded, and some of the resulting peptide fragments are loaded into MHC class II (forming pMHC class II) molecules in a process called **antigen presentation**. Some pathogens avoid phagocytotic and macropinocytic mechanisms altogether or infect cells that do not express MHC class II molecules. Such antigens are broken down, and their peptide fragments are loaded into MHC class I (forming pMHC class I) molecules (Fig. 10.2).

A. Presentation by MHC class II

Dendritic cells located at potential microbial portals of entry (e.g., skin and mucous membranes) and in other tissues and organs serve as sentinels (see Fig. 4.5). **Immature dendritic cells** are voracious eaters that ingest large amounts of soluble and particulate matter by phagocytosis and macropinocytosis. **Phagocytosis** involves the engagement of cell surface receptors (e.g., Fc receptors, heat shock proteins, and low-density lipoprotein-binding scavenger receptors) associated with specialized regions of the plasma membrane called **clathrin-coated** pits (Fig. 10.3). Receptor engagement induces actin-dependent phagocytosis and receptor internalization to form small **phagosomes** or endocytic vesicles. Immature dendritic

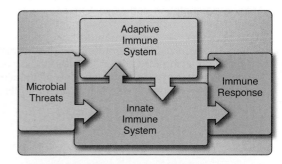

Figure 10.1
Interactions of the innate and adaptive immune systems.

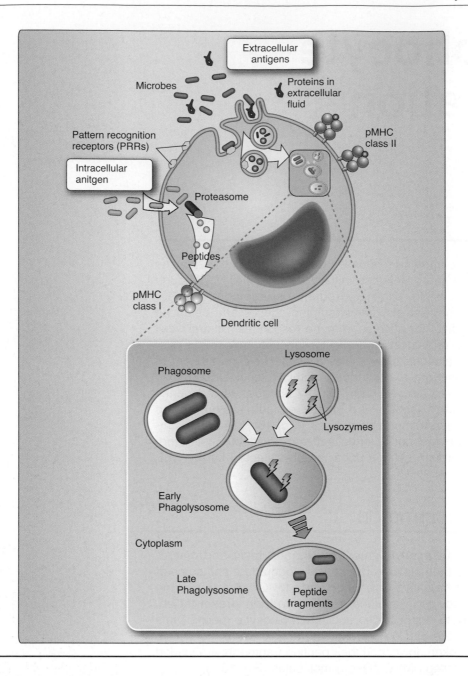

Figure 10.2

Antigen presentation pathways. **Extracellular antigens** (e.g., bacteria, cells, and many soluble molecules) enter the cell by phagocytosis or macropinocytosis packaged in phagocytic vesicles. **Inset:** Phagocytic vesicles fuse with enzyme- (lysozymes) containing vesicles (lysosomes) to form phagolysosomes that enzymatically degrade the ingested material. The lysosomal enzymes proteolytically degrade the ingested material into peptides in the late phagosome. The late phagosome will fuse with vesicles containing MHC class II. Intracellular pathogens (e.g., viruses and certain bacteria) and some antigens directly enter the cell's cytoplasm, circumventing the phagocytic apparatus. Intracellular antigens are degraded by the proteasome into peptides that are loaded into MHC class I (pMHC class I) for display on the cell surface.

cells also sample large amounts of soluble molecules as well as particles present in the extracellular fluids by **macropinocytosis**, a process in which cytoplasmic projections (**cytoplasmic ruffles**) encircle and enclose extracellular fluids to form endocytotic vesicles (Fig. 10.4). Macropinocytosis does not require clathrin-associated receptor engagement. Enzyme-containing cytoplasmic vesicles (**lysosomes**) fuse with the endocytic vesicles derived from phagocytosis or macropinocytosis (see Fig. 10.2). Within this newly formed **phagolysosome**, ingested material is enzymatically degraded into peptides.

When an immature dendritic cell senses an invasive threat, it rapidly begins to mature. Threats are detected by the same cell surface receptors used by the innate immune system. **Direct sensing** occurs through engagement of **pattern recognition receptors** (**PRRs**) that recognize **pathogen-associated molecular patterns** (**PAMPs**) on viruses, bacteria, fungi, and protozoa. Engagement of other receptors (e.g., those that detect antibodies or complement molecules that have bound to microbes) is responsible for the **indirect sensing** of perceived threats.

Although the mechanisms responsible for dendritic cell maturation remain to be clarified, we know that threat sensing causes the dendritic cells to migrate to nearby lymph nodes, decrease their phagocytic and macropinocytic activity, and increase their MHC class II synthetic activity. MHC class II α and β polypeptides, together with an invariant chain, are assembled as a complex within the endoplasmic reticulum (Fig. 10.5). Vesicles bud off from the endoplasmic reticulum to fuse with the peptide-containing, acidic phagolysosomes. The invariant chain disintegrates in the acidic environment of the newly formed vesicle, allowing phagolysosome-derived peptides to occupy the peptide-binding groove of the MHC class II molecule. The pMHC class II complex is transported to the cell surface for display and possible recognition by CD4+ T cells. MHC class II molecules make no distinction between peptides of self and nonself origin. Self antigens displayed on the phagocyte surface usually go unrecognized because most self-reactive CD4+ T cells have been eliminated during development.

B. Presentation by MHC class I

Not all antigens enter cells by phagocytosis or macropinocytosis. Some pathogens avoid phagocytes and endocytic vesicles entirely. Intracellular microbes and viruses bind to cell membranes and directly enter the cytoplasm of the host cell (Fig. 10.6). These pathogens are processed differently.

Nucleated cells normally degrade and recycle cytoplasmic proteins. Both self and nonself cytoplasmic proteins targeted for destruction are covalently tagged with **ubiquitin**, a highly conserved 76-amino-acid protein. The selection mechanisms for protein ubiquination are not known. Binding of one or more ubiquitin molecules to a protein selects it for destruction by the **proteasome**, a large proteolytic enzyme complex within the cytoplasm. Proteasome-generated peptides of 6 to 24 amino acids are transported to the endoplasmic

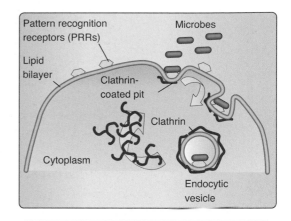

Figure 10.3

Phagocytosis. Cells, particles, and molecules are captured by PRRs associated with clathrin-coated pits. Clathrin-associated membrane invaginates and pinches off to form a phagosome. Clathrin is recycled back to the cell membrane to help form new coated pits.

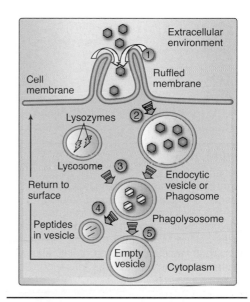

Figure 10.4

Macropinocytosis. **1.** Cytoplasmic protrusions or ruffles engulf and surrounds microbes, particles, or molecules to form a cytoplasmic vesicle **2.** that fuses with a lysosome **3.** to form a phagolysosome. **4.** Vesicles containing enzymatically degraded the material fuse with vesicles containing MHC class II (see Fig. 10.6). **5.** Empty phagolysosomes are recycled back to the cell membrane.

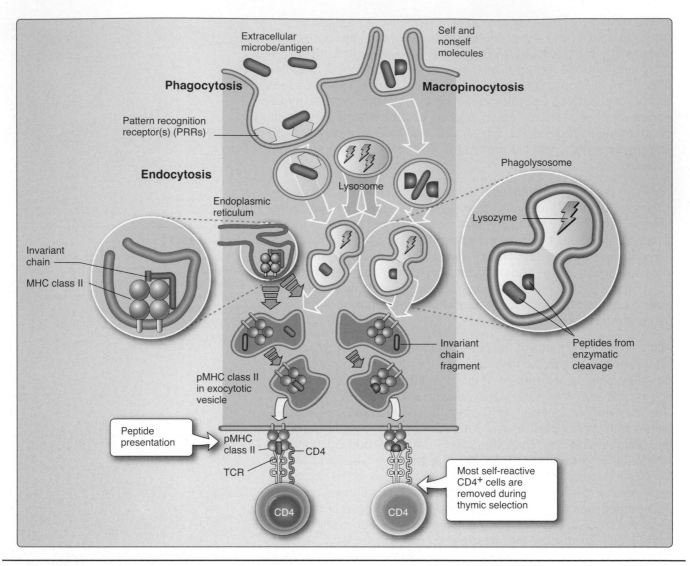

Figure 10.5
Presentation of extracellular antigens. Antigens of extracellular origin (left side of diagram) or of self origin (right side) are degraded within phagolysosomes. MHC class II αβ heterodimers together with invariant chain are assembled within the endoplasmic reticulum. Vesicles containing MHC class II + invariant chain bud off from the endoplasmic reticulum to fuse with peptide-rich vesicles that bud off from the phagolysosome. The acidic environment of the fused vesicle causes the invariant chain to disintegrate, allowing (appropriate) peptides to occupy the peptide-binding groove of the MHC class II molecule. Invariant chain-lacking MHC class II molecules that do not bind a peptide disintegrate in the acidic environment of the vesicle. The exocytotic vesicle containing pMHC class II fuses with the cell's plasma membrane, and the pMHC class II molecules are displayed on the cell surface for recognition by TCRs of CD4⁺ T cells.

reticulum by the **transporter associated with antigen processing** (**TAP-1** and **TAP-2**). The TAP heterodimer allows peptides to load into MHC class I (pMHC class I). Special transport exocytic vesicles containing pMHC class I bud from the Golgi and are rapidly transported to the cell surface for display and recognition by the appropriate CD8⁺ T cells. MHC class I molecules make no distinction between peptides of self and nonself origin. However, self peptides displayed on the phagocyte surface usually go unrecognized because CD8⁺ T cells that are potentially reactive to self peptides are removed during thymic selection.

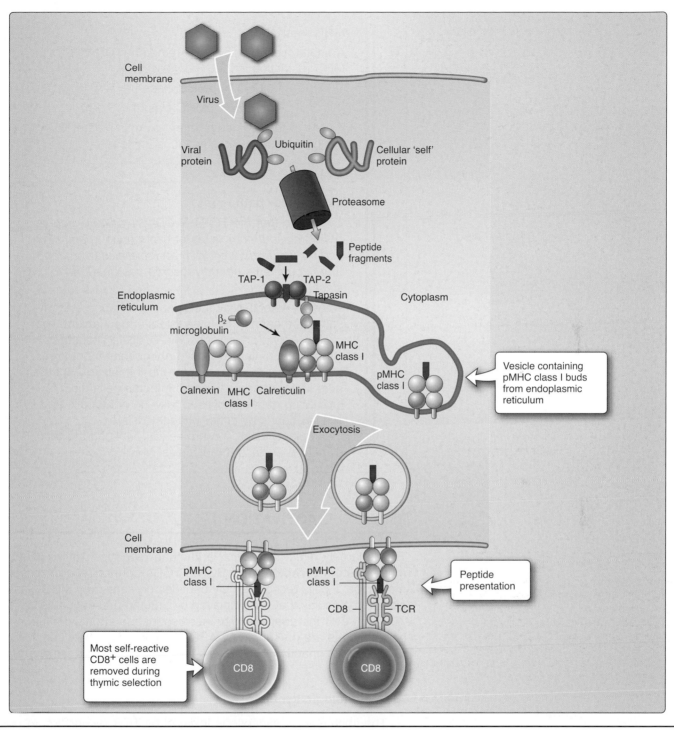

Figure 10.6
Presentation of intracellular or cytoplasmic antigens. Cytoplasmic proteins of both self and nonself origin may be marked for destruction by the covalent attachment of ubiquitin, which targets them for proteolytic degradation by the proteasome enzyme complex. Proteasome-generated peptide fragments within the cytoplasm are transported into the endoplasmic reticulum by gatekeeper TAP-1 and TAP-2 heterodimers. Calnexin, a chaperone molecule, binds to newly synthesized MHC class I molecules to allow β_2 microglobulin to form a MHC class I:β_2 complex. Calnexin is replaced by another chaperone molecule, calreticulin. A third chaperone molecule, tapasin, associated with the TAP heterodimer, assists possible loading into the peptide into the MHC class I:β_2 complex. The MHC class I:β_2 complex rapidly disintegrates if a suitable peptide is not loaded. Exocytotic vesicles containing the newly formed pMH7 class I complexes bud off from the endoplasmic reticulum and are transported for display on the cell surface by CD8+ T cells with the appropriate TCR.

> ## MHC restriction
>
> A useful memory device to remember CD4/CD8 MHC restriction is the "*Rule of eight*":
>
> $$CD4 \times pMHC\ class\ II = 8$$
> $$CD8 \times pMHC\ class\ I = 8$$
>
> T cells of the γδ lineage often express neither CD4 nor CD8, and their restriction is unclear.

> ## Intracellular pathogens
>
> *I just read that the TCRs of CD4⁺ T cells recognize pMHC class II complexes of exogenous origin. How can a peptide derived from an intracellular pathogen that circumvents phagolysosome vesicles load into a class II molecule?*
>
> To avoid detection by the adaptive immune system, some pathogens employ a "stealth mechanism" by circumventing phagolysosome vesicles altogether. Others may enter the cell in phagosomes but are able to leave them and enter the cytoplasm. But their ruse is not perfect, as some infected cells die, prompting dendritic cells to take up dead cells and cellular debris by either phagocytosis or macropinocytosis. The proteolytic peptides are then displayed in class II molecules. Mystery solved.

III. T CELL ACTIVATION

T cells largely direct the adaptive immune response. Unlike innate immune system receptors and BCRs, TCRs cannot recognize soluble molecules. T cells recognize only peptides presented by MHC class I or class II molecules that are displayed by antigen-presenting cells (APC). The nature of the adaptive immune response is strongly influenced by how epitopes are presented by APCs. The interface between APC and a previously unactivated (naïve) T cell is called the **immunologic synapse**.

A. Immunologic synapse

The immunologic synapse is initiated by TCR recognition of pMHC (Fig. 10.7). The weak interaction of TCR with pMHC is stabilized by the interaction with CD4 or CD8 molecules that bind to the "constant" nonpeptide-binding portions of pMHC class II and class I, respectively. Formation of the pMHC:TCR:CD(4 or 8) complex provides a **first signal** though the TCR-associated CD3 complex to the T cell. This first signal is necessary but not sufficient to stimulate a naïve T cell to proliferate and differentiate. A **second signal** (or more properly a group of signals) provided by one or more **costimulatory molecules** is also required for T cell activation. The first and second

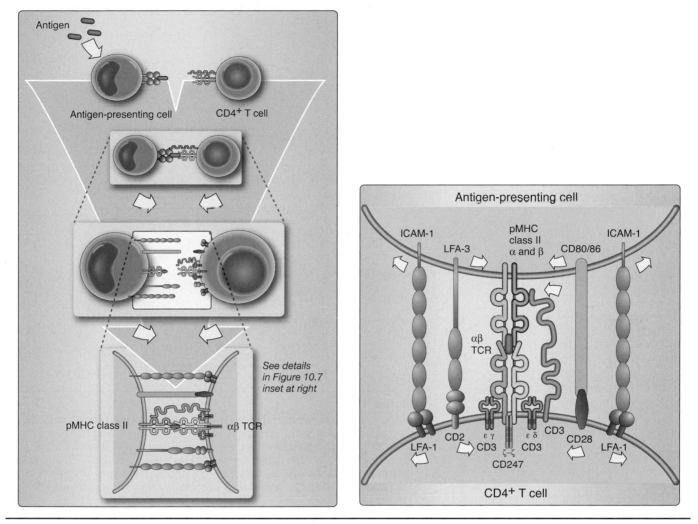

Figure 10.7

Immunologic synapse. Extracellular antigens are displayed (presented) by MHC class II molecules by APC. TCRs of circulating CD4$^+$ T cells that recognize peptide and MHC class II (pMHC class II) form a weak bond that is stabilized by the noncovalent interaction of the T cell's CD4 molecule with the nonpeptide-binding portion of MHC class II. **Inset.** Adhesion molecules expressed by T cells (leukocyte function antigen-, LFA-1, or CD11a/CD18) interact with ICAM-1 (immune cell adhesion molecule-1 or CD54) on APC. LFA-1:ICAM-1 complexes move away from the pMHC:TCR:CD4 complex. At the same time CD2:LFA-3 (CD2:CD58) and costimulatory complexes (e.g., CD28:CD80/86) move toward the pMHC:TCR:CD4 complex.

signals initiate intracellular signaling cascades activating one or more transcription factors leading to specific gene transcription. Without costimulation, T cells either become selectively unresponsive, a condition known as **anergy**, or undergo apoptosis.

B. T cell signal transduction

The immunologic synapse stabilizes T cell-APC interaction and promotes the migration of molecules within the T cell membrane. Cytoplasmic tails of some of these molecules contain **immunoreceptor tyrosine-based activation motifs (ITAMs)** that initiate a signaling cascade when brought into close proximity (Fig. 10.8). The cytoplasmic tails of CD3 complex molecules (CD3ε, γ, δ, and CD247 ζ) bear ITAMs. In contrast, the cytoplasmic tails of the TCR

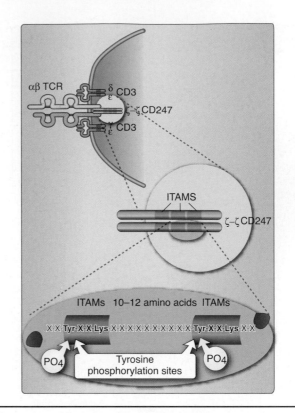

Figure 10.8
Immunoreceptor activation motifs (ITAMs). Ligand engagement leads to
polypeptide dimerization, activation of tyrosine kinases, and the phosphorylation of tyrosine residues within specialized intracellular portions of receptor or accessory polypeptides. These ITAMs contain four amino acids (indicated as two X's flanked by tyrosine (Tyr) and lysine (Lys)). Multiple ITAMs
are located at 10- to 12-amino-acid intervals along the cytoplasmic tail.

lack ITAMs. Signals transduced following TCR through the CD3
complex provide the first signal for T cell activation (Fig. 10.9). Costimulatory molecules provide the second signal for T cell activation
(Fig. 10.10).

C. CD4$^+$ T cell maturation

The initial encounter of T cells with antigen is called **priming**, and
the nature of this encounter is crucial to the development of the subsequent adaptive immune response. Primed CD4$^+$ T cells are termed
T helper or **Th** cells because they are instrumental in "helping" other
leukocytes respond (Fig. 10.11). Upon activation, naïve CD4$^+$ **Th
precursor** (**Thp**) cells are stimulated to secrete a variety of cytokines and express cell-surface cytokine receptors, becoming path-
way-uncommitted **Th0** cells (Fig. 10.11). CD4$^+$ Th0 cells may mature
along one of two functional pathways. The developmental pathway
that the Th0 follows depends upon the nature of signals it receives at
the time it interacts with the APC. In the presence of microbe-derived
lipopolysaccharide, APCs secrete IL-12 and other cytokines that
increase leukocyte recruitment and activation. CD4$^+$ T cells generally respond to these signals by recruiting and activating phagocytic
cells or by activating cytotoxic T lymphocytes (CTL). These T cells are
known as **Th1 cells**. T cells that develop along the other pathway are

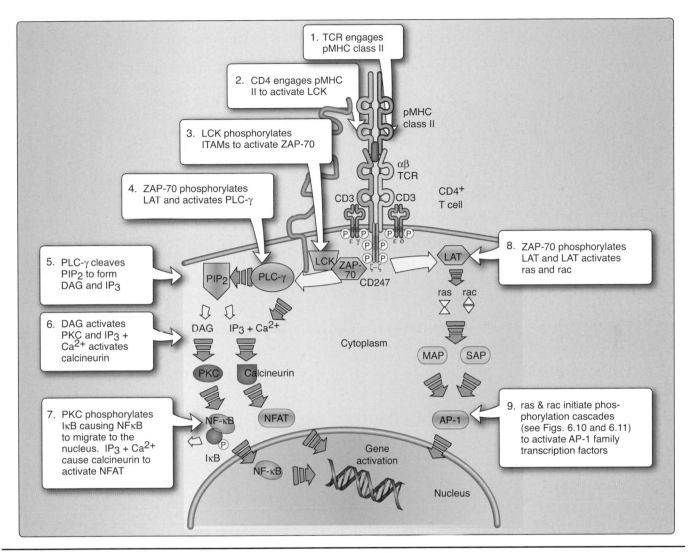

Figure 10.9
Details of T cell "first signal" transduction. **1.** The T-cell receptor (TCR) engages a peptide presented by MHC class II (pMHC II). **2.** CD4 stabilizes this complex by binding noncovalently to the nonpeptide-binding region of MHC class II, causing (**3**) the LCK tyrosine kinase to phosphorylate immunoreceptor activation motifs (ITAMs) on the cytoplasmic tails of CD3 complex molecules (CD3ε, γ, and δ and the CD247 ζ–ζ homodimer). **4.** ZAP-70 tyrosine kinase "docks" onto the phosphorylated ITAMs and phosphorylates the remaining CD247 ζ–ζ ITAMs and phosphorylates and activates phospholipase C-γ (PLC-γ). **5.** PLC-γ cleaves phosphatidylinositol 4,5-bi(s)phosphate (PIP$_2$) into diacylglycerol (DAG) and inositol tri(s)phosphate (IP$_3$). **6.** DAG activates protein kinase C (PKC) and IP$_3$ together with calcium (Ca^{2+}) activate calcineurin. **7.** PKC phosphorylates IκB (inhibitor of nuclear factor kappa B, NFκB) causing the inhibitor to dissociate from NFκB. Likewise, calcineurin activates nuclear factor of activated T cells (NFAT). Both transcription factors (NFκB and NFAT) migrate to the nucleus, where they activate genes. **8.** ZAP-70 also phosphorylates the linker of activation for T cells (LAT), which activates the guanine nucleotide exchange factors (GEFs), ras and rac. **9.** Ras and rac initiate phosphorylation cascades (see Figs. 6-10 and 6-11) to activate the AP-1 family of transcription factors.

known as **Th2 cells** and generally respond to extracellular pathogens by stimulating B cells to differentiate into antibody-secreting plasma cells. In other cases, the presence of IL-4 may lead Th0 to follow the Th2 differentiation pathway. Among the functional roles of Th2 cells is the production of cytokines responsible for the proliferation and activation of B cells and their differentiation into plasma cells or memory B cells.

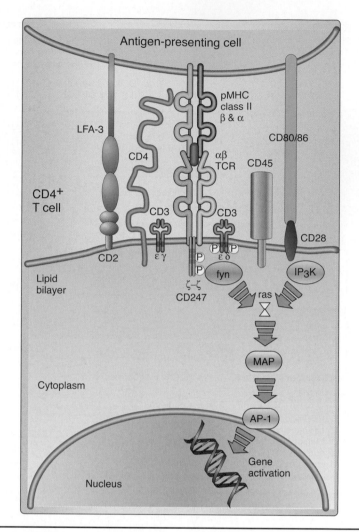

Figure 10.10

The second signal: costimulation. A second signal (costimulation) is required for T cell activation. Upon formation of the immunologic synapse (see Fig. 10.9), the common leukocyte antigen (CD45) dephosphorylates and activates Fyn kinase. Both CD28 (costimulatory molecule) and Fyn associate with inositol tri(s)phosphate kinase (IP_3K) to activate Ras and initiate a phosphorylation/activation cascade (see Figs. 6.10 and 6.11).

D. CD8$^+$ T cell maturation

Recognition of pMHC class I (first signal) displayed on the surface of an infected APC or other cell by naïve CD8$^+$ T cell(s) causes them to express IL-2 receptors (IL-2R, Fig. 10.12). Phagocytosis of the cellular debris of a virus-infected cell and display of viral pMHC class II by APC stimulates a CD4$^+$ T cell to produce IL-2 and provides a second signal to the CD8$^+$ T cell through its IL-2R. APC-CD4$^+$ T cell interaction increases CD80/86 expression by APC. Interaction of APC CD80/86 with CD28 on CD8$^+$ T cells promotes CD8$^+$ T cell differentiation. Appropriately stimulated CD8$^+$ T cells proliferate and differentiate into cytolytic effector cells called **cytotoxic T lymphocytes** (**CTL**). Fully differentiated CTLs contain two types of cytolytic granules, **perforin** (a pore-forming protein) and **granzymes** (serine

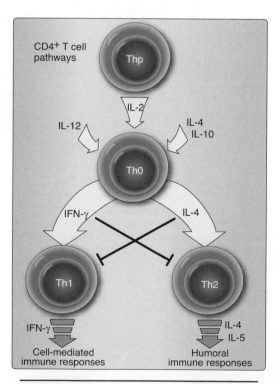

Figure 10.11

Differentiation of CD4$^+$ T helper 1 (Th1) and Th2 lymphocytes.

proteases), that are used to deliver a fatal blow to a cell expressing the appropriate pMHC class I complex (see Chapter 11).

E. Memory T cells

TCR engagement with the appropriate pMHC class II (first signal) and CD28 engagement with CD80/86 (second signal) stimulate CD4$^+$ T cells to produce IL-2, express IL-2 receptors (IL-2R), and proliferate. In most stimulated CD4$^+$ T cells, CD152 (cytotoxic T-lymphocyte-associated antigen-4, or CTLA-4), normally sequestered within the Golgi apparatus, travels to the cell membrane. There, it binds to CD80/86 with an avidity that is 100-fold greater than that of CD28 (Fig. 10.13). CD152 engagement inhibits T cell IL-2 mRNA expression and halts cell proliferation, thus ensuring that CD4$^+$ T cell-mediated responses are self-limiting. However, if all CD4$^+$ T cells were unable to respond upon second exposure, the body would be at severe risk to subsequent encounters with the same infectious organism. Fortunately, some CD4$^+$ T cells enter into a **memory** state. Memory T cells typically express CD28, increase their adhesion molecule expression, and decrease their surface expression of CD62L

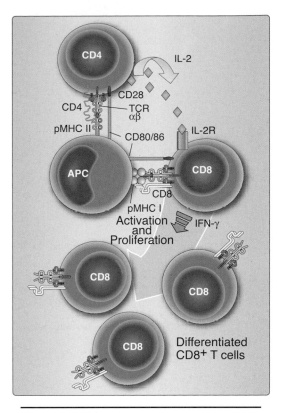

Figure 10.12
CD8$^+$ T cell activation.

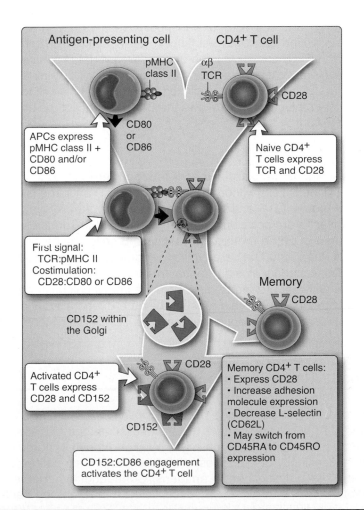

Figure 10.13
Generation of memory T cells.

(L-selectin). By increasing their expression of CD28, memory T cells are more likely to respond rapidly to CD80/86 displayed by APC. By decreasing L-selection expression (CD62L), memory T cells no longer home to lymph nodes but home to sites of inflammation because of increased expression of other adhesion molecules. For some CD4$^+$ T cells, the memory phenotype results in a change in their surface expression of CD45 from the naïve CD45RA to the memory CD45RO isoform.

IV. B CELL ACTIVATION

In contrast to TCRs, BCRs recognize and bind epitopes on either cell-bound or soluble molecules. The BCR complex of mature B cells contains membrane-bound immunoglobulin monomers associated with Igα and Igβ molecules (Fig. 10.14). Similar to the CD3 complex, the cytoplasmic tails of Igα and Igβ molecules contain ITAM motifs. BCR cross-linking initiates intracellular signaling. Because all of the immunoglobulins on a given B cell have the same specificity, an antigen must contain multiple identical epitopes for cross-linking to occur (Fig. 10.15). Cross-linking of BCRs induces tyrosine kinases such as lyn, lck, fyn, and blk to phosphorylate the Igα and Igβ ITAMs. ITAM phosphorylation allows docking of Syk and activation of phospholipase C-γ (PLC-γ) to initiate a signal transduction cascade resulting in the activation of transcription factors (e.g., NF-κB and NFAT) and gene activation. BCR binding initiates endocytosis, enzymatic degradation, and subsequent display of peptide fragments as pMHC class II complexes and cause the B cell to express costimulatory molecules. This allows the B cell to function as an APC for TCR recognition by a CD4$^+$ T cell.

A. T-independent activation

Some antigens are classified as **T-independent (TI)** to indicate that they activate B cells without help from T cells. TI antigens fall into two distinct groups (TI-1 and TI-2) based upon how they activate B cells. TI-1 antigens are polyclonal activators that bind to surface structures other than BCRs. Therefore, they activate B cells irrespective of BCR epitope specificity They are typically microbial in origin, such as the lipopolysaccharide. In high concentration, TI-1 antigens stimulate B cells to activate, proliferate, and increase immunoglobulin production and secretion, and for this reason, they are often called **B cell mitogens**. In low concentrations, TI-1 antigens stimulate antigen-specific T

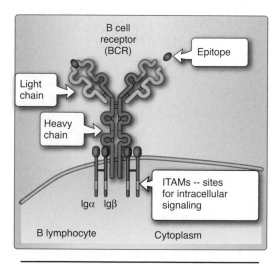

Figure 10.14
B cell receptor (BCR). Surface-bound immunoglobulin functions as the epitope-specific BCR. All BCRs expressed by a single B cell have identical epitope specificity. Epitope binding causes conformational change in the BCR that transduces a signal to the cytoplasm via Igα and Igβ accessory molecules.

CLINICAL APPLICATION
Wiskott-Aldrich syndrome

The capsular polysaccharide of *Haemophilus influenzae* B is a TI-2 antigen. Antibody responses to *H. influenzae* are essential for protective immunity. Individuals with Wiskott-Aldrich syndrome, an immunodeficiency disease, respond poorly to protein antigens and not at all to polysaccharide antigens. Consequently, people with Wiskott-Aldrich syndrome are susceptible to infections by bacteria that have polysaccharide capsules.

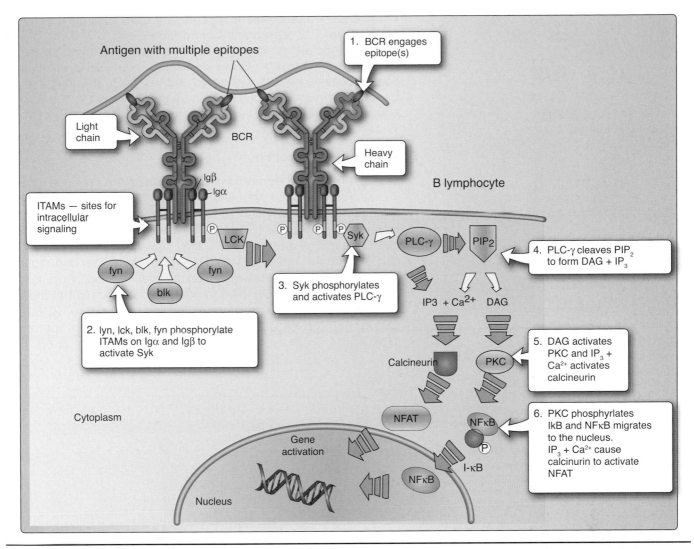

Figure 10.15
Details of the B cell signaling cascade. Cross-linking leads to BCR aggregation, and the close proximity of the cytoplasmic tails of the Igα and Igβ allows phosphorylation of their ITAMs by tyrosine kinases (lyn, blk, lyn, and lck). Syk docks, phosphorylates, and activates phospholipase C-γ (PLC-γ) and leads to the signal transduction cascade (see Figs. 6.10 and 6.11).

cells. TI-2 antigens contain repetitive epitopes and are often multivalent polysaccharides. In contrast to TI-1 antigens that stimulate both mature and immature B cells, TI-2 antigens specifically activate only mature B cells. Repetitive epitopes on polysaccharides bind to and cross-link specific BCRs (Fig. 10.15). The close proximity of Igα and Igβ cytoplasmic tail results in phosphorylation and initiation of a signal transduction cascade. It is not clear whether immune responses to TI-2 antigens are totally T-independent. Addition of even small numbers of T cells increases antibody production to TI-2 antigens.

Sometimes, a second T-independent signal is provided to the B cell coreceptor complex in conjunction with complement components (Fig. 10.16). C3d or C3b binds to an antigen (e.g., a microbe) that is also bound to the BCR through epitope recognition. CD21 (type 2 complement receptor, or CR2) binds to antigen-bound C3d or

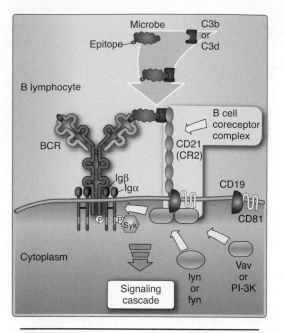

Figure 10.16

B cell coreceptor complex. Second signaling may be provided to a B cell through its complement receptor 1 (CR1, CD35) or CR2 (CD21). A microbial epitope is bound by the BCR. Complement fragment C3b or C3d also binds to the microbe. CR35 (CR1) binds to the bound C3b and CR21 (CR2) binds to the bound C3d fragment. CD19 and CD81 rapidly associate with the CR. CD19, CD21, and CD81 collectively form the B cell coreceptor complex. Tyrosine kinases (lyn, fyn, Vav, or PI-3K) are activated to phosphorylate ITAMs on Igα and Igβ, allowing Syk docking and the initiation of signaling cascades.

CD35 (type 1 complement receptor, or CDR1) binds to antigen-bound C3b. Cell-membrane-bound CD19 and CD18 (or TATA-1) rapidly associate to form the B cell coreceptor complex (CD21: CD19:CD81). Once the B cell coreceptor complex is established, several tyrosine kinases (lyn or fyn and Vav or PI-3K) phosphorylate the cytoplasmic tail of CD19. At the same time, fyn, lyn, and/or blk phosphorylate ITAMs on Igα and Igβ to allow docking of Syk tyrosine kinase and the initiation of a signal transduction cascade.

B. T-dependent activation

Most often, second signals for B cell activation are provided by CD4[+] T cells. This is especially true for epitopes found on protein antigens. Engagement of the TCR of a CD4[+] T cell and the formation of an immunologic synapse (Fig. 10.17) result from the presentation of pMHC class II by a B cell or APC (first signal). Costimulation through CD28:CD80/86 and/or CD40:CD154 provides a second signal to the T cell, resulting in the production of T cell–derived cytokines such as IL-4. The B cell is signaled through the engagement of the BCR (via Igα and Igβ), costimulatory molecules (e.g., CD40, CD80, and CD86), and the encounter of pMHC class II with the appropriate TCR. These B cell events cause the B cell to express IL-4R. Once

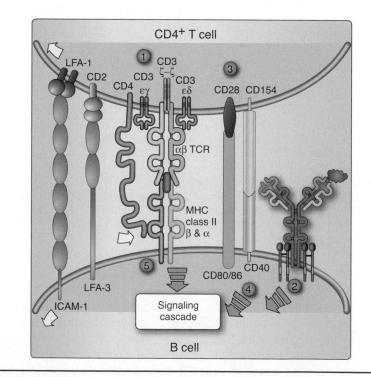

Figure 10.17

Most B cell responses require CD4[+] T cell help. **1.** Engagement of pMHC class II with the TCR:CD3:CD4 complex is a first signal to a CD4[+] T cell. **2.** BCR interaction with its obligate epitope is a first signal to a B cell. CD28 and/or CD154 engagement with CD80/86 and CD40, respectively, provides costimulation to the **3.** CD4[+] T cell and to **4.** the B cell. **5.** Interaction of pMHC class II with the αβ TCR and CD4 molecules may provide additional B cell stimulation. Signaling events lead to IL-4 secretion by the T cell and display of IL-4R by the B cell.

the IL-4R encounters its ligand (IL-4), the B cell will proliferate and, in the presence of additional T cell–derived cytokines, differentiate into an antibody-secreting plasma cell.

C. Plasma cells and memory B cells

Plasma cells are terminally differentiated B cells (see Chapter 9) that actively secrete immunoglobulins (Fig. 10.18). The epitope specificity of the immunoglobulins secreted by plasma cells is the same as the surface immunoglobulin of the B cell from which it differentiated. Not all B cells differentiate into plasma cells. Following stimulation, some become memory B cells, poised for reencounter with the same epitope.

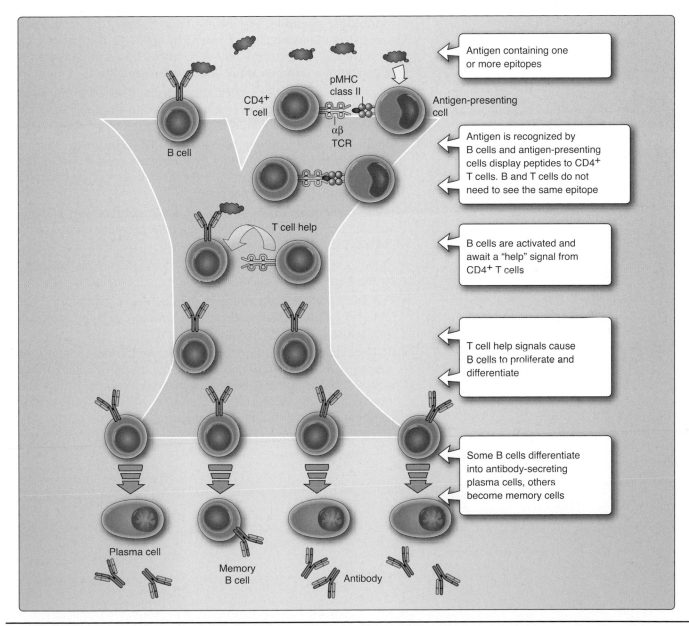

Figure 10.18
Cell interactions leading to antibody secretion.

Chapter Summary

- Dendritic cells sample their environment by phagocytosis and pinocytosis, enzymatically degrade what they ingest, and load the peptide fragments into MHC class II (forming pMHC class II) molecules in a process called **antigen presentation.**

- Dendritic cells detect threats either directly or indirectly through the same cell surface receptors that are used by the innate immune system.

- Pathogens such as intracellular microbes and viruses bind to cell membranes and directly enter the cytoplasm of the host cell.

- The interface between APC and naïve T cell is called the **immunologic synapse**. The initial step in building the immunologic synapse is the recognition of pMHC by the TCR. The immunologic synapse both stabilizes T cell–APC interaction and promotes the migration of molecules within the T cell membrane.

- The initial encounter of T cells with antigen is called **priming**, and the nature of this encounter is crucial to the development of the subsequent adaptive immune response

- Upon activation, antigen-naïve $CD4^+$ **Th precursor** cells are stimulated to secrete a variety of cytokines, express cell-surface cytokine receptor, and become **Th0** cells that are not yet committed to either the Th1 or Th1 pathway.

- Some pathogens, such as viruses, avoid contact with endocytic vesicles entirely by directly entering and replicating within the host cell's cytoplasm.

- Naïve $CD8^+$ T cells recognize pMHC class I (first signal) displayed on the surface of an infected cell.

- The BCR complex of mature B cells contains membrane-bound IgM and IgD monomers associated with $Ig\alpha$ and $Ig\beta$ molecules Cross-linking of BCRs initiates signaling.

- BCR binding initiates endocytosis, enzymatic degradation, and subsequent display of peptide fragments as pMHC class II complexes and cause the B cell to express costimulatory molecules, thus allowing the B cell to function as an APC for TCR recognition by a $CD4^+$ T cell and may mature as a plasma cell.

Study Questions

10.1 T cells recognize epitopes they have never before encountered by

A. randomly generating enormous numbers of TCRs prior to antigenic encounter.
B. sampling the environment using phagocytosis and pinocytosis.
C. synthesizing immunoglobulins specific for a wide variety of epitopes.
D. selecting widely expressed molecules as TCR ligands.
E. using genomically encoded pattern recognition receptors.

The correct answer is A. T cell receptors are randomly generated prior to any engagement with antigens. Phagocytic cells use phagocytosis and pinocytosis to internalize antigens without regard to the specificity of the ingested material. T cells do not synthesize immunoglobulins. The selection for receptors recognizing a widely expressed set of microbial molecules is a property of toll-like receptors, not of T cell receptors. The genomically encoded pattern recognition receptors are toll-like receptors.

10.2 Which of the following naïve cells load peptide fragments into MHC class II molecules?

A. CD4$^+$ T cells
B. CD8$^+$ T cells
C. dendritic cells
D. $\gamma\delta$ T cells
E. neutrophils

The correct answer is C. Of those cell types listed, only dendritic cells can process peptide fragments and load them onto MHC II molecules for presentation. Lymphocytes, whether of the CD4$^+$, CD8$^+$, or $\gamma\delta$ type, cannot do this. Neutrophils can ingest peptides and degrade them but do not synthesize MHC II molecules.

10.3 Fragments of a cytoplasmic pathogen are presented to T cells by

A. direct engagement of cell surface pattern recognition receptors.
B. macropinocytosis into $\gamma\delta$ T cells.
C. MHC class I molecules to CD8$^+$ T cells.
D. phagocytosis and presentation to CD4$^+$ T cells.
E. placement into endocytic vesicles and complexing with MHC class II molecules.

The correct answer is C. Cytoplasmically derived peptides are presented by MHC I molecules. Pattern recognition receptors do not present peptides to T cells, nor do $\gamma\delta$ T cells. CD8$^+$ T cells recognize peptide fragments presented by class I MHC molecules. They are not processed in endocytic vesicles for presentation by MHC II molecules to CD4$^+$ T cells.

10.4 The term *immunologic synapse* refers to

A. PAMP recognition by pattern recognition receptors.
B. restriction of CD4$^+$ T cells to MHC class I.
C. selective unresponsiveness of T cells.
D. T cell recognition of soluble molecules.
E. the interface between antigen-presenting cells and T cells.

The correct answer is E. The immunologic synapse is the interface between T cells and antigen presenting cells. It does not refer to the recognition and binding by pattern recognition receptors. CD4$^+$ T cells are restricted to the recognition of peptide presented by MHC II molecules. The selective unresponsiveness of T cells is called *tolerance* or *anergy*. T cell receptors do not recognize soluble molecules.

10.5 CD4$^+$ T cells that respond to intracellular pathogens by recruiting and activating phagocytic cells are termed

A. antigen-presenting cells.
B. cytotoxic T lymphocytes.
C. Th0 cells.
D. Th1 cells.
E. Th2 cells.

The correct answer is D. CD4$^+$ Th1 cells recruit and activate macrophages to destroy intracellular pathogens. Antigen-presenting cells are not T cells. Cytotoxic T lymphocytes are CD8$^+$. Th0 and Th2 cells, while also being CD4$^+$, do not engage in this activity.

10.6 In the presence of microbe-derived lipopolysaccharide,

    A. antigen-presenting cells may secrete IL-12.
    B. release of cytokines results in leukocyte activation.
    C. stimulation of IFN-γ secretion activates leukocytes.
    D. Th0 cells further differentiate into Th1 cells.
    E. all of the above

The correct answer is E. All of these activities can follow activation of phagocytic cells by the recognition and binding of lipopolysaccharide via their toll-like receptors. Activated phagocytes can secrete a variety of cytokines that can be involved in chemotaxis and activation of other leukocytes. Among these cytokines is IL-12, which stimulates natural killer cells to increase their production of IFN-γ, which, in turn, promotes the differentiation of CD4$^+$ Th0 cells into Th1 cells.

10.7 Upon encountering an appropriate pMHC I on an infected cell,

    A. B cell receptors become cross–linked, and signaling ensues.
    B. CD4$^+$ cells release IL-4.
    C. CD8$^+$ cytotoxic T cells destroy the infected cell.
    D. naïve Th1 cells secrete cytokines.
    E. Th0 cells differentiate into Th2 cells.

The correct answer is C. Once activated, cytotoxic T lymphocytes can bind and destroy infected cells expressing pMHC I complexes recognized by their T cell receptors. Neither B cells nor CD4$^+$ T cells recognize pMHC I. T helper cells—whether Th0, Th1, or Th2—are CD4$^+$ and do not recognize pMHC I.

10.8 Activation of an individual naïve B cell involves binding of membrane-associated epitopes leading to

    A. dendritic cell presentation of MHC class I.
    B. recognition of different epitopes by surface IgD and IgM.
    C. signaling from both the B cell receptor and a CD4$^+$ Th2 cell.
    D. the isotype switch.
    E. ubiquitination and destruction of antigen by proteasomes.

The correct answer is C. Activation of a naïve B cell requires both the engagement of its B cell receptor (immunoglobulin) and the receipt of secondary signals from CD4$^+$ Th2 cells. The B cell does not require interaction with antigen-presenting cells such as dendritic cells. The IgD and IgM on its surface have the same epitope specificity. Turnover of cytoplasmic molecules by proteasomes is a normal ongoing activity but is not involved in the naïve B cell's activation. The isotype switch occurs only during the reactivation of memory B cells, not during the initial activation of naïve B cells.

Lymphocyte Effector Functions

11

I. OVERVIEW

The innate immune system uses both humoral and cellular means to surround, phagocytize, enzymatically degrade, or otherwise kill microbial intruders (Fig. 11.1). The adaptive immune system also uses humoral and cellular defenses. In contrast to the innate immune system, the responses of the adaptive immune system are more narrowly targeted and directed and can be adjusted to deal with the persistence of the threat.

One arm of the adaptive immune system uses soluble molecules (fluids or "humors"), including antibodies and complement, to target and destroy invasive threats. **Humoral immunity** may be thought of as arrows or missiles in the immune system's armory. Produced and secreted by plasma cells, antibodies are soluble molecules that travel throughout the body to find and bind to their targets. The binding of an antibody to a microbial epitope can inhibit or prevent microbial spread by several means: immobilization, prevention of microbial attachment to host cells, promotion of increased phagocytosis, and targeting microbes for destruction by other soluble molecules or by leukocytes such as natural killer (NK) cells and eosinophils.

The other arm of the adaptive immune system, called **cell-mediated immunity**, is akin to hand-to-hand combat in which leukocytes directly engage invaders or infected cells harboring the invaders. Cell-mediated adaptive immune responses are controlled and regulated by T cells. Some T cells, such as cytotoxic T lymphocytes, make direct contact with infected cells and proceed to destroy the "nest" within which the microbes are multiplying, by damaging their cell membranes or inducing them to undergo apoptotic deaths. Other T cells summon and direct other leukocytes to assault and destroy the microbes or infected cells, a response called delayed (-type) hypersensitivity (DTH), which will be discussed further in Chapter 14.

II. HUMORAL IMMUNITY

Humoral immunity is based on the actions of antibodies and complement. Although cells produce both, it is the binding of these soluble molecules that is responsible for the humoral immune responses of the adaptive immune system. One of these responses, neutralization, is directly due to the binding by antibodies, while opsonization, complement activation (more specifically, the classical pathway of complement activation), and antibody-dependent cell-mediated cytotoxicity involve the use of antibodies

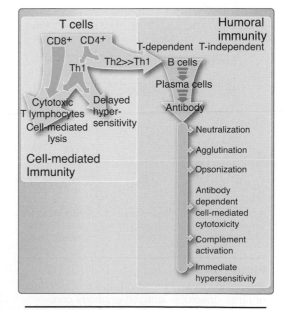

Figure 11.1
Lymphocyte effector functions—an overview.

to "tag" cells or molecules for destruction by other elements of the immune system.

A. Antigen-antibody reactions

Antigen (Ag) -antibody (Ab) interactions are some of the most specific noncovalent biochemical reactions known and can be represented by the simple formula

$$Ag + Ab \rightleftharpoons AgAb$$

Although the reaction is driven to the right, favoring binding and formation of Ag-Ab complexes, notice that the process is reversible. The strength of interaction (i.e., Ag-Ab association, right arrow, over the dissociation of Ag from Ab, left arrow) is called **affinity**. Different immunoglobulins within an individual show a wide range of affinity. **Valence** refers to the number of epitope-binding sites on an immunoglobulin molecule and varies from two (monomeric forms of all isotypes) to four (secretory IgA) to ten (for pentameric IgM). The term **avidity** is often used to describe the collective affinity of multiple binding sites (affinity + valence) of an immunoglobulin.

The **precipitin reaction** is the term applied to the interaction of soluble antigen with soluble antibody that results in the formation of Ag-Ab complexes (**lattices**) large enough to **precipitate** from solution. To understand Ag-Ab reactions, you must understand the **quantitative precipitin reaction**.

The quantitative precipitin curve can be demonstrated by mixing and incubating varying amounts of antigen (in a constant volume) with equal and constant volumes of antiserum (containing antibodies) (Fig. 11.2). Precipitate formation in a series of tubes can be measured and used to describe the three distinct zones of the quantitative precipitin curve. The amount of precipitate that is formed depends on the ratio of the antigen to antibody and is also affected by the antibody's avidity. A similar curve can be generated by keeping the antigen constant and varying the amount of antibody added.

The three zones of the quantitative precipitin curve are as follows:

- **Zone of Ag excess**. There is insufficient antibody to form large lattices. The antigen-antibody complexes are too small to precipitate. The net result is the formation of soluble complexes.
- **Equivalence zone**. Optimal precipitation occurs in this area of the curve. Large lattices can be formed, and visible precipitating complexes are formed.
- **Zone of Ab excess**. Not enough antigen is present to form large lattices, and the net result is formation of soluble complexes.

These principles of the quantitative precipitin curve apply to all antigen-antibody reactions and form the basis of many clinical diagnostic tests (see Chapter 20).

B. Agglutination

Antibodies can also bind to and cross-link cells or particles, causing an aggregate formation in the **agglutination** reaction. Agglutination has the effect of entrapping microbial invaders within a molecular net,

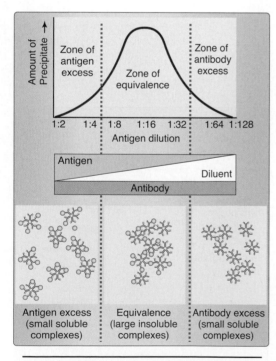

Figure 11.2
Precipitin curve. Formation and precipitation of large, insoluble antigen-antibody complexes occur at optimal ratios of antigen and antibody. The ratio depends upon the complexity of the antigen and the avidity of the antibody.

inhibiting their mobility (Fig. 11.3), and rendering them more susceptible to destruction. Antibodies of the IgM and IgA isotypes are particularly adept at this because they contain 10 and 4 binding sites,
respectively. However, IgG antibodies in sufficient concentrations can
also agglutinate cells or particles. Antibodies can also agglutinate
nonmicrobial cells, as is commonly demonstrated by the use of IgM
antibodies for ABO typing of erythrocytes (see Chapters 17 and 20).

C. Neutralization

Neutralization is the binding of antibodies to microbial epitopes or
soluble molecules (e.g., toxins) in a manner that inhibits the ability
of these microbes or molecules to bind to host cell surfaces. Binding
to host cell surfaces is a necessary step for microbes and toxins
to enter and damage host cells. Antibodies generated against the
microbes (or toxins) often include some that block their interaction
with the host cell surface, thus preventing the microbe (or toxin) from
entering the cell (Fig. 11.4). Neutralizing antibodies are usually of the
IgG and IgA isotypes. It is the presence of neutralizing antibodies
generated during the initial infections that provides the greatest protection against subsequent reinfection by the same organism.

D. Opsonization

Sometimes the binding of an antibody (usually of the IgG1 or IgG3
isotype) to a microbial surface is enough to "whet the appetite" of a

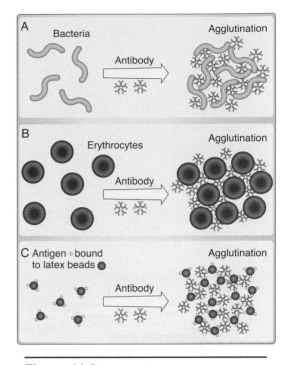

Figure 11.3
Agglutination. Antibodies can crosslink infectious agents (**A**), host cells (**B**) or antigen
bound the surface of particles (**C**).

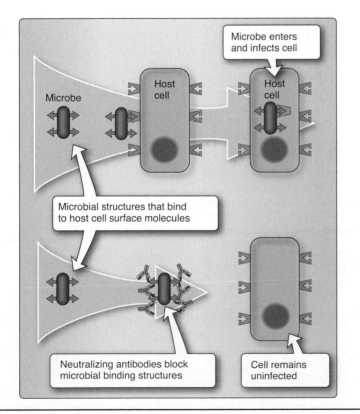

Figure 11.4
Neutralization. Neutralization occurs when antibodies block the structures
on infectious agents or toxin molecules that are used to attach to and enter
host cells.

phagocyte, making the microbe a more attractive "meal." This process is known as **opsonization.** In essence, antibodies binding to microbes "tag" them for subsequent destruction by phagocytic cells. Upon binding, the antibody molecules undergo conformational changes that include the Fc region (see Fig. 6.6). Macrophages, dendritic cells, and neutrophils bear surface receptors (FcR) for the Fc portion of bound immunoglobulin. Table 11.1 presents the types and distribution of Fc receptors. FcRs on phagocytic cells recognize antigen-bound antibody molecules, tethering the "tagged" microbe to the phagocytic cell and stimulating its engulfment and destruction (Fig. 11.5). Binding and engulfment via the FcγRI receptor is facilitated by the simultaneous use of complement receptors (CR) (Fig. 11.6; also see Fig. 5.3). Thus the roles of bound antibody and bound

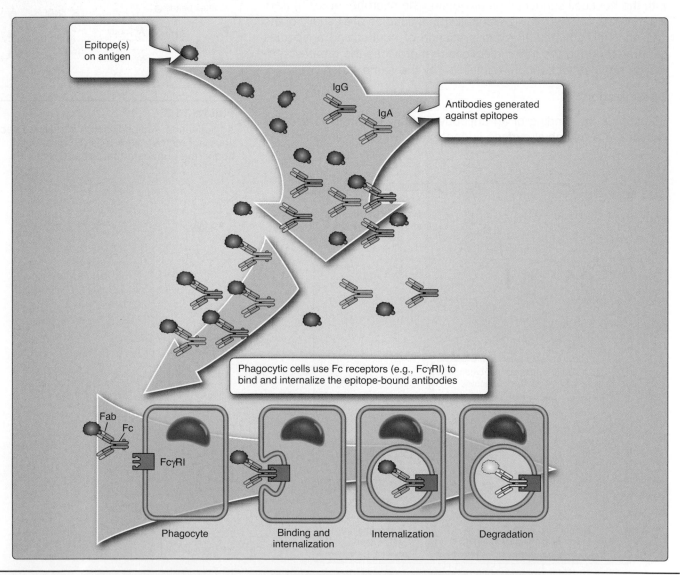

Figure 11.5

Uptake and opsonization via Fc receptors. Fc receptors (FcR) allow attachment of epitope-bound antibodies to cells for internalization. There are multiple types of Fc receptors that are specialized for different antibody isotypes (see Table 1).

Table 11.1
FC RECEPTORS

Receptor	Isotype Bound	Expressed On	Binding Promotes
FcγRI	IgG1 > IgG3 > IgG4 > IgG2	Mast cells, dendritic cells, eosinophils, neutrophils	Internalization, opsonization, induction of killing
FcγRII-A	IgG1 > IgG2 > IgG3 > IgG4	Macrophages, dendritic cells, eosinophils, neutrophils, platelets	Internalization, degranulation
FcγRII-B1	IgG1 > IgG3 > IgG4 > IgG2	B cells, mast cells	Inhibits stimulation of B cells and mast cells
FcγRII-B2	IgG1 > IgG3 > IgG4 > IgG2	Macrophages, eosinophils, neutrophils	Internalization
FcγRIII	IgG1 > IgG3	NK cells, eosinophils, macrophages, neutrophils, mast cells	Induction of killing
FcαRI	IgA1, IgA2	Macrophages, neutrophils, eosinophils	Internalization, induction of killing
Fcα/μRI	IgA, IgM	Macrophages, B cells	Internalization
FcεRI	IgE prior to epitope binding	Mast cells, eosinophils, basophils	Degranulation

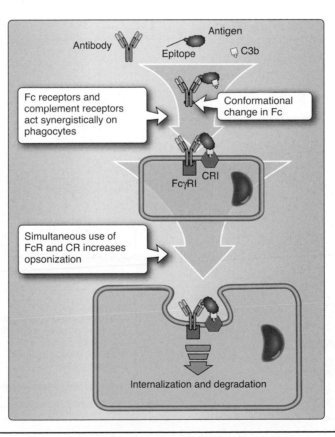

Figure 11.6
Synergy of Fc receptors and complement receptors for opsonization. Simultaneous use of Fc receptors (FcR) and complement receptors (CR) to tether antigens bound by both antibodies and complement fragments synergistically increases opsonization.

complement fragments such as C3b are synergistic in serving as **opsonins** to stimulate phagocytosis.

E. Antibody-dependent cell-mediated cytotoxicity

The "tagging" of an invasive organism can attract phagocytic cells and other cytolytic cells. FcRs on **NK cells** (FcγRIII) and **eosinophils** (FcγRI and FcαRI) are IgG- and IgA-specific (see Table 11.1). The bound cells may be bacteria, protozoa, or even some parasitic worms. As with phagocytic cells, these receptors allow the cytolytic cells to bind invasive organisms "tagged" with IgG or IgA antibodies, but rather than engulfment, they utilize cytolytic mechanisms to kill the "tagged" organisms (Figs. 11.7A, 11.7B). This process is termed **antibody-dependent cell-mediated cytotoxicity** (**ADCC**). The cytolytic mechanisms used by NK cells and eosinophils in ADCC are similar to some of those utilized by cytotoxic T cells to kill the intruder.

F. Complement activation

The **classical pathway of complement** is activated by conformational changes that occur in the Fc portion of antibodies upon epitope binding. Antibodies (usually of the IgM and IgG isotypes) facilitate the sequential binding of the C1, C4, C2, and C3 components of the complement system (Fig. 11.8). Like the alternative and mannan-binding lectin pathways (see Figs. 5.7 and 5.10), completion

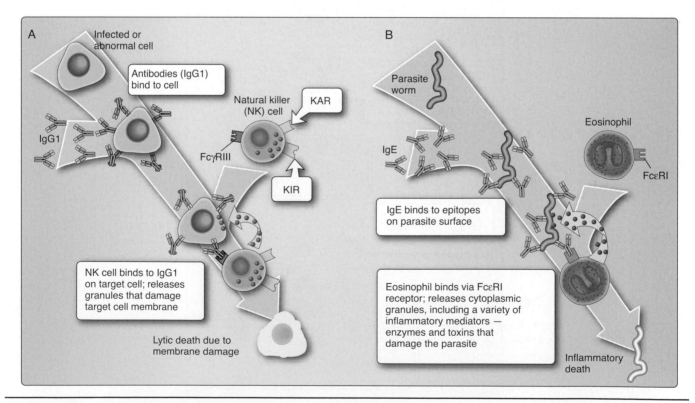

Figure 11.7

Antibody-dependent cell-mediated cytotoxicity (ADCC). Fc receptors on natural killer cells (**A**) and on eosinophils (**B**) allow them to attach to and destroy, by direct cellular attack, cells that have been "tagged" by antibodies. On NK cells, these are distinct from the KAR and KIR receptors used to detect stress molecules and MHC I molecules.

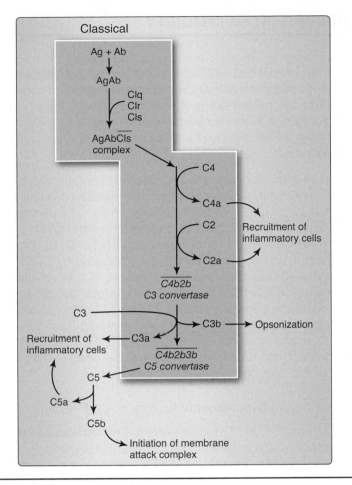

Figure 11.8
Classical pathway of complement activation. The classical pathway of complement activation is triggered by the binding of antibodies to antigen to form antigen-antibody (Ag-Ab) complexes that permit the subsequent binding of the C1 component.

of the classical complement pathway results in the production of **C3b**, a "sticky" fragment of C3 that readily binds to surfaces (of cells, microbes, or particles; see Fig. 20.12) as a highly effective opsonin (see Fig. 5.4), the release of small pro-inflammatory fragments such as **C5a**, **C4a**, and **C3a**, and the assembly of the **membrane attack complex** (see Figs. 5.8 and 5.9).

G. Immediate hypersensitivity

Mast cells and basophils have surface receptors that bind the Fc portion of IgE molecules that have not yet bound to their epitopes. Thus these cells acquire a set of receptor-bound immunoglobulins that function as epitope-recognizing surface receptors. When the surface IgE is cross-linked by appropriate epitopes, the mast cell/basophil is triggered to degranulate. This release of cytoplasmic granules triggers a set of events known as *immediate hypersensitivities*. Immediate hypersensitivity responses, including asthma and allergies, are discussed in detail in Chapter 14.

III. CELL-MEDIATED IMMUNITY

Innate and adaptive immune responses can be viewed as a form of warfare at the cellular and molecular levels against potential invasive organisms. Antibodies and complement can be effective weapons against microbes that are caught out in the open. However, microbes are not solely dependent on their numbers but also employ evasive tactics, including hiding within host cells where antibodies and complement cannot reach them.

Cell-mediated immune responses are directed to curtail microbial stealth by determining whether infectious agents are sheltered within host cells and are thus beyond the reach of humoral immunity. Cell-mediated responses resemble cavalry charges and hand-to-hand combat and take two basic forms: **delayed (-type) hypersensitivity** (**DTH**), mediated by CD4$^+$ Th1 cells, and **cell-mediated lysis**, mediated by CD8$^+$ cytotoxic T lymphocytes (CTLs). Cell-mediated immunity is a life-or-death struggle at close quarters. In DTH, some T cells act as "scouts" and "senior officers," identifying sites of infection, calling in reinforcements (mostly macrophages and other leukocytes), and ordering them to kill the infectious foe and/or the host cell sheltering the foe. CTLs, by contrast, engage in direct cell-to-cell combat to actively destroy their infectious opponent or the host cell in which that opponent is hiding.

A. Delayed (-type) hypersensitivity: role of CD4$^+$ T cells

Once activated, CD4$^+$ Th1 cells leave the lymph nodes in which they were activated and prowl through the vasculature, body tissues, and lymphatic system, seeking host cells displaying the same pMHC class II combination that originally triggered their activation. If, in the course of recirculating through body tissues, a previously activated Th1 cell reencounters the appropriate pMHC class II displayed on a phagocytic cell (e.g., at the site of an infection), it binds and interacts. Access to the infectious site is facilitated by the secretion of phagocyte-derived cytokines such as IL-1, IL-8, and TNF-α that activate local vascular endothelium and promote vascular permeability. The phagocyte, as an APC, can **reactivate** the Th1 cell to proliferate anew and gain the ability to activate macrophages (Fig. 11.9). Thus T cells from the adaptive immune system direct the activities of cells of the innate immune system.

In the DTH response, macrophage activation by CD4$^+$ Th1 cells is mediated by direct contact (binding of CD40 and CD154) and by IFN-γ secreted by the T cells. Once activated, macrophages increase their phagocytic activity as well as the production and release of destructive enzymes and reactive oxygen intermediates. Activated macrophages become blind, enraged killers that attack not only infectious agents and infected cells, but also normal uninfected cells in the vicinity (see Chapter 5). They also secrete cytokines that attract other leukocytes, especially neutrophils, to the site of infection. Together, the activated macrophages and neutrophils rampage through the site of infection, damaging cells, ingesting and killing microbes, and removing cellular debris.

The DTH response can be a double-edged sword. Because activated macrophages are not antigen-specific, they injure friend and foe alike,

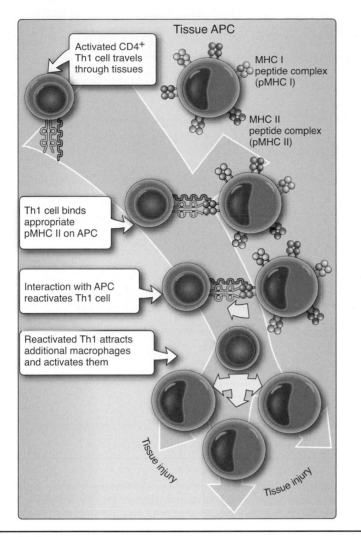

Figure 11.9
Delayed (-type) hypersensitivity. Activated CD4$^+$ Th1 cells can, upon subsequent reactivation through interaction with antigen-presenting cells (APC) in body tissues, secrete cytokines that activate local macrophages to engage in a nonspecific destruction of local cells and tissues.

that is, normal tissue along with infected cells. DTH responses, in fact, have two phases: a specific phase based on the Th1 T cell activity and a nonspecific phase based on the activity of the newly activated macrophages (Fig. 11.10). Reactivation of each Th1 cell is epitope-specific (e.g., a peptide derived from *Leishmania*) and requires stimulation by the precise pMHC II specific to its TCR. However, the macrophages that are subsequently activated by the Th1 cell are not epitope-specific and are able to destroy not only *Leishmania*, but also any other available microbes. Thus a response stimulated by a single microbe can (within the context of the local infectious site) provide protection against a variety of microbes. As long as the DTH response eliminates the threat and subsides so that proper tissue repair and healing can follow, it is an extraordinarily beneficial defense mechanism. Excessively active or chronic DTH responses often inflict permanent damage on host tissues that may impair normal function and, in some cases, may be fatal. For example, much or most of the pulmonary injury sustained in

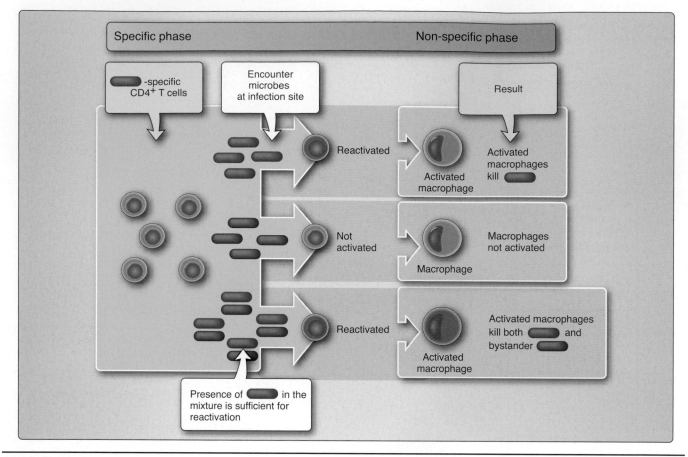

Figure 11.10
Specific and nonspecific phases of delayed (-type) hypersensitivity. Although DTH responses are epitope-specific in their initiation because they involve binding of TCR by pMHC II, the local macrophage-mediated destruction that ensues is not limited by the triggering epitope. Activated macrophages destroy not only the infectious agents that initiated the DTH, but also other microbes in the immediate vicinity.

response to *M. tuberculosis* is inflicted by activated macrophages that surround the bacteria to form nodules (or tubercles, from which the organism derives its name) and not by the infectious agent itself.

B. Cytotoxic T lymphocytes: role of CD8⁺ T cells

Only a small proportion of the cells of the body express MHC class II molecules, although all nucleated cells express MHC class I molecules. Thus CD8⁺ T cells can scan nucleated cells throughout the body to see what cytoplasmically derived peptides are being presented on those MHC I molecules.

1. **Target cell recognition:** Like activated CD4⁺ T cells, activated CD8⁺ CTLs circulate throughout the body, "sampling" pMHC class I complexes on body cells to determine whether the same pMHC I that led to its own activation can be found. If the CTL detects this same complex on the surface of another cell, it recognizes that it has contacted an infected cell (Fig. 11.11). CTLs bind directly to pMHC I on infected cells and destroy them.

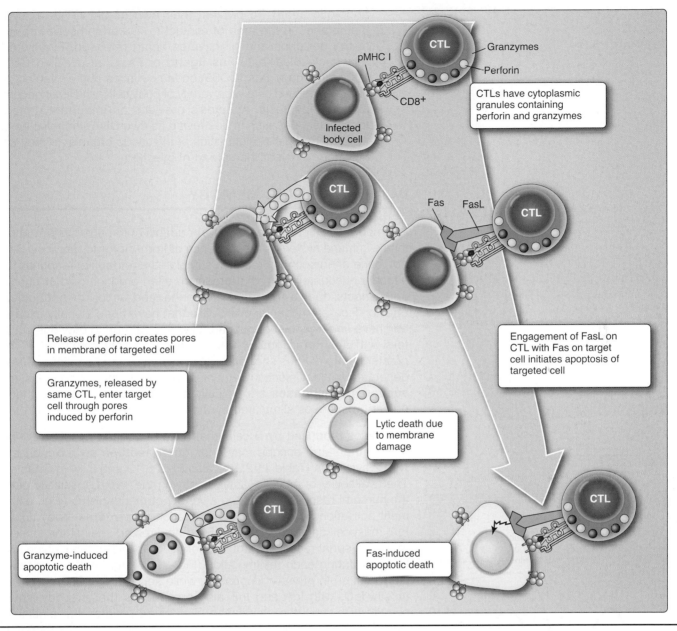

Figure 11.11
Recognition, binding, and cytolysis by cytotoxic T lymphocytes. Cytotoxic T lymphocytes (CTLs) utilize their TCRs to recognize and bind specific pMHC I that are presenting appropriate cytoplasmically derived peptides (e.g., from viruses multiplying in the cytoplasm). Direct attachment to the infected cell permits the CTL to destroy the infected cell through the induction of membrane damage by perforins or through the induction of apoptosis by either granzymes or engagement of the Fas and FasL surface molecules.

2. **Target cell destruction:** Once attached to a cell that needs to be eliminated, CTLs can use multiple mechanisms to destroy those targeted cells (see Fig. 11.11). They release **perforins** that puncture the cell membranes of the infected cells, effectively lysing them. CTLs also release **granzymes** that enter the cytoplasm through the membrane lesions caused by the perforins and induce the infected cell to degrade its own DNA and thus undergo an

apoptotic death. To prevent their own death, CTLs alter their membranes in the area of contact to make themselves resistant to the perforins and granzymes being released. Finally, CTLs bear molecules (e.g., **Fas ligand** or **FasL**, also called CD178) that can engage **Fas** (CD95) on the surfaces of the infected cells. Fas is expressed on a wide variety of body cells, and its engagement induces apoptosis. Apoptosis provides an important protective mechanism because in destroying its own DNA, the infected cells also destroy the nucleic acids of infectious organisms they carry, helping to prevent the spread of infection.

IV. IMMUNOLOGIC MEMORY

An important difference between the adaptive immune system and the innate immune system is the presence of **immunologic memory**. Simply put, once an infectious organism stimulates an adaptive response, subsequent encounters with that organism often produce mild or unnoticeable effects due to the rapid and enhanced action of antibodies or effector T cells. Antigen-specific cells that have been clonally expanded and have undergone some degree of activation during previous encounters with antigen (**memory cells**) can be rapidly mobilized in much greater numbers, thus shortening the response time to antigen. Whether generated against infectious organisms or other types of antigens, these **secondary responses** are typically faster and more vigorous than the primary responses stimulated by the initial exposure (Fig. 11.12).

Antibodies produced by B cells that have prolonged or repeated exposure to the same epitope may undergo an **isotype switch** induced by type 2 cytokines (Table 11.2; see also Figs. 8.13 and 8.14 in Chapter 8). The availability of multiple isotypes having the same specificity permits the humoral response to initiate a variety of mechanisms (e.g., complement activation by IgM and IgG, secretion into external body fluids by IgA, mast cell degranulation by IgE) to be directed against the same epitope. The serial reactivation of memory B cells allows the isotype switch to occur during each restimulation (Fig. 11.13). IgM is the predominant isotype seen in primary responses, while secondary responses include mostly IgG, with IgA and IgE also present. As the antibody isotypes change with repeated stimulation by a given antigen, the binding efficiency of the antibodies changes as well, owing to the incorporation of small mutations in the DNA encoding the variable regions of the light and heavy chains (Fig. 11.14; also see Fig. 8.15). B cells bearing mutations that result in tighter binding of epitopes by their surface immunoglobulins are stimulated to proliferate more rapidly, while those binding less well do not proliferate as vigorously. As a result, the antibody response is continuously dominated by the B cells that produce the highest-affinity antibodies against the epitope in question, a process known as **affinity maturation** (see Chapter 8).

The development of immunologic memory can be artificially exploited through **vaccination**. Deliberate exposure to an infectious organism in a form that is unable to cause full-blown disease can thus provide protection against a subsequent exposure to a fully virulent form of that organism. Likewise, deliberate exposure to a nontoxic form of a toxin (e.g., heat-denatured tetanus toxoid) can provide protection against future exposure to the natural form of that toxin. During the **primary**

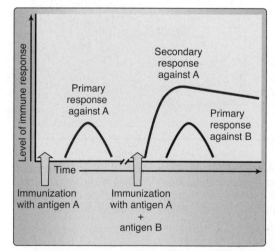

Figure 11.12
Primary and secondary adaptive immune responses. Upon initial antigen encounter, both humoral and cell mediated adaptive responses are of limited in intensity and duration (primary response). Subsequent exposures to antigen (secondary response) are characterized by increased intensity and duration. Each epitope elicits a separate response.

Table 11.2
**CYTOKINES RESPONSIBLE FOR HUMAN
ISOTYPE SWITCHES**

Type 1 or 2 Cytokines	Promotes Switch To
IL-4	IgG1, IgG3, IgG4, IgE
IL-10	IgG1, IgG3
TGF-β	IgA
IFN-γ	IgG1, IgG3

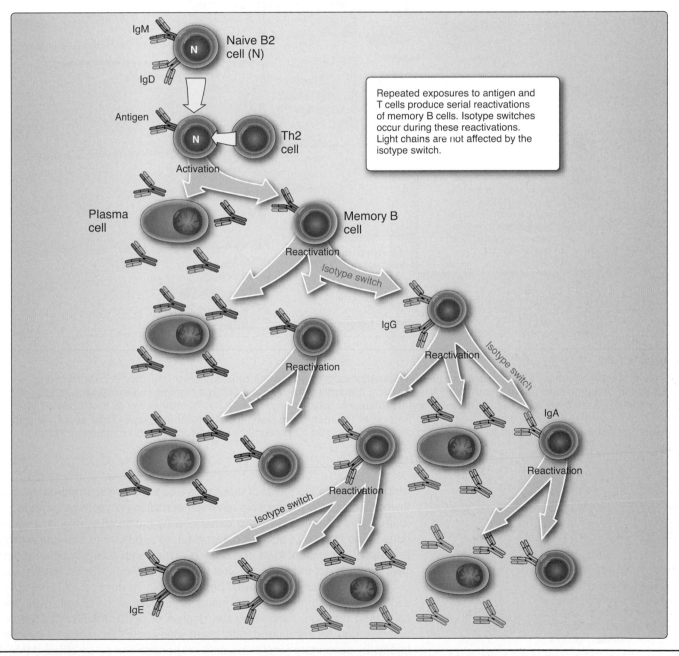

Figure 11.13
Isotype switch in memory B cells. Isotype switches occur during the sequential reactivations and proliferations of memory B cells that occur when they are periodically reexposed to antigen and T cell signals.

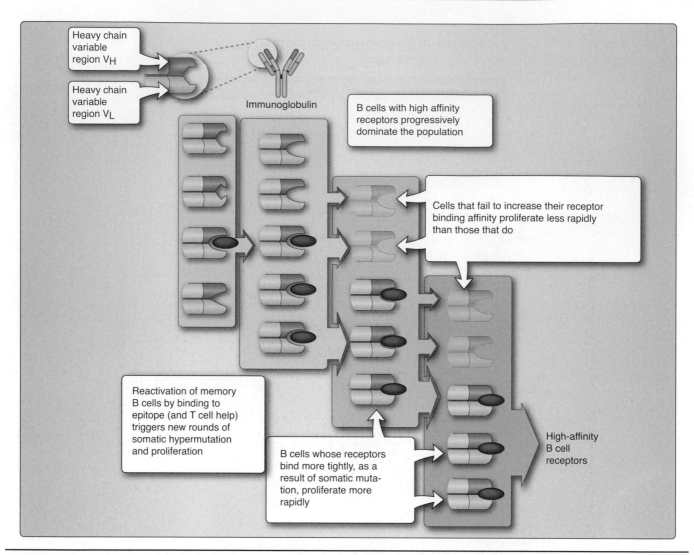

Heavy chain variable region V_H

Heavy chain variable region V_L

Immunoglobulin

B cells with high affinity receptors progressively dominate the population

Cells that fail to increase their receptor binding affinity proliferate less rapidly than those that do

Reactivation of memory B cells by binding to epitope (and T cell help) triggers new rounds of somatic hypermutation and proliferation

B cells whose receptors bind more tightly, as a result of somatic mutation, proliferate more rapidly

High-affinity B cell receptors

Figure 11.14

Affinity maturation in memory B cells. Somatic hypermutation occurs during the proliferation of memory B cells following reactivation. Accumulated mutations in the DNA encoding the antigen-binding regions may cause changes in the affinity of the synthesized antibody for its epitope. Mutations that cause increased affinity drive the memory cells to proliferate even more rapidly so that they represent an increased fraction of the memory B cells specific for the epitope. Thus over time and repeated exposure, the response to a given epitope is characterized by production of antibodies with increasing affinity.

response, while the threat of disease is lessened by the "crippled" microbe, the body can build a defensive reservoir consisting of memory lymphocytes (both T and B) that have been expanded by proliferation and have undergone some degree of activation. Upon future exposure to that same organism, even in a virulent form, the body is armed with a large pool of reactive cells that can act more quickly and with greater vigor against the organism during a **secondary response**. The opportunity to develop IgG and IgA antibodies against the microbes enables an individual to neutralize the reencountered microbe, minimizing the degree of actual infection to the point where it can be eliminated with great efficiency. Clearance of infectious agents by secondary (or subsequent) responses can be so efficient that the individual is unaware of the reinfection altogether.

Although we think of immunologic memory primarily in the sense of enhancing the response against subsequent exposures to an infectious organism or other antigen, this is not always the case. In some cases, responses to future exposures can be diminished, a state known as **tolerance**. This phenomenon is important in preventing the immune system from producing superfluous (and potentially injurious) responses against harmless organisms and molecules in the environment, as well as against the body's own cells and molecules. These important considerations are discussed in upcoming chapters.

Chapter summary

- Humoral immunity is based upon the actions of soluble antibodies and complement.

- The precipitin reaction is the interaction of soluble antigen with soluble antibody that results in the formation of Ag-Ab complexes (lattices) large enough to fall out of solution as a visible precipitate.

- Antibodies can bind and cross-link cells or particles, causing an aggregate formation in a reaction known as **agglutination.**

- **Neutralization** is the binding of antibodies to microbial epitopes or soluble molecules (e.g., toxins) in a manner that inhibits the ability of those microbes/molecules to bind to host cell surfaces.

- Macrophages, dendritic cells, and neutrophils bear surface receptors (FcR) for the Fc portion of bound immunoglobulin. With the exception of FcRε that binds free IgE, FcRs recognize and bind only those antibodies that have already bound to their epitopes. The binding of FcRs to antibodies on microbes tethers the "tagged" microbes to the phagocytic cell and stimulates their engulfment and destruction. Bound immunoglobulin and bound complement fragments such as C3b are synergistic in serving as **opsonins** to stimulate phagocytosis.

- The **classical pathway of complement** is activated by conformational changes that occur in antibodies upon epitope binding (usually of the IgM and IgG isotypes) to facilitate the sequential binding of the C1, C4, C2, and C3 components of the complement system.

- Cell-mediated responses include two basic forms: **delayed (-type) hypersensitivity (DTH)**, mediated by CD4$^+$ Th1 cells, and **cell-mediated lysis**, mediated by CD8$^+$ cytotoxic T lymphocytes (CTLs).

- In the DTH response, macrophage activation by CD4$^+$ Th1 cells is mediated by direct contact (binding of CD40 and CD154) and by IFN-γ secreted by the T cells. Once activated, macrophages increase their phagocytic activity as well as the production and release of destructive enzymes and reactive oxygen intermediates.

- In cell-mediated lysis, activated CD8$^+$ CTLs search out cells that have the same pMHC complex that stimulated their own activation. Once such a cell is found, CTLs can use multiple mechanisms to destroy those targeted cells. These include lysis resulting from the infliction of membrane damage and the induction of apoptosis.

- Immunologic memory is an adaptive response. Once an infectious organism stimulates an adaptive response, the immune response to subsequent exposures is altered. Future encounters with that organism may produce mild or unnoticeable effects due to the rapid and enhanced action of antibodies or effector T cells.

Study Questions

11.1 Following a motor vehicle accident, a 25-year-old male requires a blood transfusion. Blood type tests done prior to the transfusion involve the use of IgM antibodies against A and B antigens on erythrocytes. A positive reaction is an aggregate formation that is known as

A. agglutination.
B. complement activation.
C. neutralization.
D. opsonization.
E. precipitin reaction.

> The correct answer is A. Agglutination is the aggregation or clumping of cells or particles bound together by antibodies (usually IgM or dimeric IgA). Complement activation is initiated by the attachment of the C1 component of complement to epitope-bound antibody (IgM or IgG). Neutralization is the blocking by antibody of structures on microbes and toxins that allow them to bind to host cell surfaces. Opsonization is the increased phagocytic uptake of cells or molecules tagged by antibodies (usually IgG1). The precipitin reaction results from the assembly of large antigen-antibody complexes causing them to precipitate from solution.

11.2 The process that is synergistically enhanced by the binding of both antibodies and complement fragments such as C3b by phagocytes is known as

A. agglutination.
B. complement activation.
C. neutralization.
D. opsonization.
E. precipitin reaction.

> The correct answer is D. Opsonization is the increased phagocytic uptake of cells or molecules tagged by antibodies (usually IgG1). Agglutination is the aggregation or clumping of cells or particles bound together by antibodies (usually IgM or dimeric IgA). Complement activation is initiated by the attachment of the C1 component of complement to epitope bound antibody (IgM or IgG). Neutralization is the blocking by antibody of structures on microbes and toxins that allow them to bind to host cell surfaces. The precipitin reaction results from the assembly of large antigen-antibody complexes that precipitate from solution.

11.3 The term applied to the interaction of soluble antigen with soluble antibody that results in the formation of insoluble antigen-antibody complexes is

A. agglutination.
B. complement activation.
C. neutralization.
D. opsonization.
E. precipitin reaction.

> The correct answer is E. The precipitin reaction results from the assembly of large antigen-antibody complexes that precipitate from solution. Agglutination is the aggregation or clumping of cells or particles bound together by antibodies (usually IgM or dimeric IgA). Complement activation is initiated by the attachment of the C1 component of complement to epitope-bound antibody (IgM or IgG). Neutralization is the blocking by antibody of structures on microbes and toxins that allow them to bind to host cell surfaces. Opsonization is the increased phagocytic uptake of cells or molecules tagged by antibodies (usually IgG1).

11.4 The binding of antibodies to microbial epitopes or soluble molecules in a manner that inhibits the ability of these microbes/molecules to bind to host cell surfaces is termed

A. agglutination.
B. complement activation.
C. neutralization.
D. opsonization.
E. precipitin reaction.

> The correct answer is C. Neutralization is the blocking by antibody of structures on microbes and toxins that allow them to bind to host cell surfaces. Agglutination is the aggregation or clumping of cells or particles bound together by antibodies (usually IgM or dimeric IgA). Complement activation is initiated by the attachment of the C1 component of complement to epitope bound antibody (IgM or IgG). Opsonization is the increased phagocytic uptake of cells or molecules tagged by antibodies (usually IgG1). The precipitin reaction results from the assembly of large antigen-antibody complexes that precipitate from solution.

11.5 Which of the following antibody isotypes facilitate the sequential binding of the C1, C4, C2, and C3 components of the complement system?

A. IgA and IgD
B. IgA and IgE
C. IgA and IgM
D. IgE and IgG
E. IgG and IgM

> The correct answer is E. The classical pathway of complement is initiated by the interaction of C1 (followed by C4, C2, and C3) with epitope-bound IgG or IgM. IgA, IgD, and IgE do not bind to C1.

Regulation of Adaptive Responses

12

I. OVERVIEW

What happens when the immune system goes awry? When functioning properly, the innate and adaptive immune systems recognize and attack nonself while leaving self relatively undisturbed. The innate immune system expresses a finite number of genomically "hard-wired" receptors that recognize molecules widely expressed by potentially pathogenic organisms but not by the host (self). The adaptive immune system faces a daunting task because its receptors are somatically and randomly generated. Selection mechanisms in the thymus and bone marrow eliminate overtly self-reactive T cells and B cells during development. However, these mechanisms cannot eliminate all potentially self-reactive cells, because the adaptive immune system often encounters self molecules that were not present during receptor selection within the thymus or did not appear until a later point of development (e.g., those arising during and after puberty). **Autoimmunity** is a condition in which the immune system perceives self as nonself. Many serious and potentially fatal diseases, such as multiple sclerosis, some forms of diabetes, and systemic lupus erythematosus, are caused by autoimmune reactions.

Fortunately, the adaptive immune system has evolved several mechanisms to deal with potentially self-reactive lymphocytes. Unregulated adaptive immune responses are harmful. Without immune regulation, the adaptive immune response would be in a constant state of immunologic outrage, lashing out at nonself epitopes to which we are constantly exposed (e.g., food, drink, cosmetics), many of which pose no threat, and at those vital epitopes to which we are infrequently exposed (e.g., maternal-fetal interactions).

II. TOLERANCE

Normally, the immune system's offensive machinery is reserved for use against external threats. Positive and negative thymic selection ensures that mature T cells recognize self MHC I or II molecules (positive selection) but are not overtly self-reactive against self peptides (negative selection). Thymocytes that are unable to make these distinctions meet an apoptotic death. However, no system is perfect; not all self peptides are presented within the thymus, and some self peptides arise after the waning of thymic function. In addition, some peptides are restricted to anatomic sites that are not easily accessible to the immune system. Consequently, some potentially autoreactive T cells slip through positive and negative selection. As a result, the adaptive immune system must use additional means to avoid self reactivity. Selective nonresponsive-ness or **tolerance** requires that when the adaptive immune system does recognize self, it should adopt a nondestructive strategy. Several toler-ance mechanisms have evolved to minimize potential harm caused by postdevelopmental selection autoreactive cells.

A. Anergy

Anergy is a state of lymphocyte nonresponsiveness. It occurs follow-ing peptide + major histocompatibility complex (pMHC) engagement (T cells) or free epitope engagement (B cells). In the absence of additional "instruction" from antigen-presenting cells (APC) in the case of T cells) or from CD4$^+$ cells in the case of B cells, the immune system does not respond. Anergy is therefore a form of regulation imposed upon the activation of naïve T and B cells.

In Chapter 10, we saw that naïve T cells require interaction with both pMHC and a set of costimulatory second signals from an APC (usually a dendritic cell) to become activated. The importance of this two-signal activation can be understood by considering what might happen, in the absence of such regulation, with T cells that escape negative selection in the thymus. Since all nucleated cells of the body express MHC I molecules presenting self peptides, naïve CD8$^+$ T cells specific for self pMHC class I could become activated by simply recognizing, via their T cell receptor (TCR, first signal), appro-priate pMHC I complexes on any normal nucleated body cell. Once so activated, they would be able to bind and kill other normal body cells. The need for second signals from APCs minimizes this risk. TCR binding of self-reactive naïve CD8$^+$ T cells with normal non-APC body cells (that are unable to provide the appropriate second signals) causes the CD8$^+$ T cell to become anergic rather than acti-vated. In other words, receipt of signal 1 in the absence of simulta-neous receipt of signal 2 removes the T cell from the immunologic arena. How CD4$^+$ T cells are anergized remains unclear, primarily because their interaction is almost always with APCs.

B cells, too, require a second signal following B cell receptor (BCR) engagement. If they fail to receive a second signal, they become unresponsive to the combined restimulation by both first and second signals. Anergized cells are not killed but remain in circulation and cannot, under normal circumstances, be reactivated.

B. The role of CD152 (CTLA-4) in anergy

T cells constitutively express CD28 that engages CD80 (B7.1) or CD86 (B7.2) costimulatory molecules displayed by APCs (see Chapter 10). TCR engagement of the appropriate pMHC (first signal) + CD28:CD80/86 (second signal) stimulates the T cell to produce IL-2, express IL-2 receptor (IL-2R), and enter into the cell cycle. After activation of the T cell, CD152 (cytotoxic T-lymphocyte-associated antigen 4, or CTLA-4), which is normally sequestered within the Golgi apparatus of naïve T cells, moves to the cell membrane, where it binds with CD80/86 with an avidity that is 100-fold greater than that of CD28. CD152 engagement inhibits IL-2 mRNA expression by the T cell and its progression through the cell cycle. This mechanism ensures that activated T cells do not continue to act once they are

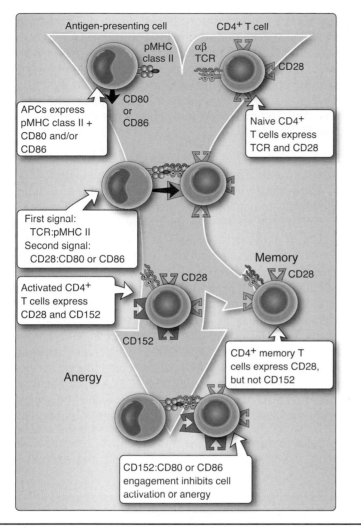

Figure 12.1
CD152 (CTLA-4) in T cell regulation. The expression of CD152 by T cells
begins only after they have been activated. CD152 competes with CD28
for binding to CD80/CD86 and does so with a greater affinity than CD28.
Binding of CD152 by CD80/86 provides a signal for anergy that inactivates
the T cell, providing a means for imposing a finite period of activity on each
activated T cell.

no longer needed. The T cells provide their own mechanism for turn-
ing themselves off after a period of time. If the stimulus remains, the
anergic T cells are replaced by newly activated ones. If the antigenic
stimulus has been removed, the response ends. The reactive T cells
disappear, with the exception of quiescent memory cells (Fig. 12.1).

B. Regulatory T cells

Regulatory T cells may also maintain tolerance. Characteristically,
they inhibit the activity of autoreactive lymphocytes. The molecular
basis for their regulatory action is still unclear, but they appear to fall
into one of two categories: T regulatory (T_{reg}) and T suppressor (Ts)
cells. T_{reg} cells express both CD4 and CD25 molecules and are
thought to be important inhibitors of immune-mediated inflammatory

diseases such as inflammatory bowel disease. Ts cells are CD8$^+$ and inhibit the activation and proliferation of CD4$^+$ T cells, including Th1 cells. Both T$_{reg}$ and Ts may inhibit specific antibody production by B cells. One additional mechanism for minimizing unwanted reactivity may be apparent in the cytokines produced by Th1 and Th2 cells. Th1-produced IFN-γ inhibits the maturation of Th0 cells into Th2 cells, and Th2-produced IL-4 inhibits the differentiation of cells along the Th2 pathway.

1. **CD4$^+$ T$_{reg}$ cells:** These cells express both CD4 and CD25 (the α chain of the IL-2 receptor, IL-2R) molecules. The β and γ chains form a low-affinity IL-2R, and the addition of the α chain confers a high affinity for binding IL-2. These CD4$^+$CD25$^+$ T cells, estimated to constitute 5% to 10% of peripheral CD4$^+$ T cells, have been identified in a variety of tissues and have been implicated in the prevention of some autoimmune responses and some responses against nonself as well (Fig. 12.2). They are present in the absence of intentional immunization and are therefore sometimes called natural T$_{reg}$s. Although their activation requires TCR engagement, the inhibitory effects of T$_{reg}$s appear to be nonspecific and seem to inhibit the activation of CD4$^+$CD25$^+$ T cells specific for a variety of epitopes. A subset of CD4$^+$CD25$^+$ T cells also express the RO isoform of CD45 (CD45RO), glucocorticoid-induced tumor necrosis factor receptor (GITC), and CD152 (CTLA-4) molecules on their surface and the Foxp3 transcription factor within their nuclei. These cells are believed to be the actual suppressive subpopulation.

T$_{reg}$ cells undergo positive and negative selection within the thymus, possibly involving interaction with the epithelial cells of

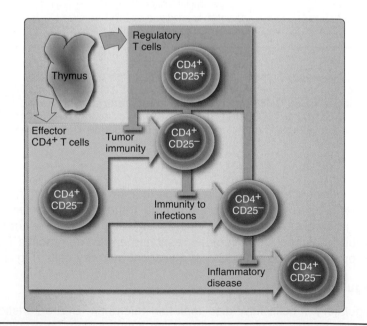

Figure 12.2
CD4$^+$25$^+$ T$_{reg}$ cells. Thymus-derived CD4$^+$CD25$^+$ T$_{reg}$ The ability of Th1 or Th2 cells to mutually inhibit one another's activity through cytokine signals provides a model system for studying regulatory arrangements among lymphocyte subpopulations.

the thymic Hassall's corpuscles. Reportedly, T_{reg}s do not proliferate rapidly; nor do they produce high levels of IL-2, IL-4, IL-10, or TGF-β following stimulation. Their presence has been demonstrated, in vivo and in vitro, to be associated with the suppression of several autoimmune diseases (e.g., autoimmune gastritis, chronic colitis). Recent evidence suggests that T_{reg} cells can also inhibit responses against some infectious agents (e.g., *Leishmania*). The means by which T_{reg} cells exert their effects on other lymphocytes and perhaps on APCs as well are still unclear, as are the means by which they themselves may be regulated.

2. **CD8$^+$ suppressor cells:** These cells are an inhibitory subpopulation of CD8$^+$ T cells. These **suppressor T cells (Ts)** do not express CD28 surface molecules (CD8$^+$CD28$^-$). Their presence has been associated with the suppression of graft rejection and the inhibition of some autoimmune diseases (e.g., experimental autoimmune encephalomyelitis). Their mode of action is still under investigation, but there is evidence that some of their effect might occur through their influence on APCs. Their activation requires interaction with CD4$^+$ T helper cells. They also express the Foxp3 nuclear transcription factor that is a distinct characteristic of T_{reg} cells.

III. THE Th1/Th2 PARADIGM

Immune responses often represent states of balance between different sets of response mechanisms. Often, whether an immune response is increasing or decreasing depends upon the particular activity being examined. Production of Th2 cytokines against a specific antigenic stimulus may increase, while Th1 cytokines production stimulated by that same antigen may decrease, and vice versa. In other cases, both types of responses may increase or decrease at the same time. The mutual inhibition by CD4$^+$ Th1 and Th2 cells provides a model for analyzing the regulatory interactions of different T cell subpopulations (Fig. 12.3). IL-4, IL-10, and TGF-β secreted by Th2 cells promote antibody-mediated responses not only by stimulating antibody production and isotype

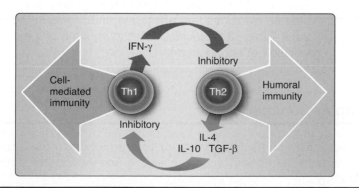

Figure 12.3
The Th1/Th2 paradigm. The ability of Th1 or Th2 cells to mutually inhibit one another's activity through cytokine signals provides a model system for studying regulatory arrangements among lymphocyte subpopulations.

Table 12.1
REGULATORY CYTOKINES

Cytokine	Source	Target	Action
IL-2	T cells	T cells	Proliferation and growth
IL-4	Th2 cells NKT cells Mast cells	B cells	Proliferation and growth, isotype switch to IgG1, IgG3, IgG4, IgE
		Th0 cells	Inhibit maturation along Th1 pathway
IL-10	Th2 cells CD8 T cells Macrophages B cells	B cells	Isotype switch to IgG1, IgG3
		Th0 cells	Promotes maturation along Th2 pathway and inhibits Th1 pathway maturation
IL-12	Dendritic cells	NK cells	Stimulates production of IFN-γ that in turn drives development of Th0 to Th1
	Macrophages	Th0 cells	Promotes maturation along Th1 pathway and inhibits Th2 pathway maturation
TGF-β	Th2 cells	B cells	Isotype switch to IgA
		Th1 cells	Inhibits activity
IFN-γ	NK cells	Th0 cells	Differentiation into Th1 pathway
	Th1 cells	B cells	Isotype switch to IgG1, IgG3
		Th2 cells	Inhibition of Th2 cells

switches, but also by simultaneously diminishing the activity of cells of the Th1 pathway. Conversely, Th1 cells promote cell-mediated responses in part by the secretion of IFN-γ that stimulates macrophage activation but also stimulates the isotype switch to IgG1 and IgG3 (the primary opsonizing antibodies promoting phagocytosis). At the same time, IFN-γ inhibits Th2 cells promoting other isotype switches.

IV. REGULATORY CYTOKINES

Much of the regulation of lymphocyte activation and subsequent activity is mediated through cytokines. For example, T cell–derived cytokines are critical for B cell activation and isotype switching, while B cells (acting as antigen presenting cells) can utilize cytokines to influence T cell activation. Even within the T cell compartment, different subsets of lymphocytes secrete cytokines that affect one another as in the case of Th1 and Th2 cells. Table 12.1 provides a listing of some of the cytokines involved in regulation of lymphocytes.

Chapter Summary

- In selective nonresponsiveness or **tolerance,** when the adaptive immune system does recognize self, it adopts a nondestructive strategy.
- Naïve lymphocyte unresponsiveness or **anergy** results from T cell or B cell receptor (TCR or BCR) engagement without second signal instruction from an antigen-presenting cell or CD4$^+$ T cell, respectively.

- T cell surface CD152 (CTLA-4) binds more avidly than CD28 with CD80 (B7.1) and/or CD86 (B7.2) to inhibit interleukin-2 (IL-2) production, IL-2 receptor (IL-2R) expression, and entry into cell cycle by CD4$^+$ T cells to promote a state of anergy.

- **T regulatory (T$_{reg}$) cells** express both CD4 and CD25 (IL-2 receptor α chain) molecules. T$_{reg}$s have been implicated in the prevention of autoimmune responses (e.g., inflammatory bowel disease) and in the prevention of some nonself responses.

- T$_{reg}$ cells undergo positive and negative selection within the thymus, possibly involving interaction with the epithelial cells of the thymic Hassall's corpuscles.

- Some subpopulations of CD8$^+$ T cells also appear able to suppress immune responses. These **suppressor T cells (Ts)** are negative for the CD28 surface molecule (CD8$^+$CD28$^-$). Their presence has been associated with the suppression of graft rejection and the inhibition of some autoimmune diseases (e.g., multiple sclerosis, systemic lupus erythematosus).

Study Questions

12.1 A state of T lymphocyte nonresponsiveness that occurs following peptide + major histocompatibility complex (pMHC) engagement is known as

A. allergy.
B. apoptosis.
C. anergy.
D. autoimmunity.
E. hypersensitivity.

The correct answer is C. Anergy is a state of nonreactivity that occurs when a lymphocyte receives a stimulus through its TCR or BCR in the absence of the additional appropriate signals provides by antigen-presenting cells or T cells. Allergy involves the degranulation of mast cells following binding of antigen to IgE molecules already affixed to the mast cell surfaces. Apoptosis is the programmed death of a cell through degradation of its nucleic acids. Autoimmunity is the active response of the immune system against self epitopes. Hypersensitivity is a response mediated by activated lymphocytes or their products. Allergy is one form of hypersensitivity.

12.2 Which of the following cells have been implicated in the prevention of autoimmune responses (e.g., inflammatory bowel disease) and in the prevention of some nonself responses?

A. antigen-presenting cells
B. anergized T cells
C. CD4$^+$CD25$^+$ T$_{reg}$ cells
D. follicular dendritic cells
E. naïve T cells

The correct answer is C. CD4$^+$CD25$^+$ T$_{reg}$ cells inhibit a variety of responses against self epitopes as well as some responses against epitopes associated with infectious agents and tumors. Antigen-presenting cells do not have this capacity. Anergized cells are inactive. Follicular dendritic cells are involved in the display of antigen to B cells and T cells in the lymph node follicles. Naïve T cells require activation before they can begin to carry out any of their effector functions.

12.3 Which of the following cells require interaction with both pMHC and a set of costimulatory second signals from an antigen-presenting cell (usually a dendritic cell) to become activated?

A. anergized T cells
B. B cells
C. mast cells
D. naïve T cells
E. natural killer cells

The correct answer is D. Dendritic cells are the usual participants in the activation of naïve cells. Anergized T cells remain refractory to subsequent engagement of pMHC and remain quiescent. B cells do not require binding of pMHC for activation. Mast cells become activated and degranulated via the binding of antigen to IgE molecules already affixed to the mast cell surfaces. Natural killer cells do not have receptors for binding pMHC.

12.4 The Foxp3 nuclear transcription factor is expressed within

A. B cells.
B. CD4$^+$/CD8$^+$ (double positive) thymocytes.
C. CD8$^+$ cytotoxic cells.
D. CD4$^+$CD25$^+$ T regulatory cells.
E. Th2 cells.

12.5 In activated T cells, CD152 (CTLA4)

A. becomes sequestered within the Golgi.
B. binds to the appropriate surface pMHC.
C. induces progression through the cell cycle.
D. stimulates transcription of IL-2 mRNA.
E. begins to move to the membrane and bind CD80/86.

The correct answer is D. Expression of the Foxp3 nuclear transcription factor is a distinctive feature of CD4$^+$CD25$^+$ T$_{reg}$ cells. *Foxp3* is not expressed by any of the other cell types indicated.

The correct answer is E. Following activation of a T cell, CD152 begins to move from the Golgi apparatus out onto the cell surface, where it competes with CD28 for binding of CD80/CD86 on antigen-presenting cells. It does not remain sequestered in the Golgi, nor does it bind to pMHC. Its binding induces an inhibition of IL-2 mRNA and the progression of the T cell through the cell cycle.

UNIT IV
Clinical Aspects of Immunity

"To let the punishment fit the crime."
Sir William Gilbert, *The Mikado*, 1885

The immune system normally functions smoothly to protect us from the vast numbers of microbes that surround us, many of which would like nothing more than to make a meal of us. We notice those times when it stumbles, when it faces an onslaught by an intruder with which it is unfamiliar and requires some extra time to accelerate from zero to sixty. This is when we become clinically ill from infection. But far more frequently, our immune system identifies, confronts, and eliminates infectious threats without our notice.

Microbes have to be tracked to their hiding places, and they may employ their own weaponry that the immune system has to defend against. The immune system must cope with their evasive tactics. Once they have been apprehended, however, the immune system may choose from among a variety of possible punishments. Death may be inflicted by destroying the nurseries in which microbes are reproducing. It may be inflicted by impalement or by a thousand small cuts that destroy the ability of the microbes to keep their cells intact. Sometimes microbes are poisoned, and sometimes they are forced to commit suicide. Often, they end up as a phagocyte's meal.

No system functions perfectly all of the time—not automobiles, not computers, and not the immune system. Sometimes parts are missing or become damaged, and we are left open to increasing risk of infectious disease. On other occasions, the immune system misidentifies its targets. Instead of picking the guilty microbe out of the lineup, it mistakenly identifies its innocent neighbor and inflicts corporal punishment upon its own body.

And sometimes the immune system adopts the martial policy that "collateral damage" is unavoidable in time of war. In the hot pursuit of the microbial targets, the immune system may lay waste to innocent bystanders along the way. The pursuit may end with a shootout in which the offending microbes are killed but at the cost of a trail of extensive death or damage to normal cells and tissues.

When the immune system performs too weakly or too vigorously, medical intervention may be necessary. Missing or damaged parts can be replaced. Tonics may be administered to invigorate parts of the immune system. And through vaccination, it can be placed on red alert, poised to act with lightening speed and overwhelming force when next needed. On the other hand, an overheated immune system might need to be calmed by soothing potions. And sometimes, rogue elements need to be identified and neutralized or eliminated.

The Well Patient: How Innate and Adaptive Immune Responses Maintain Health

13

I. OVERVIEW

The human body is a fortress. It is always surrounded by organisms that have the potential to enter and do harm. For strategic defense, the perimeter is mined with microcidal molecules, mucous secretions, and neutralizing antibodies. Its walls and borders—the skin and mucosal membranes—comprise tightly packed cells (living and dead) that form a barrier against the entry of invaders. Despite these defenses, the barriers can be breached through cuts, abrasions, injections, and so on. Sentries posted along the borders—phagocytes, natural killer (NK) cells, and complement components—are like watchdogs that attack intruders while also raising an alarm to the rest of the immune system that an invading force has landed and must be repelled.

In the face of this incessant barrage of hostile invaders, how do we remain healthy? Cells and molecules of the immune system must be mobile to communicate with each other, to patrol the body for evidence of invasion, and to congregate in areas where they are needed. When the invading threat has been located, it must be contained and ultimately destroyed. The immune system can unleash a diverse "arsenal" of weaponry at intruders. Depending upon the defensive strategies of the enemy and their ability to "return fire," only some of the host "artillery" will be successful. However, by unleashing a diverse attack, the immune system ensures that a fatal blow is usually dealt to the enemy in one way or another.

Environmental antigens in the air we breathe and the food and liquids we ingest do not necessarily pose threats to us, even though they are nonself. We also live in symbiotic relationships with numerous commensal microbes, as long as they remain outside of our body (the lumenal surfaces of the digestive and respiratory tracts are topologically outside of the body). By necessity, some environmental molecules, such as food and drink, must enter the body through the mucosal tissues. The immune system must distinguish between friend and foe; otherwise, eating would inevitably lead to massive intestinal inflammation. That part of the immune system associated with mucosal surfaces uses a variety of methods to prevent or dampen inflammatory responses except where pathogenic stimuli intrude.

A good defense can be made even better by advance preparation. Vaccination is an attempt to deliberately stimulate a primary immune response in a way that presents a low risk of injury and infection. The goal of vaccination is to ensure that subsequent encounters with potentially injurious or lethal microbes or toxins are met with secondary immune responses: neutralizing antibodies, increased antibody levels, and heightened cell-mediated responses to meet and eliminate the threat with far greater vigor and speed than would be possible in an initial exposure. Successful vaccination requires consideration of the structure and lifestyle of the threat (microbe or toxin) as well as strategies to provoke the most beneficial types of immune responses.

II. CELLULAR RECIRCULATION AND HOMING

Microbes may use stealth to attempt to enter the body undetected. Like sentries, leukocytes continually monitor the body for these unwanted visitors. Immature dendritic cells are strategically located to serve as sentinels of the immune system. Upon perceiving a threat (see Chapter 10), dendritic cells mature and migrate to nearby lymph nodes. There, they act as messengers to convey immunologic intelligence to T and B lymphocytes. When this information is placed into the right "hands" (receptors), the lymphocytes aggressively respond and rush to the site of the threat. Leukocyte mobility is essential to instigating rapid and effective immune responses.

Leukocytes and their products use two circulatory systems (see Chapter 7). A system of lymphatic vessels carries lymphatic fluid composed of cellular debris, live and dead microbes, and leukocytes to lymph nodes, where its contents are scrutinized by leukocytes. Leukocytes also use the cardiovascular system to carry "warrior" leukocytes to sites of invasion. Chemokines and cell adhesion molecules, expressed by endothelial cells that line the blood and lymph vessels, control leukocyte migration.

A. Adhesion molecules: the glue that binds

Adhesion molecules are grouped into several families: selectins, addressins, integrins, and immunoglobulin supergene family molecules (Table 13.1). Their cell surface expression is upregulated or downregulated depending upon the nature of the stimulatory signal and serves to bind or glue cells together temporarily. One important role for adhesion molecules is to stabilize the weak interaction of pMHC molecules with TCRs, allowing the cells time to "decide" whether offensive action needs to be taken to ward off a potential threat (Fig. 13.1). Adhesion molecules also determine where and which leukocytes will migrate to a particular organ or tissue.

Table 13.1
ADHESION MOLECULES

Family	Name	Synonym(s)	Expressed By	Ligand(s)	Adhesion Structure
Selectins	E-selectin	CD62E	Activated endothelium	Sialyl Lewis x	
	L-selectin	CD62L	Leukocytes	CD34 GlyCAM-1 MadCAM-1 Sulfated sialyl Lewis x	
	P-selectin	CD62P	Platelets, activated endothelium	Sialyl Lewis x, PSGL-1	
Addressins	CD34	gp105-120	Endothelium	L-selectin	
	GlyCAM-1		High endothelium venules (HEV)		
	MadCAM-1		Mucosal lymphoid tissue venules		
Integrins	LFA-1	CD11a:CD18	Phagocytes, neutrophils, T cells	ICAM-1, -2, -3	
	Mac-1	CD11b:CD18	Neutrophils, macrophages, monocytes	ICAM-1 iC3b Fibrinogen	
	CR4	CD11c:CD18	Dendritic cells, neutrophils, macrophages	iC3b	
	VLA-4	CD49d:CD29	Lymphocytes, macrophages, monocytes	VCAM-1	
Immunoglobulin supergene family	CD2	LFA-2	T cells	LFA-3	
	ICAM-1	CD54	Activated endothelium, lymphocytes, dendritic cells	LFA-1 Mac-1	
	ICAM-2	CD102	Dendritic cells	LFA-1	
	ICAM-3	CD50	Lymphocytes	LFA-1	
	LFA-3	CD58	Antigen-presenting cells, lymphocytes	CD2	
	VCAM-1	CD106	Activated endothelium	VLA-4	

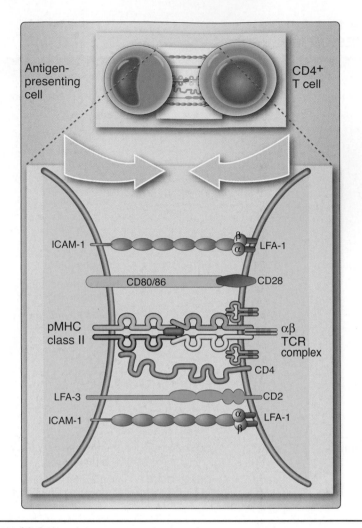

Figure 13.1
Adhesion molecules stabilize cell-to-cell interactions. Adhesion molecules expressed by antigen-presenting cells interact with costimulatory (e.g., CD28) or integrin (e.g., LFA-1) molecules expressed by CD4+ T cells to stabilize the otherwise week interaction between pMHC class II and the TCR.

B. Between vasculature and organs/tissues

At sites of microbial invasion, leukocytes and other cells send out distress signals by releasing cytokines or chemokines. These pro-inflammatory signals activate local cardiovascular endothelium (e.g., IL-1 and TNF-α) to express selectin molecules, increase expression of chemotaxic molecules (e.g., IL-1 and IL-8), and activate leukocytes (IL-1, IL-6, IL-8, IL-12, and TNF-α; Fig. 13.2). All of these activities attract leukocytes to sites of infection and facilitate development of inflammation.

C. To sites of infection and inflammation

Leukocytes migrate out of the blood vessels to underlying sites of inflammation using a four-step process known as **extravasation**.

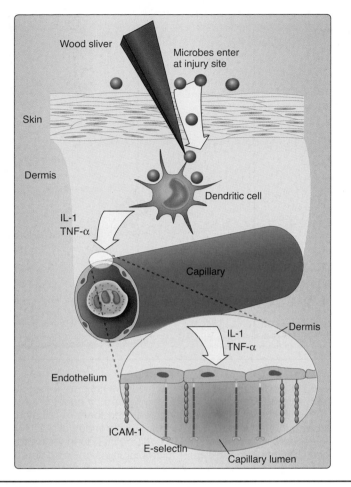

Figure 13.2
Adhesion molecules: indicators of invasion. Microbes and/or their products that enter through a breach in the dermis induce phagocytes to secrete pro-inflammatory cytokines, which in turn induce the expression of adhesion molecules by vascular endothelium.

First, endothelial cells express P-selectin (CD62P) within minutes of receiving pro-inflammatory signals (e.g., LTB4, C5a, or histamine). Within a few hours, the cells also express TNF-α. In addition, the presence of bacterial lipopolysaccharide (LPS) induces E-selectin (CD62E) expression by the endothelium. These adhesion molecules make contact with molecules on leukocytes, gradually slowing them down until they roll to a stop on the endothelial surface (part 1 of Fig. 13.3). The second step, called *tight binding*, entails interaction of leukocyte integrins such as LFA-1 (CD11a:CD18) and Mac-1 (CD11b:CD18) with TNF-α-induced ICAM-1 (CD54) expressed by endothelial cells (part 2 of Fig. 13.3). In the third step, the leukocyte crosses through the wall of the blood vessel, a process known as **diapedesis** (part 3 of Fig. 13.3). Finally, leukocytes migrate to the site of microbial invasion, attracted by chemokines (part 4 of Fig.13.3).

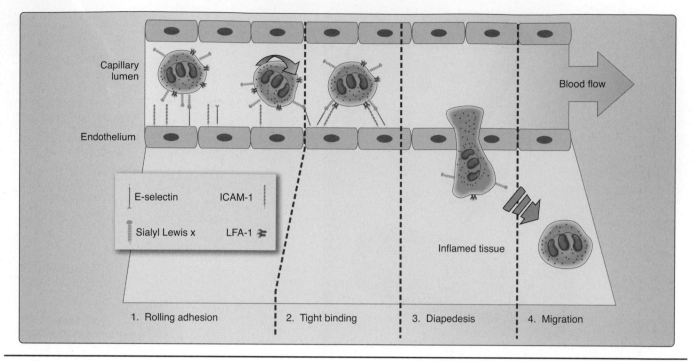

Figure 13.3
Adhesion molecules: directors of leukocyte migration. Activated leukocytes migrate from the blood vessels by a four-step process known as extravasation. **1.** *Rolling adhesion.* P- (CD62P) then E-selectin (CD62E) expressed by endothelium in response to TNF-α or to lipopolysaccharide (LPS) interacts with sialyl Lewis x on leukocytes causing them to roll along the endothelial surface. **2.** *Tight binding.* Interaction between leukocyte integrins (e.g., LFA-1, Mac1) with endothelial ICAM-1 causes leukocytes to tightly adhere to the endothelium. **3.** *Diapedesis.* A process in which endothelial-bound leukocytes enter tissues underlying the endothelium. **4.** *Migration.* Leukocytes migrate to the site of microbial invasion, attracted by chemokines.

III. RESPONSES TO INFECTIOUS AGENTS

The innate and adaptive immune systems provide protection against an array of infectious organisms that vary in size, method of entry into the body, tropisms, reproduction, and pathologies. Many microbes have structural features or lifestyles that enable them to evade or actively subvert the immune responses directed against them. Fortunately, the immune system has a built-in redundancy that activates several different types of responses against a particular invader. As long as at least one of these responses is effective, the infection can be eliminated or controlled.

A. Humoral responses

The innate humoral responses are preexisting and begin acting against infectious agents upon initial contact. Activation of the complement system, through either the mannan-binding lectin pathway or the alternative pathway, provides an almost immediate and highly effective barrier to microbial growth and reproduction. Not only does protection involve the direct lysis of microbial cells via assembly of the membrane attack complex, but the generation of certain complement fragments serves to heighten the activity of other immune mechanisms. C3b and C4b act as opsonins to accelerate the phagocytic ingestion and destruction of microbes, while C3a, C4a, and C5a help to initiate inflammation by attracting and activating leukocytes.

With the subsequent involvement of the adaptive immune response, antibodies augment the role of complement by initiating the classical pathway. Antibodies also tag infectious agents for destruction by phagocytes (opsonization) or by natural killer cells and eosinophils (antibody dependent cell-mediated cytotoxicity). IgE can trigger the release of inflammatory mediators by mast cells and basophils, an important element in immunologic resistance to parasitic worms. Finally, antibodies can inhibit entry of microbes into the body and into cells by neutralization. The effectiveness of humoral responses against infectious organisms varies, depending upon the localization and specific structural features of each organism.

B. Cell-mediated responses

Many infectious agents not only enter the body, but once inside, go on to enter individual cells. Some may be taken up by phagocytes utilizing toll-like receptors or Fc receptors and complement receptors. However, many microbes, such as viruses and some bacteria, facilitate their own entry into host cells as part of their natural life cycle. Once inside, they are sheltered from the actions of antibodies and complement, and cell-mediated responses are required to clear the infection.

Within cells, viruses persist and reproduce in the cytosol. Most intracellular bacteria live within endosomes formed during their entry into the cells (Fig. 13.4). However, the cytosolic and endosomal compartments are not completely isolated from one another. Extracellular viruses (and cellular debris containing viral particles) can be taken up by endosomes via phagocytosis. In addition, some intracellular bacteria can exit endosomes and enter the cytosol, as can some of their products or fragments (Fig. 13.5).

Regardless of the route taken, the localization of the infectious organism/material in the cytosolic or endosomal compartments determines the type of cell-mediated response they elicit. Infectious organisms or products in the cytosol will be processed and presented on MHC class I molecules, eliciting responses by CD8$^+$ T cells. Infectious organisms and fragments present in endosomes (phagolysosomes) will be processed there and presented by MHC class II molecules, generating CD4$^+$ T cell responses. The cytotoxic T cell responses (CD8$^+$) and delayed (-type) hypersensitivity (CD4$^+$) responses that are generated are then capable of destroying the infected cells, disrupting the reproduction of the invasive organisms, and destroying the remaining microbes.

C. Effective responses to pathogens

As part of the ongoing struggle between pathogen and host, infectious organisms are specialized to take advantage of specific niches in the host environment, intracellular or extracellular. They become

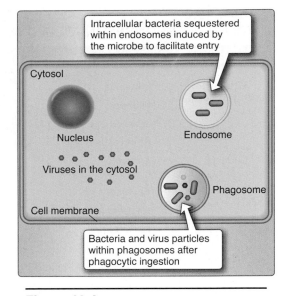

Figure 13.4
Cytosolic and endosomal localization of intracellular microbes determines the way in which microbes are processed and presented to the immune system.

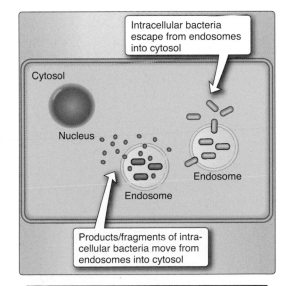

Figure 13.5
Some endosomal and cytosolic intracellular bacteria or their products may escape from endosomes.

Table 13.2

INNATE RESPONSES INVOLVED IN CLEARANCE OF ACTIVE INFECTIONS

Organisms	Representatives	Phagocytosis[a]	Neutrophils	Complement[a,b]	NK Cells[c]
Viruses (intracellular, cytoplasmic)	Influenza	■			■
	Mumps	■			■
	Measles	■			■
	Rhinovirus	■			■
Bacteria (intracellular)	*Listeria monocytogenes*		■		■
	Legionella spp.		■	■	■
	Mycobacteria		■		■
	Rickettsia				■
Bacteria (extracellular)	*Staphylococcus* spp.	■		■	
	Streptococcus spp.	▨		▨	
	Neisseria spp.	▨		▨	
	Salmonella typhi	■		■	
Protozoa (intracellular)	*Plasmodium malariae*				
	L. donovani				
Protozoa (extracellular)	*Entamoeba histolytica*	■		■	
	Giardia lamblia	■		■	
Fungi (extracellular)	*Candida* spp.			■	
	Histoplasma			■	
	Cryptococcus			■	

[a]Normal responses ■ ; reduced effectiveness because of bacterial capsules ▨ .

[b]Initiating lysis and/or opsonization.

[c]NK cells can be activated to secrete interferon-γ, which boosts phagocytic cell activity.

"guerrilla fighters" within these niches, taking advantage of the local terrain and adapting their "camouflage," "defense maneuvers," and "weaponry" to the conditions in which they find themselves. The host immune system, in turn, must be versatile enough to detect, contain, and attack the invasive organisms wherever they have "set up camp" and to strike through the camouflages and defenses to the heart of the enemy camp. The types of immune responses that will be most effective are determined by the nature of the infectious agents (Tables 13.2 and 13.3).

1. **Viruses:** Resistance to viral infection begins with the innate immune system (see Chapter 5, especially Figs. 5.4 and 5.14). Virally infected cells can produce type I interferons (IFN-α and IFN-β) that induce resistance in neighboring cells. In addition, natural killer cells detect stress molecules produced by virally infected cells and can bind and kill those cells in which the infection leads to reduced expression of MHC I molecules. The participation of phagocytic cells in the destruction of microbes and infected cells and the ingestion and degradation of the resulting cellular debris lead to activation and participation of the adaptive immune response.

Table 13.3
ADAPTIVE RESPONSES INVOLVED IN CLEARANCE OF ACTIVE INFECTIONS

Organisms	IgM, IgG, IgA				IgE	CTL	DTH
	Complement Activation	Opsonization	ADCC	Neutralizing Antibody			
Viruses				■		■	
Bacteria (intracellular)				■		■	■
Bacteria (extracellular)	■	■		■			
Protozoa (intracellular)				■			■
Protozoa (extracellular)	■	■	■	■			
Fungi							■
Flatworms					■		
Roundworms			■		■		

Immune defense against viral infection (and against infectious agents in general) has two aspects: clearance of active infections and inhibition of subsequent infections. Initial infections occur in the absence of virus-specific antibodies that can neutralize free virus and prevent infection. As a result, the body has to rely on cell-mediated responses to clear initial infections. Because viruses are localized in the cytosol, their presence within a cell is "broadcast" to the immune system by the presentation of virally derived peptides on surface MHC I molecules. In addition, the death of infected cells generates cellular debris containing both host and viral material that is ingested, processed and presented by MHC class II molecules on antigen-presenting cells. As a result, both CD4$^+$ and CD8$^+$ T cells can be generated. The CD4$^+$ T cells are important in assisting the activation and proliferation of CD8$^+$ T cells and in the subsequent activation of B cells, but it is the CD8$^+$ T cells that become the primary agents for destroying the infected cells (see Chapters 10 and 11). CD4$^+$ T cells can bind only peptides presented by the limited subset of body cells that express MHC class II molecules. However, because MHC class I molecules are expressed by all nucleated cells of the body, the display of viral peptides by MHC class I molecules provides a way for CD8$^+$ T cells to identify all virally infected cells—antigen-presenting cells (APC) and non-APCs—in the body, with a few exceptions that we will discuss later.

Once activated, CD8$^+$ cytotoxic T cells (CTLs) proceed to identify, bind, and kill infected cells throughout the body, destroying the nests within which the viruses are breeding. In addition to causing lysis of the infected cells, the ability of CTLs to induce the apoptotic death of infected cells leads to the destruction of nucleic acids of both host and viral origin within the infected cells. This provides an important means of stemming the spread of infectious particles from the disrupted cells. Together, the destruction of both the infected cells and their viral inhabitants results in the clearance of the initial infection.

CLINICAL APPLICATION
Rhinovirus

A 50-year-old female presents with rhinorrhea and sore throat of four days' duration. She also has malaise, headache, and dry cough associated with sneezing and nasal congestion. On examination, the patient is afebrile. Her nasal mucosa is mildly erythematous and edematous with clear watery nasal discharge. Her pharynx is normal in appearance without any erythema or exudate. Mild, nontender anterior cervical lymph nodes are palpable. Her lungs are clear, and cardiac examination is normal.

This patient has clinical symptoms and signs consistent with the common cold (upper respiratory infection) associated with rhinovirus infection. Rhinovirus binds to ICAM-1 adhesion molecules on respiratory epithelial cells to facilitate entry and infection. Because rhinovirus is an obligate intracellular (cytosolic) parasite, the body must generate cell-mediated innate (NK cells) and adaptive (CTLs) responses that destroy the infected cells to terminate viral replication. Treatments for the common cold are mainly supportive measures that include rest and drinking plenty of fluid. Medications such as decongestants, antitussives, and analgesics may be helpful in lessening the symptoms. Antibiotics are not useful in eliminating rhinovirus, although they may be useful against bacterial infections secondary to the viral infection.

Clearance of the initial infection provides the basis for protection against future infection as well. In addition to the generation of increased numbers of virus-specific CD4$^+$ and CD8$^+$ T cells, generation of virus-specific antibodies also occurs, although usually too late to participate in clearance of the original infection. However, the generation of neutralizing antibodies to inhibit viral infectivity is the primary means of limiting or preventing reinfection (see Chapter 11). During reexposure to a particular virus, the number of viral particles able to enter host cells is drastically reduced by neutralizing antibodies, and viruses that do succeed in entering host cells are rapidly dealt with by heightened secondary cell-mediated responses. Resistance to reinfection can be so effective that no noticeable signs or symptoms develop.

2. **Bacteria:** Most bacteria spend their entire existence in a fluid extracellular environment. Others spend much of their time within host cells (intracellular), although they must spend some time in an extracellular environment as they establish an initial infection or move on to infect additional cells.

   a. **Extracellular bacteria.** Many extracellular pathogenic bacteria, including *Staphylococcus*, *Streptococcus*, *Neisseria*, *Bordetella*, and *Yersinia*, infect humans. These organisms, once they are within the host, are constantly exposed to humoral host defenses (complement and antibodies) as well as becoming prey for phagocytes (Fig. 13.6). These responses are usually adequate for clearance. Sometimes, however, bacteria that are normally extracellular may generate substrains that gain the ability to invade host cells. When this occurs, additional immunologic responses are needed for clearance—the same responses that are involved in the clearance of bacteria that normally enter host cells.

b. **Intracellular bacteria.** Pathogenic bacteria that normally invade human cells include *Mycobacteria, Shigella, Salmonella, Listeria,* and *Rickettsia.* In addition, pathogenic strains of normally extracellular bacteria such as *Escherichia coli* occasionally gain the ability to become intracellular pathogens. During infection, these organisms spend much of their time within host cells (usually phagocytes), where antibodies and complement can no longer have access to them. Some enter the host cell via phagocytosis but have mechanisms that allow them to escape destruction and persist within the host phagocyte (Fig. 13.7). In some cases (e.g., *Legionella*), fusion of the endosome with lysosomes is inhibited. In others (e.g., *Mycobacterium*), the microcidal environment of the phagolysosome can be inhibited by microbial actions such as modifying the pH. Other bacteria (e.g., *Brucella*) can direct their own entry into host cells by inducing the formation of vacuoles that are distinct from the usual phagolysosome formation pathway. Whatever the route of entry and persistence, their clearance, like that of viruses, requires adaptive cell-mediated responses. Because most intracellular bacteria live, at least initially, within intracellular endosomes, the earliest adaptive responses for clearance are often delayed (-type) hypersensitivity (DTH) responses generated by CD4+ T cells. Activation of infected macrophages by CD4+ T cells, mediated by CD40/CD154 engagement and IFN-γ, boosts their capacity to destroy internalized microbes and promotes more active and destructive phagocytic activity. The activation of macrophages carrying intracellular bacteria may also be facilitated by NK cells. IL-12, produced by phagocytes following uptake of bacteria, boosts the activity of NK cells. These activated NK cells, in turn, produce IFN-γ that can activate the infected macrophages.

Subsequently, some intracellular bacteria and/or their products may enter the cytosol. For example, *Listeria* and *Shigella* remain within endosomes for a rather short time, then escape into the cytosol. Others (e.g., *Chlamydia*) modify the endosomal walls to permit an exchange of molecules between the endosomal compartment and the cytosol. The presence of bacteria or bacterial products in the cytosol permits proteasomal degradation and the production of bacterially derived peptide fragments that can be loaded onto MHC class I molecules for surface presentation to CD8+ T cells and the subsequent generation of CTL responses for clearance. The generation of antibodies against intracellular bacteria, while ineffective against bacteria sequestered within host cells, can nevertheless

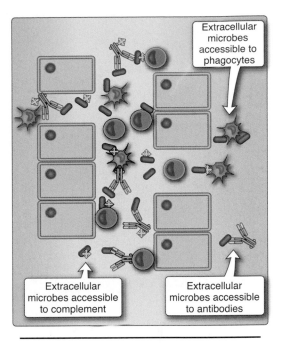

Figure 13.6
Extracellular bacteria. Extracellular bacteria are exposed to the actions of complement, antibodies, and phagocytes.

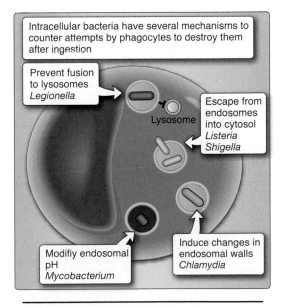

Figure 13.7
Intracellular bacteria.

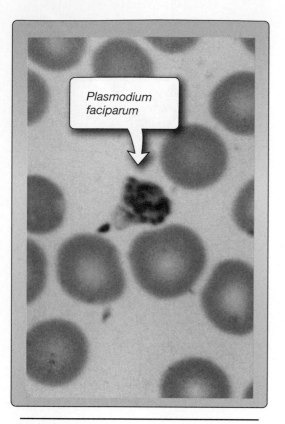

Figure 13.8
Erythrocyte infection by *Plasmodium falciparum*. *P. falciparum* is visible within erythrocytes on blood smears.

be highly effective in the neutralization and prevention of reinfection.

3. **Protozoa, fungi, and worms:** Like bacteria, infectious **protozoa** can be either extracellular or intracellular within the host. Extracellular protozoa are susceptible to the actions of antibodies, although unlike bacteria, their antibody-mediated destruction appears to be predominantly based on opsonization and phagocytosis, with a lesser role for complement-mediated lysis.

CLINICAL APPLICATION
Malaria

A 40-year-old female presents with fever, chills, sweats, headaches, muscle pains, nausea, and vomiting persisting for several days. Physical examination reveals elevated temperature, perspiration, and tiredness. According to the patient, she had returned to the United States two weeks earlier after visiting Nigeria. Prior to her travel, she was prescribed medication that could be taken to prevent the onset of malaria. However, she misunderstood the instructions and thought that the pills should be used only for treatment after developing malaria, not to prevent infection.

In addition to ordering routine blood tests, her physician examines her blood smear on a microscopic slide. It reveals several red blood cells infected with *Plasmodium falciparum* (Fig. 13.8). Her physician confirms that she has malaria and promptly treats her with anti-malaria drugs. Active infection by *P. falciparum* causes a significant destruction of erythrocytes, accounting for her clinical signs. Several days after initiating treatment, her symptoms resolve and the patient recovers. Malaria causes 500 million infections and 2 million deaths per year worldwide. It is the most common infection causing illness and death in travelers.

Intracellular protozoa (e.g., *Plasmodium, Toxoplasma*) are cleared by the same methods that are effective for intracellular bacteria. They enter host cells by the same methods (erythrocytes and liver cells for *Plasmodium* and several cell types by *Toxoplasma*) and use a similar array of methods to persist once inside. Some of them modify the endosomes or vesicles around them to exchange materials with the cytosol or, as with *Trypanosoma cruzi*, to escape into the cytosol. As a result, cell-mediated immune responses by both CD4$^+$ and CD8$^+$ T cells can become involved in clearance.

Fungi (e.g., *Candida, Histoplasma, Aspergillus*) can trigger a variety of immune responses, including the production of high levels of specific antifungal antibodies. However, antibodies appear to be ineffective in clearing fungal infections, although they can become the basis for hypersensitivity responses triggered by fungal infection. Instead, inflammatory cell-mediated DTH responses are the primary means for clearing fungal infections.

Inflammatory responses are involved in resistance to infections by **flatworms** (e.g., tapeworms and flukes) and **roundworms** (e.g., *Ascaris*, hookworms, filarial nematodes). IgE-mediated type I hypersensitivities and cell-mediated DTH responses create inflammation at the site of infection that may disrupt or inhibit the anchoring of these worms to tissues such as the intestinal epithelium. The binding of IgG and IgA antibodies to worm surfaces can also attract eosinophils that are capable of binding and killing some types of worms through antibody-dependent cell-mediated cytotoxicity.

D. Microbial evasion of immune responses

Infectious agents do not always meekly succumb to the host immune responses that are sent against them. As part of the spiraling "arms race" between host and pathogen, they develop mechanisms for evading, disrupting, and even destroying host immunity.

1. **Evasion:** Many infectious agents adopt strategies to slip by the surveillance of the host immune system (Fig. 13.9). Some, such as influenza and HIV, have inefficient DNA repair systems that permit the frequent incorporation of random mutations into their antigenic surface molecules. As a result, by the time a host generates an efficient immune response against the original influenza infection, viral variants with new coat proteins have been produced that are different enough to be unaffected by that response. In time, new responses will be generated against the new variants, but in the meantime, yet more variants will have been produced that are again different enough to escape the newly generated immune responses. This process, termed **genetic drift**, accounts for the frequent changes that occur in the influenza virus from one "flu season" to the next and for the high antigenic diversity that is found among HIV isolates within a single infected individual (Fig. 13.10A). Genetic drift is distinct from a second process called **genetic shift**, also seen in the influenza virus (Fig. 13.10B). Genetic shift occurs when influenza viruses from different species (e.g., pig and duck) infect the same cell. Under these circumstances, genetic exchange between the two types of viruses can generate new hybrid viruses with characteristics that are considerably different from those of either of the two original types. Genetic shift is usually the source of the occasional highly virulent strains of influenza that arise and cause severe illness or death in large numbers of infected hosts. Genetic drift and genetic shift are not the only means by which infectious organisms change their antigenic molecules to stay ahead of developing host responses. Bacteria such as *Neisseria gonorrhoeae* and protozoans such as *Trypanosoma brucei* carry multiple, slightly variant copies of the genes that encode their major surface antigen molecules and periodically change the gene being actively transcribed.

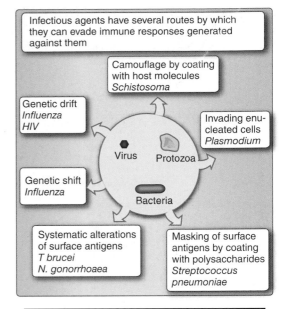

Figure 13.9
Immune evasion. Infectious agents can employ a variety of mechanisms to evade immune responses directed against them.

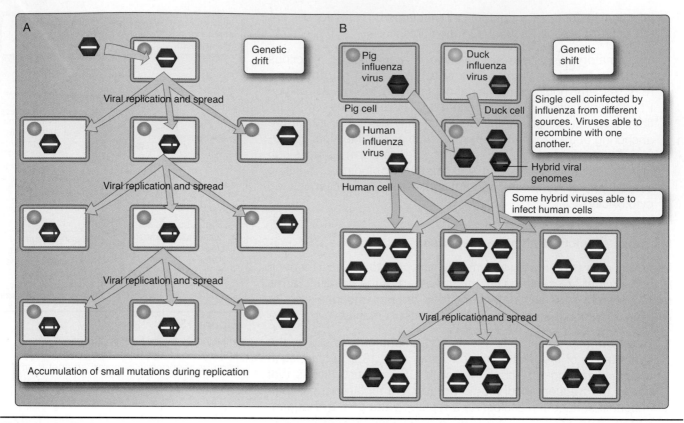

Figure 13.10
Genetic drift and genetic shift. **A.** Genetic drift results from the accumulation of small mutations in genes encoding immunogenic molecules of the microbe. **B.** Genetic shift results from recombination between different strains of a microbe, creating new hybrid forms that may be more virulent than the parental strains involved in the recombination.

CLINICAL APPLICATION
Avian flu

Xin C., a 20-year-old male, presents with sore throat, cough, muscle aches, and high fever for several days. According to the patient, he has just returned to the United States after visiting his relatives in China. While in China, he spent some time at a poultry farm. Although Xin might have the typical influenza viral illness, he might have avian influenza (bird flu). Other symptoms of bird flu include pneumonia, acute respiratory distress, respiratory failure, and life-threatening complications. Exposure to and close contact with infected poultry are risk factors for becoming infected with bird flu.

Human infections with avian influenza A (H5N1) have been reported in Asia, Africa, and Europe. This viral infection can be transmitted from direct contact with infected poultry. To date, H5N1 viral infection from human to human is rare. However, there is a concern that the virus could change (e.g., via genetic shift) and that, since the human immune system has yet not been extensively exposed to the virus, a worldwide outbreak of the disease could occur in humans. Scientists around the world are closely monitoring the situation.

Some microbes are able to prevent the immune system from detecting potentially immunogenic molecules on their surfaces. Certain bacteria form polysaccharide capsules that coat other surface molecules such as LPS and peptidoglycan and resist attachment of complement components that trigger opsonization, or formation of the membrane attack complex. Two additional types of evasion by stealth and camouflage are particularly interesting. *Plasmodium*, the protozoan that is responsible for malaria, infects erythrocytes. Being enucleated, erythrocytes express neither MHC class I or II molecules on their surfaces. Thus, once within the erythrocyte, *Plasmodium* is sheltered not only from antibodies and complement, but also from the surveillance of CD4$^+$ and CD8$^+$ T cells. The larval and adult forms of *Schistosoma*, a blood fluke, are able to coat themselves with a variety of molecules, including MHC molecules, taken from host cells, disguising themselves as host cells to elude the host immune system.

2. **Disruption:** A variety of infectious agents secrete products that interfere with the immune responses generated against them. For example, *Mycobacteria* can alter phagolysosomal pH levels, and *Legionella* can inhibit the fusion of endosomes with lysosomes. Numerous viruses (including cytomegalovirus, adenovirus, and HIV) inhibit the development of CD8$^+$ T cell responses by using a variety of methods to disrupt the presentation of cytosolic peptide fragments by MHC class I molecules (Fig. 13.11). In addition, some infectious organisms (e.g., some species of *Neisseriae*, *Haemophilus*, and *Streptococcus*, as well as *Schistosoma*) secrete enzymes that degrade immunoglobulins or complement components in the local environment, and some (e.g., Epstein-Barr virus) secrete mediators that inhibit the activities of local leukocytes.

3. **Destruction:** The ultimate act of resistance by an infectious agent against a host immune system is to destroy it. A dramatic example of this approach is HIV/AIDS (see Chapter 15). Initially infecting dendritic cells and macrophages and eventually spreading to T cells as well (especially CD4$^+$ T cells), HIV gradually destroys these leukocytes with a particularly devastating effect on the CD4$^+$ T cell population. As these cells, which are so critical to the initiation and maintenance of a broad range of immune responses, are lost, the affected individual becomes increasingly susceptible to a variety of opportunistic infections that eventually become the predominant cause of death.

IV. INFLAMMATION

Inflammation is not a singular event; instead, it is the composite of multiple immune responses elicited against a particular stimulus (Fig. 13.12, also see Fig. 5.15). In a sense, it is a "battle" in which the immune system uses every weapon in its "arsenal" in the hope that at least one of them will be effective. Inflammation is characterized by four cardinal signs: swelling, redness, warmth, and pain. Each of these results from simultaneous and ongoing multiple responses. Swelling (edema or *tumor*) results from changes in local vascular permeability that permit an influx of

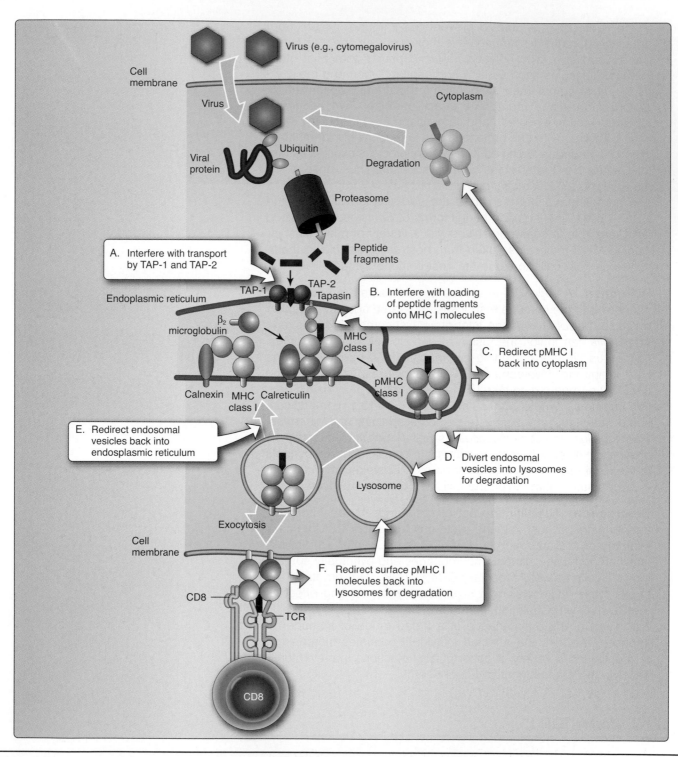

Figure 13.11

Viral mechanisms for disruption of MHC class I presentation. Numerous viruses have developed mechanisms to evade CTL responses by disrupting the presentation of viral (and other) epitopes by MHC class I molecules. These can include interfering with the transport and loading of peptides (**A**, **B**); redirection of pMHC I (or vesicles containing pMHC I) into the cytoplasm, into lysosomes or back into the endoplasmic reticulum (**C**, **D**, **E**) where they are degraded or lost; redirection of pMHC I from the surface back into lysosomes where they are degraded (**F**).

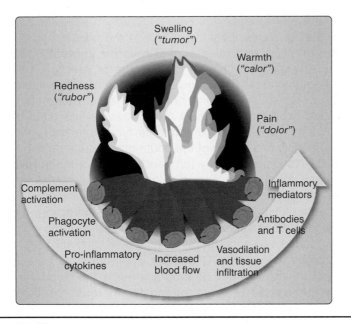

Figure 13.12
Inflammation. Inflammation results from the composite effects of multiple simultaneous responses by the innate and adaptive immune responses.

cells and fluid into the tissues. The redness (*rubor*) and heat (*calor*) are produced by increased blood flow to the affected area. Pain (*dolor*) is the result of the release of multiple chemical mediators by mast cells, basophils, and eosinophils, some of which stimulate pain receptors.

Among the many immune responses contributing to inflammation are the following:

- chemoattraction and activation of neutrophils, phagocytes, and lymphocytes
- complement activation
- degranulation of mast cells, basophils, and eosinophils to release inflammatory mediators
- heightened NK cell activity
- increased body temperature
- increased vascular permeability
- infiltration of tissues by fluids (containing antibodies and complement) and cells (particularly phagocytes and T lymphocytes)
- secretion of acute phase proteins
- secretion of pro-inflammatory cytokines and chemokines
- secretion of type I interferons

The presence of microbial products (e.g., lipopolysaccharide) at a site of injury and infection induces local phagocytes to release a variety of pro-inflammatory cytokines (e.g., IL-1, IL-6, IL-8, IL-12, and TNF) that recruit additional players to the immunologic team (see Fig. 5.15 and Table 5.1 in Chapter 5). Pro-inflammatory cytokines such as TNF-α and

IL-1 from activated phagocytes cause increased vascular permeability and stimulate increased local blood flow to the affected area. IL-6 promotes the synthesis and release of **C-reactive protein (CRP)** by the liver. Increasing greatly within 24 to 48 hours of infection, CRP readily binds to phosphocholine (a molecule expressed on some microbes) and acts as an opsonin. CRP is one of a set of serum proteins known as **acute phase proteins** that inhibit the spread of infectious organisms and also include complement components, type I interferons, fibronectin, and protease inhibitors. Some of the acute phase proteins can act on the hypothalamus to increase body temperature and produce **fever**, an effective means of inhibiting microbial growth. IL-12 stimulates NK cell activity, resulting in increased production of INF-γ. IL-8 is involved in recruitment of neutrophils to sites of inflammation and infection. Neutrophils are drawn to sites of inflammation and infection in large numbers, attracted by chemokines secreted by activated phagocytes (e.g., IL-8) and by anaphylatoxins (e.g., C5a, C4a, C3a). Their numbers increase rapidly during infection, and elevated neutrophil levels in the blood are evidence of infection in the body. They are the most numerous leukocytes infiltrating inflammatory sites and are major contributors to the clearance of infectious organisms and cellular debris.

CLINICAL APPLICATION
Cellulitis

A 25-year-old female presents with an erythematous, warm, indurated streak on her left lower leg associated with intermittent fever and mild pain. Several days previously, she had a bike accident and sustained mild trauma to her lower leg. Her examination is remarkable for an elevated temperature of 38°C and a warm, erythematous, edematous, and tender streak on her lower extremity consistent with cellulitis. She is treated with an intravenous antibiotic followed by a regimen of an oral antibiotic. The patient recovers without any complications.

Cellulitis is a common inflammation of the skin and subcutaneous tissue associated with bacterial invasion of disrupted skin. In normal healthy individuals, the most common bacteria involved are group A *Streptococci* and *Staphylococcus aureus*.

Inflammation continues until the stimulus is eliminated and healing begins. Sometimes, inflammatory stimuli cannot be eliminated, and the inflammation becomes chronic. Under such circumstances, it can cause permanent damage that is the basis for some immune-mediated diseases (e.g., rheumatoid arthritis and systemic lupus erythematosus) (see Chapters 14 and 16).

Most of the actual destructive actions that occur during inflammation are carried out by elements of the innate immune response, such as complement and phagocytic cells (see Chapter 5). Inflammation is an excellent example of how the innate system and adaptive immune system can work together, the adaptive system acting to focus and intensify the innate response. Antibodies, in initiating the classical pathway of complement activation, can target the resulting inflammation at specific microbes, molecules, or sites. Anaphylatoxins (C3a, C4a, C5a) resulting from complement activation can act as chemical signals promoting vascular permeability as well as attracting leukocytes to the site and activating them (see Table 5.2 in Chapter 5).

Similarly, elements of the innate and the adaptive systems interact in producing cell-mediated inflammation. CD4$^+$ T cells initiate DTH responses, targeting the wrath of activated macrophages at sites that are selected because of the presence of specific stimuli. However, the innate responses that the adaptive responses unleash do not have the same degree of specificity and can inflict collateral damage on normal cells and tissues that are innocent bystanders. Likewise, antibodies attached to cells can mark them for destruction but may trigger more extensive destruction, for example, by activating complement. Activated phagocytes engage in a frenzy of destruction, killing friend and foe alike, whether activated by CD4$^+$ T cells, by engagement of their Fc receptors with cells tagged by antibody, or by engagement of their complement receptors. In a sense, the T cells and antibody are the "spotters" provided by the adaptive system to direct the "artillery" provided by the innate system, but the "artillery rounds" do not land with absolute precision.

V. MUCOSAL IMMUNITY

Although IgA accounts for only 10% to 20% of serum immunoglobulin, it actually makes up about 60% to 70% of all of the immunoglobulin produced daily by normal, healthy individuals. Most of the IgA is secreted, via specialized epithelial cells, into the external environment at mucosal surfaces (see Chapter 6). Large amounts of IgA are associated with the vast mucosal surfaces of the gastrointestinal, respiratory, lachrymal, and urogenital tracts and are also present in secretions such as tears, saliva, breast milk, and some urogenital fluids.

The part of the immune system associated with the mucosal surfaces is often thought of as a separate and independent part of the overall immune system: the **mucosa-associated lymphoid tissue** (**MALT**). The immune system functioning in nonmucosal tissues, in contrast, is sometimes referred to as the **parenteral** or **peripheral immune system**. MALT contains secondary lymphoid structures with lymphoid follicles that are comparable to the spleen and lymph nodes of the parenteral system. These are the **tonsils** of the pharynx and the **Peyer's patches** of the small intestine. Despite some significant differences between the MALT and parenteral systems, they are not completely isolated from one another and can interact and influence one another. We will illustrate the nature of the mucosal immune system by examining the part of it that is associated with the gastrointestinal (GI) tract more closely.

The mucosal immune system of the GI tract contains distinct regions: the intestinal epithelium and the lamina propria (Fig. 13.13). The cells of the **intestinal epithelium** are not only capable of certain immune functions, but also include specialized **M cells** that participate in sampling antigens within the intestinal lumen and infiltrating **intraepithelial lymphocytes** (**IELs**). The **lamina propria**, lying below the epithelium, contains Peyer's patches and a large collection of B and T lymphocytes, dendritic cells, macrophages, and other leukocytes.

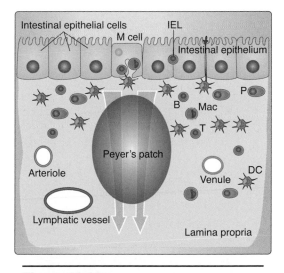

Figure 13.13
Immune environment of the GI tract. The mucosal immune system of the GI tract lies in two zones: (1) the intestinal epithelium layer, including M cells and intraepithelial lymphocytes (IELs), and (2) the underlying lamina propria, containing phagocytes, lymphocytes, Peyer's patches, and blood and lymphatic vessels. DC = dendritic cells, T = T cells, B = B cells, Mac = macrophages, P = plasma cells.

A. Epithelial layer

The intestinal epithelial layer contains the cells that have most of the initial contact with antigens from the intestinal lumen. The epithelial cells express not only MHC class I molecules, but also MHC class II and class Ib molecules (see Chapter 6). They can ingest, process, and present molecular material from the lumen and thus act as antigen-presenting cells to the IELs scattered among them. In addition to antigen presentation, intestinal epithelial cells secrete cytokines including IL-7 that aids in the development of the IELs, and TGF-β and IL-10 that inhibit cellular inflammatory responses.

IELs have a limited variability among their T cell receptors, and about two thirds of them express CD8. About 10% of them are γδ T cells, and the remainder are αβ T cells that for the most part have unusual phenotypes. Only a minor proportion of the αβ T cells among the IELs are "typical"; most have unusual or atypical characteristics. These include αβ T cells with CD8 molecules composed of two α chains instead of an α and a β (TCRαβ:CD8αα), and NKT cells that express both T cell receptors (TCRαβ) and NK cell receptors (NKG2D). Each of these atypical types of T cells appears to have a distinct function (Fig. 13.14) but jointly contribute to the removal of infected cells and initiate healing. In many cases, the information comes largely from experimental animal models (usually the mouse). Where known, the equivalent human genes or molecules are given.

- Some T cells (with either αβ or γδ TCRs) that express CD8αα recognize TL (human equivalent not yet identified), a stress molecule that appears on a variety of cell types when they are injured or infected. Binding to TL increases their cytokine production but not their cytotoxic activity.
- αβTCR:CD8αα T cells can also recognize Qa-2 stress molecules (the human equivalent is HLA-G) expressed on injured or infected host cells. αβTCR:CD8αα T cells can kill the Qa-2 expressing cells to which they bind.
- γδTCR:CD8αβ cells appear to recognize and bind fragments of glycolipids or lipopolysaccharides presented by CD1c (same terminology in humans and mice), an MHC class Ib molecule involved in presentation of nonpeptide molecular fragments by a variety of APCs, including intestinal epithelium.
- NKT cells utilize their NKG2D (same terminology in humans and mice) receptors to recognize stress molecules such as MICA and MICB (same terminology in humans and mice) on injured or infected cells and proceed to kill them if they are also expressing subnormal levels of MHC class I molecules. NKT cells among the IELs begin to secrete IL-4 and other cytokines following this activity.

The IELs act at the epithelial border to eliminate injured and infected cells, contributing to the healing of the intestinal epithelium. The IL-4, TGF-β, and IL-10 produced by NKT cells and intestinal epithelial cells create an environment at the epithelial surface that is inhibitory to development of inflammatory cell-mediated immune responses.

The scattered microfold or M cells of the intestinal epithelium are derived from cells that migrate from the crypts of the small intestine. They are located over Peyer's patches and are irregularly shaped,

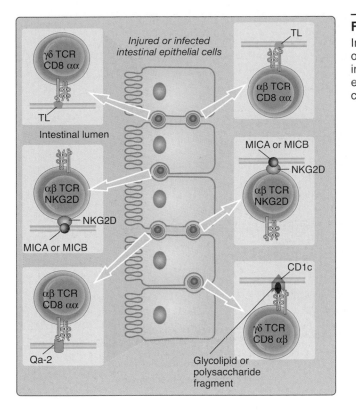

Figure 13.14

Intraepithelial lymphocytes (IELs). The IELs include several types of lymphocytes that recognize various molecules expressed by infected or injured epithelial cells or that recognize nonprotein epitopes presented by MHC class Ib molecules on the epithelial cell surfaces.

with tunnels or passageways that allow lymphocytes and dendritic cells from the underlying lamina propria to work their way closer to the luminal surfaces of the M cells (see Fig. 13.13). M cells endocytose material from the intestinal lumen and transport it to their nonlumenal surfaces, where awaiting lymphocytes and dendritic cells can access it. There is some disagreement as to whether M cells can process and present the antigens that they transport, but the dendritic cells that take up the transported antigens from the M cells are highly active in doing so.

B. Lamina propria

In contrast with the epithelial layer, the lamina propria appears to be an oasis of normalcy, containing conventional $\alpha\beta$ T cells (mostly CD4$^+$), B cells, plasma cells, and phagocytes (see Fig. 13.13). The antigen-presenting cells, particularly the dendritic cells, ingest material transported by M cells, then process and present it to T cells. Dendritic cells in the lamina propria can also extend branches between epithelial cells into the lumen and directly sample the luminal contents. Also in the lamina propria and beneath the M cells are the Peyer's patches, where antigen-presenting cells, T cells, and B cells are exposed to antigen and interact with one another (Fig. 13.15).

Dendritic cells migrate from the lamina propria to local lymph nodes (usually mesenteric), where they can activate T cells. Although the mechanisms are not understood, it appears that these antigen-presenting cells instruct the T cells as to where they migrated from and induce a significant number of the newly activated T cells to home back to the lamina propria. Activated T cells, together with antigen carried by antigen-presenting cells, can participate in the activation

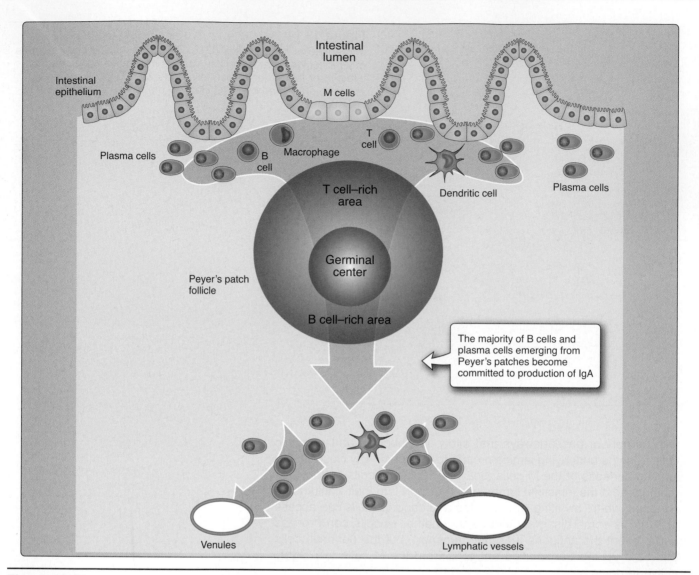

Figure 13.15

Lamina propria and Peyer's patches. Peyer's patches are collections of lymphoid tissues with follicular structures reminiscent of lymph nodes. B cells, T cells, and antigen-presenting cells circulate through and interact with Peyer's patches. Upon exiting, they may remain in the lamina propria or enter the vascular or lymphatic systems for recirculation. Plasma cells in the lamina propria cluster near the crypt areas between villi, where the antibodies they secrete (mostly secretory IgA) are transported into the mucus coating the lumenal surface of the intestinal epithelium.

of B cells in the Peyer's patches and in the local mesenteric lymph nodes. Like the T cells, the activated B cells and plasma cells can pass through the parenteral circulation before preferentially homing back to the lamina propria. B cells passing through Peyer's patches become committed primarily to production of IgA, and IgA-expressing plasma cells move to the crypts between villi, where they secrete dimeric IgA that is then transported through the specialized epithelial cells in the crypts into the mucus overlying the intestinal epithelium.

C. Mechanisms of mucosal immunity

Like other sites in the body, the mucosal immune system uses adhesion molecules and chemotactic molecules to aid in the movement of cells to the lamina propria and intestinal epithelium. For example,

T cells migrate to mucosal tissues by using L-selectin and $\alpha4\beta7$ integrin (LPAM-1) to detect MadCam-1 on vascular endothelium within MALT. The binding to MadCam-1 facilitates extravasation of the T cells into the mucosal tissues. Once in the mucosal tissues of the GI tract, the T cells use CCR9 and CCR10 chemokine receptors to detect chemotactic molecules CCL25 and CCL28 produced by the epithelium of the small and large intestine, respectively, and then use $\alpha E\beta7$ integrin (HML-1) to detect and bind E-cadherin on the vascular epithelium of the small intestine. T and B cells activated within the mucosal environment, even though they may recirculate through the body, tend to eventually return to mucosal tissues.

The mucosal environment is normally a noninflammatory one. Mechanisms have evolved to prevent the eruption of inflammatory responses, particularly cell-mediated ones. Inflammatory responses would be counterproductive in, for example, the intestinal environment, where the mucosal immune system is continually exposed to massive amounts of foreign antigens derived from food and drink. To respond vigorously to all of these nonself materials on a constant basis would create an essentially permanent state of intense chronic inflammation that would likely damage and destroy the intestinal linings. Thus, the presence of a noninflammatory "Th2-like" environment, as evidenced by the predominance of IgA over IgG and the preferential secretion of cytokines such as IL-4, IL-10, and TGF-β, contrasts with the parenteral (or peripheral) immune system by creating a setting in which tolerance to foreign antigens is the norm rather than the exception (Fig. 13.16).

Although the mucosal and parenteral systems appear to operate somewhat separately, they are not isolated from one another. Cells circulate from one into the other and back again. It has been thought that the tendency to induce tolerance within the mucosal tissues could be exploited to induce a similar tolerance in the parenteral tissue. Thus, for example, an antigen that would normally be antigenic in the parenteral tissues could be administered orally so that the initial introduction to the body's immune system is via the mucosal route, an approach termed induction of **oral tolerance**. The tolerance that is induced initially in the mucosal tissues might then influence the parenteral system to become tolerant as well. This approach has frequently been successful in experimental models, but its clinical application is still limited.

VI. VACCINATION

It was recognized long ago that individuals who survived smallpox, plague, and cholera rarely contracted the disease again, even when surrounded by others suffering from that particular disease. Early forms of vaccinations developed as attempts to confer protection from these fortunate survivors to those who still faced the risk of severe illness or death. Among ancient cultures, the Egyptians and Chinese exposed individuals to powders formed from the crusts and scales of pockmarks taken from individuals recovering from smallpox. Sometimes individuals who were treated in this way developed mild forms of the disease; on many occasions, they developed no apparent disease at all. Edward Jenner demonstrated in 1794 that intentional inoculation with material from individuals with cowpox (a mild disease in humans caused by a

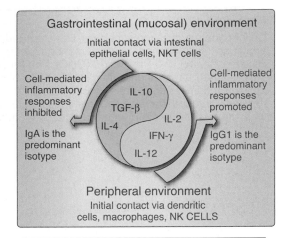

Figure 13.16
Immunologic comparison of the intestinal mucosal environment and the parenteral or peripheral environment. The peripheral immune system initially makes contact with nonself via phagocytic cells that secrete cytokines promoting a Th1-like environment. The mucosal (in this cas the GI tract) immune system initially makes contact with nonself via intestinal epithelial cells and IELs that secrete cytokines promoting a Th2-like environment.

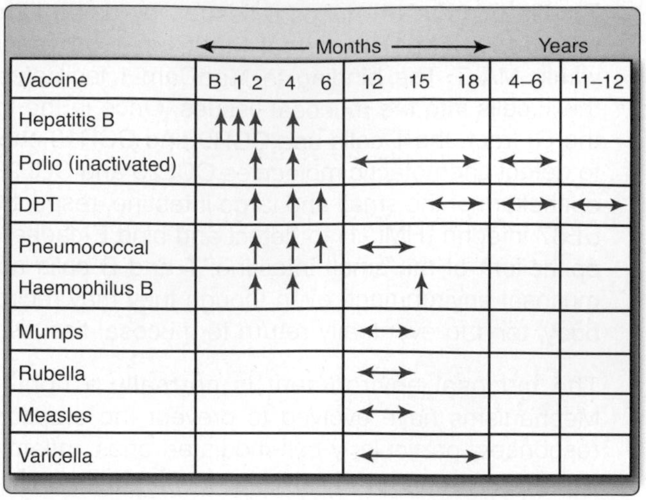

Figure 13.17

Childhood immunization schedule. The chart indicates the child-hood vaccination schedule recommended by the Centers for Disease Control and Prevention (CDC). The arrows indicate the time points or time ranges when initial vaccinations and boosters should be administered. These recommendations are periodically reviewed and updated, and readers should consult the CDC's web site to see the most up-to-date recommendations.

Vaccine	← Months →							Years	
	B 1 2 4 6				12	15	18	4–6	11–12
Hepatitis B	↑↑↑ ↑								
Polio (inactivated)	↑ ↑				←——→			←→	
DPT	↑ ↑↑						←→	←→	←→
Pneumococcal	↑ ↑↑				←→				
Haemophilus B	↑ ↑					↑			
Mumps						←→			
Rubella						←→			
Measles						←→			
Varicella						←——→			

different form of the smallpox virus that normally infects cattle) protected against smallpox (caused by a more virulent type of vaccinia virus). Jenner and his contemporaries, of course, did not know of microbes and their roles in disease. The subsequent work of Robert Koch and Louis Pasteur established that specific microbes caused specific diseases and broadened the development of effective vaccines against epidemic diseases of agricultural animals and eventually of humans. The expanded use of vaccination led to an enormous improvement in human and animal health. For both children and adults, many of the most fearful diseases throughout human history have been practically eliminated in many parts of the world. The ability to vaccinate early in life has dramatically reduced the burden of illness, crippling, and death that was once a routine part of childhood, resulting from diseases such as diphtheria, polio, and measles. Figure 13.17 presents the standard vaccination schedule in the United States recommended by the Centers for Disease Control and Prevention (CDC) at the time of writing. (These recommendations are updated regularly, and the CDC's web site should be consulted to obtain the most recent recommendations.)

Vaccination can provide excellent protection to a population, even if not every individual in a population is vaccinated, because of a phenomenon known as **herd immunity**. As the fraction of the population that is vaccinated increases, the chances of an infectious agent "finding" an unprotected individual becomes increasingly smaller, leaving the population resistant as a whole. There are limits to herd immunity, however. If a significant number of unprotected individuals become infected, the infection could spread rapidly through the unprotected members of the population. In the course of that rapid replication, new mutant forms might arise that could evade the immune response and produce disease in vaccinated individuals as well.

A. Characteristics of vaccines

Vaccines must fulfill a number of criteria to be effective in protecting large numbers of individuals:

* Effective protection against the intended pathogen must occur without significant danger of actually causing the disease or of producing severe side effects.

- The protection that is provided must be long lasting.
- The vaccine must induce the immune responses (e.g., CTLs) that are most effective against the intended pathogen across a broad range of individuals.
- Neutralizing antibodies must be stimulated in order to minimize reinfection.
- The vaccine must be economically feasible to produce.
- The vaccine must be suitably stable for storage, transport, and use.

B. Types of vaccines

Vaccines can be prepared from a variety of materials derived from pathogenic organisms.

- **Live vaccines** are based on living organisms capable of normal infection and replication. Such vaccines are not appropriate for pathogens that are capable of causing severe or life-threatening diseases.
- **Attenuated vaccines** are based on organisms that are living but have had their virulence and ability to replicate reduced by treatment with heat, chemicals, or other techniques. Attenuated vaccines typically cause only subclinical or mild forms of the disease at worst, but they do carry the possibility that mutation might enable the organisms in the vaccine preparations to revert to wild type.
- **Killed vaccines** include organisms that are dead because of treatment with physical or chemical agents. In the case of toxins, they will have been inactivated (toxoids). They should be incapable of infection, replication, or function but still able to provoke immunity. It must be understood, however, that it might be difficult to guarantee that every organism in a preparation is dead.
- **Extract vaccines** do not contain whole organisms but are composed of materials isolated from disrupted and lysed organisms but not whole organisms. These vaccines are most suitable for providing protection against diseases in which the organisms are so virulent that even killed vaccines are not used because of the risk that even a few organisms might have survived treatment.
- **Recombinant vaccines** have been made possible by molecular biology techniques that allow creation of organisms from which the removal of certain genes impairs their virulence and/or reproduction. Such organisms can infect host cells and perhaps even proliferate but cannot induce disease.
- **DNA vaccines** are those in which the host is injected with naked DNA extracted from a pathogen. The DNA is also often engineered to remove some of the genes that are critical to development of the disease. The objective is for host cells to take up the naked DNA and express the gene products from the pathogen. DNA vaccine stimulus typically lasts longer than other methods in which the vaccine is rapidly eliminated from the host.

As a rule, live vaccines are best at generating immune responses, followed by attenuated vaccines, and then by killed vaccines and extracts. Replicating organisms produce the molecules that stimulate the immune responses, but killed and extract vaccines might contain few or none of those molecules. Thus, paradoxically, the safety of a vaccine may be inversely proportional to its effectiveness. The coadministration of adjuvants can heighten the effectiveness of many vaccines.

CLINICAL APPLICATION
Poliovirus vaccine

Poliomyelitis is an acute illness involving destruction of the lower motor neurons of the spinal cord and brain stem by poliovirus, an enteric pathogen. In countries with low immunization rates, poliomyelitis continues to occur. In the United States, no case of paralytic poliomyelitis due to wild-type poliovirus has occurred in over 20 years. There are, however, a few reported cases of polio that occur (fewer than 10 per year) due to reversion to wild-type virulence of virus in the live-attenuated Sabin polio vaccine.

Vaccination is an effective method of preventing poliomyelitis. Both killed poliovirus (Salk) vaccine and attenuated live oral poliovirus (Sabin) vaccine have shown efficacy in preventing poliomyelitis.

Both vaccines have advantages and disadvantages. The advantage of the inactivated vaccine is that it can be safely used in immuno-compromised individuals; the primary disadvantage is that it is administrated by injection only, and therefore less immunity occurs in the gastrointestinal tract. The advantages of the attenuated live poliovirus vaccine include oral administration, lifelong protection, and intestinal immunity. The main disadvantage of the live virus vaccine is the small risk of polio infection due to rare incidences of reversion to normal virulence. Therefore the current recommendation is exclusive use of inactivated poliovirus vaccine.

Although vaccination now provides protection against many dangerous infectious diseases, many diseases still lack effective vaccines (e.g., HIV/AIDS and malaria). The ability to hide within cells, to camouflage themselves, to rapidly change their antigenic makeup, or to disrupt the generation of effective responses allows some of these organisms to defeat attempts to develop effective vaccines.

C. Adjuvants

Adjuvants are bacterial components or other substances, typically suspended in a medium such as oil that prolongs their dispersal into the tissues, administered together with vaccines to heighten the effectiveness of the vaccination. The bacterial (or other) material provokes a mild inflammation that attracts phagocytes and accelerates their activation and antigen presentation to T cells for development of specific adaptive immune responses. Some vaccine components themselves can serve as adjuvants. The pertussis component (from *Bordetella pertussis*) in **DTP** (Diphtheria-Tetanus-Pertussis) vaccine is also an effective adjuvant. Other adjuvants include alum and **BCG** (Bacillus Calmette Guerin). BCG includes material derived from *Mycobacterium* and is in wide use around the world as a vaccine against tuberculosis, particularly in areas of high incidence. Its use has declined in some areas where the incidence of tuberculosis has significantly declined. In the United States (and several other countries), BCG is not used routinely for human vaccinations because it interferes with the use of skin testing (creating false positives) in tuberculosis studies and because of adverse reactions (e.g., disseminated BCG infection). However, BCG is still used in the United States for certain high-risk individuals or populations.

Chapter Summary

- The innate and adaptive immune systems provide protection against an array of infectious organisms that vary in size, method of entry into the body, tropisms, reproduction, and pathologies.

- Complement is part of the innate immune system and begins resisting infectious agents upon initial contact. With the subsequent involvement of the adaptive immune response, antibodies augment the role of complement by initiating the classical pathway.

- Leukocyte mobility is the key to the immune system's ability to monitor the body for infection and to mount responses where necessary.

- Adhesion molecules stabilize cellular interactions and facilitate interactions between more specialized binding structures (e.g., TCR with pMHC).

- The expression of certain molecules on activated vascular endothelium in areas of inflammation serves to attract leukocytes to the sites of infection.

- At inflammatory sites, leukocytes can leave the vasculature and enter the tissues through a process called extravasation.

- Immune defense against infectious agents has two aspects: clearance of active infections and inhibition of subsequent infections. The most effective method of clearance depends upon the localization of the agent within the body or cells. Most resistance to reinfection is provided by neutralizing antibodies.

- Many infectious agents (e.g., *Mycobacteria, Shigella, Salmonella, Listeria,* and *Rickettsia*) enter the body and then enter individual cells. Some microbes initiate their entry into host cells as part of their natural life cycle. Microbes are also taken up by phagocytes utilizing toll-like receptors or Fc receptors and complement receptors.

- Intracellular microbes (or their products) that are in the cytosol generate CTL responses that are effective in clearing infections. Intracellular microbes within endosomes generate DTH responses responsible for clearance. Some microbes (or their products) can exist in both intracellular sites and trigger both CTL and DTH responses.

- Many extracellular pathogenic bacteria (e.g., *Staphylococcus, Streptococcus, Neisseria, Bordetella,* and *Yersinia*) infect humans but do not enter host cells. They remain in the body fluids, where they are available to antibodies, complements, and phagocytes.

- Like bacteria, infectious **protozoa** can be either extracellular or intracellular within the host. Immune responses responsible for clearance of each type are similar to those for extracellular and intracellular bacteria.

- **Fungi** (e.g., *Candida*, *Histoplasma*, *Aspergillus*) can trigger a variety of immune responses, including the production of high levels of specific antifungal antibodies. However, DTH is the response that is generally responsible for clearance of fungal infections.

- Inflammatory responses are involved in resistance to infections by **flatworms** (e.g., tapeworms, flukes) and **roundworms** (e.g., *Ascaris*, hookworms, filarial nematodes).

- **Genetic drift** occurs when random mutations in genes encoding microbial antigens create new minor variants that are sufficiently different to escape previously generated immune responses. **Genetic shift** occurs when microbes (e.g., influenza virus) from different species (e.g., pig, duck) infect the same cell, recombine and produce large changes in antigenic molecules.

- Some microbes are able to prevent the immune system from detecting potentially immunogenic molecules on their surfaces. A variety of infectious agents secrete products that interfere with the immune responses generated against them.

- Inflammation is characterized by four cardinal signs: swelling, redness, warmth, and pain.

- **Mucosal associated lymphoid tissue**, that part of the immune system associated with the mucosal surfaces, is often thought of as partly separate and independent from the remainder of the immune system.

- The ability to vaccinate early in life has dramatically reduced the burden of illness, crippling, and death that was once a routine part of childhood, resulting from diseases such as diphtheria, polio, and measles.

- **Adjuvants** are bacterial components or other substances, typically suspended in a medium such as oil that prolongs their dispersal into the tissues, administered together with vaccines to heighten the effectiveness of the vaccination.

Study Questions

13.1 A previously healthy 8-month-old girl with fever and wheezing is diagnosed with respiratory syncytial virus (RSV) infection. Assuming that this is the child's first exposure to RSV, which of the following mechanisms will most likely operate to clear the infection?

   A. CD4$^+$ T cell-mediated necrosis of infected cells
   B. complement-mediated lysis of infected cells
   C. cytotoxic T cell–induced apoptosis of infected cells
   D. MHC class I presentation of viral peptides on CD8$^+$ T cells
   E. virus-specific antibodies that neutralize free virus

The answer is C. Clearance of viral infections involves destruction of infected cells by cytotoxic T cells to prevent viral replication. CD4$^+$ T cell responses against infected cells are typically effective when the infectious agent is residing within intracellular endosomes. Complement is not effective against intracellular microbes, and sufficient levels of antibodies against the microbes are usually not yet present during primary infections. MHC presentation of viral peptides occurs on APCs, not on CD8$^+$ T cells.

13.2 In a patient with a *Salmonella* infection, which of the following mechanisms will most likely be the earliest adaptive response for clearing the infection while bacteria are present within intracellular endosomes?

A. antibody-mediated neutralization of free bacteria
B. complement-mediated lysis of infected host cells
C. CTL recognition of bacterial peptides presented by MHC class II
D. DTH responses generated by CD4+ T cells
E. type I hypersensitivity mediated by IgE antibodies

The correct answer is D. DTH responses are generally the first effective responses involved in clearance of intraendosomal microbes. Later in such infections, the microbes or their molecules may escape into the cytoplasm, making it possible for CTL responses to develop. Complement does not clear active intracellular infections. Antibodies may be effective in inhibiting reinfection but do not clear active intracellular infections.

13.3 A 25-year-old man is exposed to the roundworm *Ascaris* but does not develop clinical signs of infection. Which of the following mechanisms is likely to be responsible for his resistance to infection?

A. antibody-mediated destruction of worm-infected host cells
B. CTL-induced apoptosis of worm-infected host cells
C. complement-mediated lysis of worm attached to host tissues
D. IgE-mediated type I hypersensitivity disrupting worm attachment
E. phagocytosis of worms followed by necrosis of phagocytes

The correct answer is D. Local inflammatory responses, such as that induced by IgE, can inhibit attachment of roundworms to the intestinal wall. *Ascaris* is a large worm (adults reach 12 to 20 inches in length) and is not damaged by antibodies directed at it or by complement, CTLs, or phagocytes.

13.4 Despite having recovered fully from influenza the previous winter, a 56-year-old man becomes ill after being exposed to a colleague with influenza virus. Which of the following mechanisms permits his reinfection despite previous exposure to influenza virus?

A. Neutralizing antibodies against influenza disappear rapidly.
B. Insufficient time has passed for CD4+ T cells to develop memory.
C. Intracellular viral particles escape immune surveillance.
D. Type 1 hypersensitivity responses occur on second exposure to influenza.
E. Viral variants evade the immune response against the original virus.

The correct answer is E. The immunogenic antigens on the surface of influenza virus can change as a result of mutation or recombination so that new influenza viruses arise that might not be recognized by the immune responses generated against previous exposures. Neutralizing antibody levels (especially IgG) remain elevated for a long period of time. The time interval described is also certainly sufficient for the development of immunologic memory. Intracellular viruses do not escape notice by the immune system, as fragments of their proteins are presented by MHC class I molecules on the surface of the infected cell. IgE-mediated type I (immediate) hypersensitivity responses are not generally associated with viral responses.

13.5 A 35-year-old woman left the United States for the first time and traveled to Brazil, where she contracted malaria, a protozoan infection of erythrocytes. Which of the following describes the state of immunity resulting from this infection?

A. Antibody-mediated neutralization of the protozoa clears the infection.
B. CTL-induced apoptosis of infected erythrocytes clears the infection.
C. Complement-mediated lysis of infected erythrocytes clears the infection.
D. DTH mediated by CD4+ T cells clears the infection.
E. Host immunity is evaded by protozoa reproducing within erythrocytes.

The correct answer is E. *Plasmodium*, the protozoan causing malaria, evades the host immune system by living and reproducing within erythrocytes. Once inside the cell, the protozoa are sheltered from antibodies and complement. In addition, the absence of surface MHC I and II on the enucleated erythrocytes prevents presentation of microbial peptides, so the infected erythrocytes are not recognized by T cells. Neutralizing antibodies may reduce future infections, but are not responsible for clearance. Clearance by CTLs, complement, or DTH does not occur, for the reasons stated previously.

13.6 In response to the lipopolysaccharide from a Gram-negative bacterial infection, local host phagocytes release pro-inflammatory cytokines, including IL-6, which then stimulates hepatic synthesis and release of:

A. C-reactive protein.
B. chemokines.
C. complement.
D. immunoglobulins.
E. interleukins.

The correct answer is A. IL-6 induces production of C-reactive protein by the liver. It does not induce the liver to produce chemokines, complement, immunoglobulins, or interleukins.

13.7 Which of the following is the predominant immunoglobulin isotype secreted in the human MALT?

A. IgA
B. IgD
C. IgE
D. IgG
E. IgM

The correct answer is A. The vast majority of the antibody generated in the human MALT (mucosa-associated lymphoid tissues) is of the IgA isotype. IgE, IgG, and IgM are present, but at far lower levels, and IgD is essentially absent.

13.8 Which of the following is characteristic of the mucosal immune system?

A. A vigorous response is made to all nonself antigens encountered.
B. Chronic inflammation makes an inhospitable environment for microbes.
C. IL-2 and IFN-γ contribute to a Th1-like environment.
D. Secretion of IgG predominates over secretion of IgA.
E. Tolerance to foreign antigens is the norm rather than the exception.

The correct answer is E. Because the mucosal immune system is constantly exposed to so many nonself epitopes that are essentially harmless, it is tolerant of most of them. Although it can respond to microbes that pose a pathogenic threat, the mucosal system generally avoids the development of chronic inflammation because of the damage that could be inflicted on the delicate mucosal linings. The immunologic environment is generally described as more Th2-like than Th1-like. IgG is present at far lower levels than is IgA.

13.9 A 14-month-old boy who has not received any recommended vaccines remains healthy despite his daily association with several other children for the past year at a home day care facility. Which of the following mechanisms best explains why he has not contracted diphtheria, measles, pertussis, or polio?

A. herd immunity
B. genetic drift
C. genetic shift
D. immune evasion
E. tolerance

The correct answer is A. It is likely that most or all of the other children at the day care facility have been vaccinated; thus the infant in question is less likely to be exposed to diphtheria, measles, pertussis, or polio. The remaining choices are all mechanisms by which microbes evade immune responses and would be more likely to increase the risk of infection in both the unvaccinated and vaccinated children.

13.10 Which of the following types of vaccines would most likely evoke the best and most long-lasting protective immune response against rubeola (measles)?

A. attenuated vaccine
B. DNA vaccine
C. extract vaccine
D. killed vaccine
E. recombinant vaccine

The correct answer is A. The attenuated vaccine, in which the organism is still capable of some degree of infection and reproduction, is likely to produce a stronger immune response than are the other types of vaccines, in which the virus is incapable of doing so. In general, the safer the vaccine (in terms of risk of reversion to a virulent wild type), the less effective it is (in terms of offering protection).

Hypersensitivity Reactions

14

I. OVERVIEW

Excessive or inappropriate immune responses sometimes lead to host tissue damage resulting from prolonged or repeated antigen exposure. These reactions, called *hypersensitivity reactions*, cause tissue injury by the release of chemical substances that attract and activate cells and molecules resulting in **inflammation**. These reactions are classified into four **hypersensitivity types** depending upon the mechanism(s) that underlie the tissue damage (Table 14.1); the first three types involve antigen-antibody reactions, while the fourth is antibody-independent, involving cell-mediated immune responses only:

- **Type I** (also called **immediate hypersensitivity**) reactions are rapid, occurring within minutes of exposure to an antigen, and always involve IgE-mediated degranulation of basophils or mast cells.
- **Type II** reactions are initiated by the binding of antibody to a cell membrane or to the extracellular matrix.

Table 14.1
HYPERSENSITIVITY TYPES.

Type	Synonyms	Disorders	Mediated By	Mechanism(s)
I	Atopy, anaphylactic hypersensitivity, allergy	Allergic reactions, anaphylaxis, asthma	IgE antibody, complement not involved	Cross-linking of FcRε-bound IgE antibodies on mast cells cause degranulation and release of vasoactive amines (e.g., histamine) resulting in smooth muscle contraction, vasoconstriction, and vasodilation of capillary endothelium.
II	Cytotoxic	*Erythroblastosis fetalis*, Goodpasture's syndrome, autoimmune hemolytic anemia	IgM or IgG ± complement	IgM or IgG antibody binds to epitopes on cells or other tissue components promoting phagocytosis, antibody-dependent cell-mediated cytotoxicity, antibody-mediated function disruption (receptor blocking), or complement-mediated lysis.
III	Immune complex disease	Serum sickness, Arthus reaction, systemic lupus erythematosus	IgG ± complement	Antigen-antibody complexes in tissues or serum activate complement and attract neutrophils that release lytic molecules.
IV	Cell-mediated hypersensitivity	Contact dermatitis, tuberculosis, chronic graft rejection	Cell-mediated, antibody-independent	Release of mediators by sensitized CD4$^+$ T cells provoke tissue destruction by mononuclear cells. CD8$^+$ T cells known as cytotoxic T lymphocytes (CTL) may kill chemically modified host cells and cells that display disparate MHC molecules.

- **Type III** hypersensitivity reactions involve the interaction of antibodies with soluble molecules to make soluble antigen-antibody complexes that become deposited in tissues.

- **Type IV** hypersensitivity reactions are those in which cells of the immune system directly attack host cells in the absence of antibody. These reactions include contact dermatitis (CD, also called contact sensitivity, CS); delayed (-type) hypersensitivity (DTH); and, occasionally, cytotoxic T lymphocyte (CTL) responses.

II. TYPE I HYPERSENSITIVITY

Commonly called **allergic** or **immediate hypersensitivity reactions**, type I responses occur within minutes to hours of antigen exposure. Some individuals develop IgE antibodies in response to relatively harmless environmental antigens or **allergens**. IgE molecules readily bind to Fc receptors (FcRε or CD23) on the surfaces of mast cells and basophils (Fig. 14.1). Unlike other FcRs, FcRεs bind antigen-free immunoglobulin (IgE), and the IgE-CD23 complexes function as antigen-specific cell-surface receptors. Cross-linking of surface-bound IgE molecules generates intracellular signals via CD23, leading to mast cell or basophil degranulation and the release of vasoactive amines (e.g., **histamine**) and other inflammatory mediators. Histamine and other inflammatory mediators cause vascular endothelial cell junctions to loosen (**vasodilation**) and increase vascular permeability, resulting in fluid accumulation in the tissues (**edema**). Histamine also induces smooth muscle contraction in arterial and arteriole walls (**vasoconstriction**) to accelerate fluid distribution from the central trunk of the body into peripheral tissues.

A. Localized reactions

Because mast cells accumulate in respiratory passages, intestinal walls, and the skin, type I reactions are often most pronounced in these tissues. Sites affected are typically those where the initiating antigen is most often encountered. Antigens that enter the body by inhalation localize primarily to the nasopharyngeal and bronchial tissues, where smooth muscle contraction and vasodilation increase mucous production and the constriction of respiratory passages (Fig. 14.2). In combination, these responses can produce the severe and potentially fatal disorder known as **asthma**. Allergens that contact other tissues may produce IgE-mediated inflammatory responses, causing rashes, redness, and edema—the classic "wheal and flare" appearance. Food or ingested allergens primarily affect the gastrointestinal tract.

CLINICAL APPLICATION
Asthma

Eighteen months ago, Jenny Q., a 31-year-old female, received a Persian cat (*Felis domesticus*) as a birthday present. Jenny became sensitized to the major cat allergen (the salivary protein Fel d1) and reported persistent symptoms of nasal congestion, rhinorrhea,

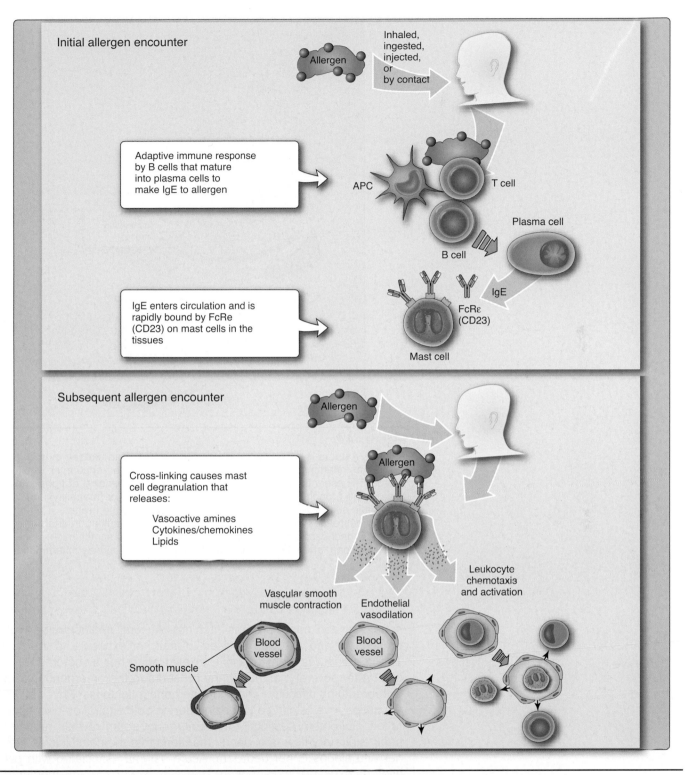

Figure 14.1

Type I reactions. These reactions result from the interaction of surface-bound IgE with antigen. Presentation of antigen (often referred to as allergen) to antigen-specific CD4$^+$ T cells allows them to provide signals to antigen-specific B cells that cause their maturation into IgE secreting plasm cells. IgE enters into the circulation, is rapidly bound by CD23 (FcRε) on tissue mast cells and basophils, and serves as antigen (allergen)-specific receptors on those cells. Subsequent encounter with multi-valent (having multiple identical epitopes) allergen cross links CD23 on mast cells and basophils inducing a signalling cascade, leading to degranulation. The released substances cause contraction of vascular (and other) smooth muscle, dilation of vascular endothelium (vasodilation), leukocyte chemotaxis and activation.

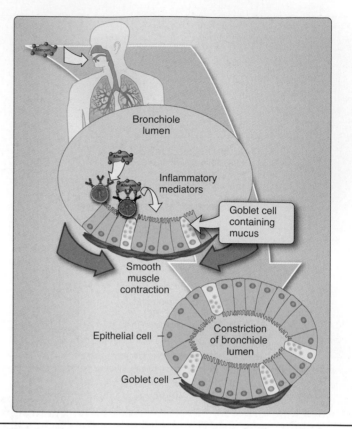

Figure 14.2

Asthma. Asthma is a reversible airway obstruction often caused by the release of inflammatory mediators from mast cells upon encounter with allergen. These inflammatory mediators cause the loosening of tight junctions in the bronchiole epithelium, increased capillary permeability, and spasmatic contraction of smooth muscle surrounding the bronchi. This temporarily decreases the size of the bronchial lumen, resulting in shortness of breath. Bronchospasms triggered by non-immunologic stimuli such as cold, viral infections, and exercise, also stimulate the same airway inflammation.

sneezing, and nasal pruritus (itching). An oral antihistamine was prescribed, and she was advised to limit her exposure to the cat. These measures were effective in alleviating her symptoms for a time. After several months, Jenny presents to the emergency room with breathing difficulty, wheezing, and chest tightness. Physical examination reveals diffuse wheezing during both expiration and inspiration. Spirometry testing in the emergency room reveals reduced peak expiratory flow rate. Jenny mentions that the cat still lives with her and sleeps in her bedroom. Acute asthma associated with cat allergen exposure is diagnosed. This is an example of IgE-mediated Type I hypersensitivity. If the cat is removed from her house or if she limits her exposure to the cat by keeping it out of her bedroom and uses her medications, her prognosis is good.

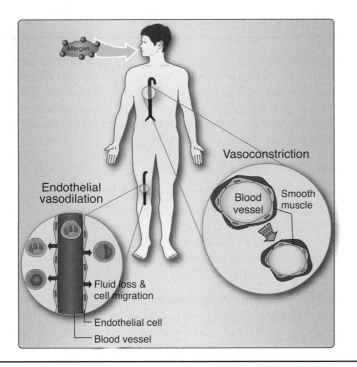

Figure 14.3
Anaphylaxis and shock. Exposure to allergen may cause the rapid release of vasoactive amines from mast cells and basophils as well as a flood of cytokines, resulting in the contraction of smooth muscle in the vasculature and vasodilation of capillary endothelium. Blood pressure decreases, resulting in vascular shock. In addition, the release of mediators increases the contraction of smooth muscle in the diaphragm and respiratory tract, making breathing difficult.

B. Systemic reactions

In some cases, such as injected allergens (e.g., venom or toxins), antigen may be disseminated by the bloodstream, resulting in systemic inflammation. In 1902, at the request and sponsorship of Albert I of Monaco, Charles Richet and Paul Portier investigated jellyfish nematocyst toxin that sometimes induced a life-threatening response. Their experiments were conducted on the Prince of Monaco's yacht (ah, the past glamour of science!). They found that initial injection of dogs with a small amount of toxin had little effect. However, when a second injection of the same amount of the toxin was administered several weeks later, the dogs suffered immediate shock and even death. Termed **anaphylaxis** ("against protection"), this clinical shock syndrome is characterized by vascular smooth muscle constriction (**vasoconstriction**) combined with gap formation between adjacent capillary endothelial cells (**vasodilation**) that results in severe fluid loss and leads to **shock** (Fig. 14.3).

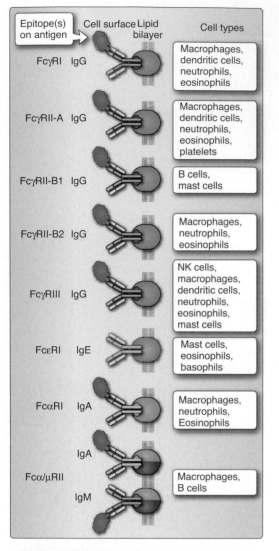

Figure 14.4
Fc receptors. Receptors for Fc portion of immunoglobulin are expressed by a variety of cell types. With the exception of FcRε (CD23), FcRs bind only antigen-bound antibody. IgE readily binds to FcRε (CD23) in the absence of antigen.

III. TYPE II HYPERSENSITIVITY

Type II hypersensitivity reactions are initiated by the interaction of antibody (IgM or IgG, not IgE) with cell membranes or with the extracellular matrix. Complement may also be involved. The antigens that are recognized may be intrinsic to the cell membrane or extracellular matrix, or they may be exogenous molecules, such as a drug metabolite adsorbed onto the cell membrane or extracellular matrix.

A. Interaction of antibody with cells

Cell-surface or extracellular matrix epitope binding by antibodies (usually IgM or IgG) results in a conformational change in the Fc portion of the antibody molecule (Fig. 14.4). The conformational change in the Fc portion of the antibody molecule is recognized by cellular FcRs and by complement, and several immune-mediated destructive mechanisms may then come into play, targeted upon the site(s) of antibody binding.

1. **Antibody-dependent cell-mediated cytotoxicity (ADCC):** This is complement independent but requires the cooperation of leukocytes (Fig. 14.5). FcR-bearing cells [e.g., monocytes, neutrophils,

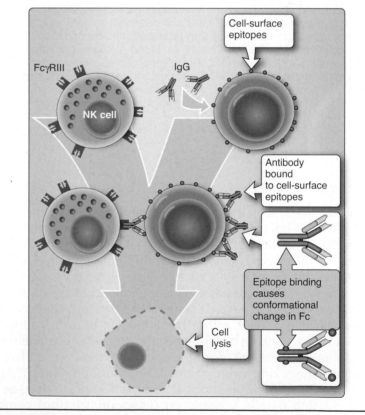

Figure 14.5
Antibody-dependent cell-mediated cytotoxicity. Specific binding of immunoglobulin to cell surface epitopes causes a conformation change in the Fc portion of the antibody molecule. FcγRIII, expressed by natural killer (NK) cells, recognize and bind the altered antibody, causing the NK cell to release perforin granules that cause lysis of the antibody-coated cell.

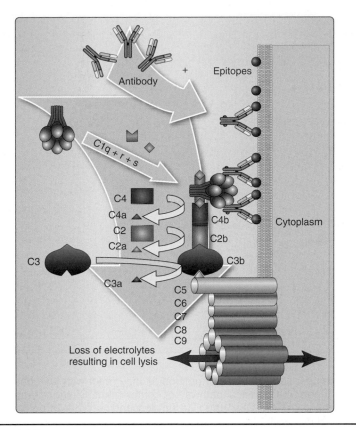

Figure 14.6
Type II hypersensitivity reactions. These reactions may involve complement-mediated lysis. Antibodies that invoke the classical and terminal or lytic pathways of complement activation recognize epitopes on cell membranes and cause formation of the membrane attack complex, transmembrane pore formation, and loss of electrolyte balance, causing lysis.

eosinophils, and natural killer (NK) cells] bind to cells that have IgG or IgM antibodies bound to surface epitopes on a cell.

2. **Complement:** Complement activated by IgM and IgG antibodies generates active components of the classical pathway, namely, C3b and C4b. These components are then deposited on the surfaces of antibody-coated cells or extracellular matrix to function as **opsonins**. Phagocytes recognize bound antibody through their FcRs and bound complement components through their complement receptors. In this manner, both complement and antibody function as opsonins to increase phagocytosis and the destruction of microorganisms (Fig. 14.6).

3. **Blood group antibodies:** These exemplify type II hypersensitivity reactions. Hemolytic anemias may result from the binding of IgM antibodies to carbohydrate structures on erythrocytes (notably anti-A or anti-B antibodies) resulting in their phagocytosis and in the presence of complement, their rapid lysis (hemolysis, Fig. 14.7). Antibodies (IgG) to certain protein molecules on erythrocytes [e.g., Rh factor(s)] do not activate complement; erythrocytes are destroyed by phagocytosis (Fig 14.7).

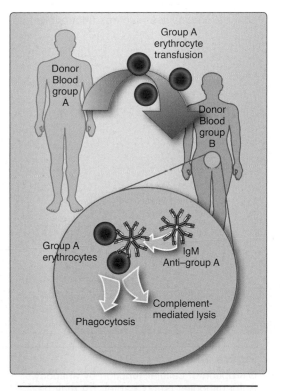

Figure 14.7
"Natural" antibodies against blood group AB antigens. These naturally occurring IgM antibodies bind to erythrocyte membranes, rendering them susceptible to phagocytosis or complement-mediated lysis.

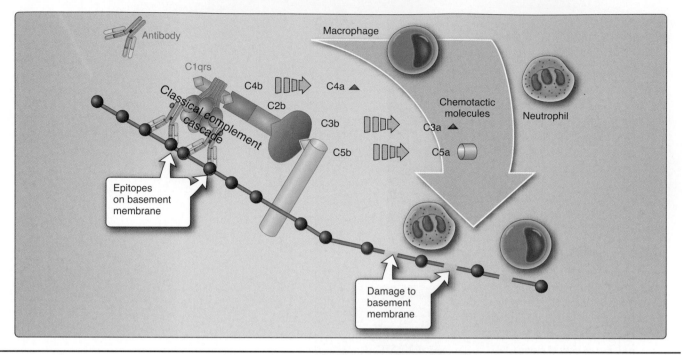

Figure 14.8
Antibodies against matrix proteins. Autoreactive IgG (autoimmune; see Chapter 16) antibodies may react with epitopes on extracellular matrix, such as the basement membrane, and trigger the classical pathway of complement. Sequential activation of complement components C4, C3, and C5 result in the release of C5a, C3a, and C4a (in descending order of potency) activate phagocytes (such as neutrophils and monocytes) to damage the basement membrane.

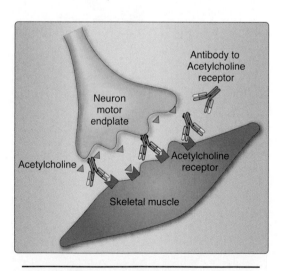

Figure 14.9
Disruption of cellular function by antibody. Autoantibodies (see Chapter 16) may be produced against the acetylcholine receptor (in a condition known as myasthenia gravis), blocking the interaction of the acetylcholine receptor with its obligate ligand (acetyl-choline) and leading to increased muscle weakness and death.

B. Interaction of antibody with the extracellular matrix

Antibodies that bind to extracellular matrix proteins (e.g., basement membrane) may activate the classical pathway of complement, generating anaphylotoxins (e.g., C5a, C4a, C3a, in descending order of potency, not in order of appearance) that recruit neutrophils and monocytes. FcR engagement with the bound antibody results in the release of reactive oxygen intermediates, resulting in inflammation and tissue injury (Fig. 14.8).

C. Antibody-mediated disruption of cellular function

Sometimes antibodies bind to cell surface receptors without activating complement or binding to FcRs. This binding blocks the receptor's ability to interact with its natural ligand (Fig. 14.9). The antibody-receptor interaction may be stimulatory (e.g., Graves disease) or inhibitory (e.g., insulin-resistant diabetes, myasthenia gravis) to the receptor's signaling pathway(s).

IV. TYPE III HYPERSENSITIVITY

Circulating antigen-antibody complexes may lead to inflammation at their sites of deposition, often resulting in blood vessel inflammation (**vasculitis**). Immune complexes may cause injury resulting from the interaction with exogenous (e.g., microbes, viruses or chemically modified self proteins) or endogenous antigens (e.g., serum proteins). Type III reactions may occur locally or systemically.

A. Localized reactions

Localized type III hypersensitivities, also known as **Arthus reactions**, result from acute immune complex vasculitis causing tissue necrosis. These reactions are elicited four to six hours after the intradermal introduction of a small amount of antigen. Antibody diffuses from the vasculature to form large immune precipitates that activate complement to induce a painful localized edematous inflammatory lesion (Fig. 14.10). Lesions range from necrotizing vasculitis with polymorphonuclear cell infiltration to the formation of a sterile abscess.

B. Systemic reactions

Systemic immune complex disease, in some cases termed **serum sickness,** occurs with the wide dissemination of antigen-antibody complexes throughout the body. Very large immune complexes are rapidly cleared from the body by phagocytic cells and are relatively harmless. Smaller, circulating immune complexes have less chance to be seen by phagocytes and remain in the circulation longer. These complexes have the greatest pathologic consequences.

1. **Exogenous antigens:** Administered either in large amounts or for a prolonged period of time, these may induce antibody responses.

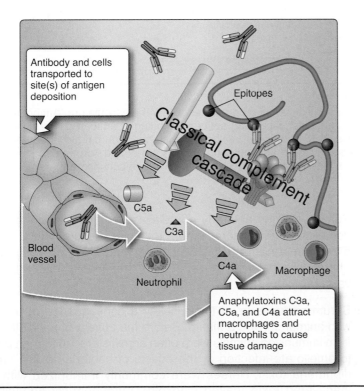

Figure 14.10

Arthus or acute immune complex vasculitis. This localized type III hypersensitivity reaction results from the tissue deposition of antigen-antibody complexes. Circulating antibodies leave the vasculature to interact with antigens introduced into the tissue.

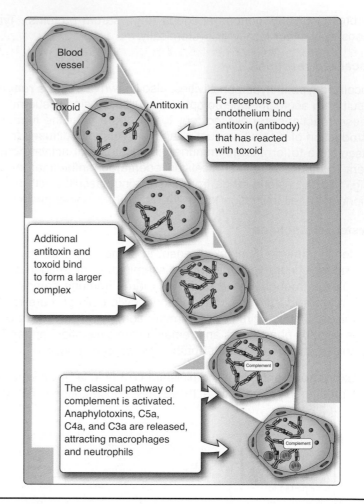

Figure 14.11

Accumulation of immune complexes within the vasculature. Antibodies are produced against circulating antigens. Binding of antigen conformationally changes the Fc portion of antibody, which can then bind to endothelial Fc receptors. More antibody and antigen are bound, forming an immune complex that activates the classical pathway of complement.

Soluble antigen-antibody complexes immobilized along the endothelium activate complement to cause vascular injury. Complement components (e.g., C5a, C4a, and C3a) attract polymorphonuclear cells to the site, and these cells exacerbate the vascular injury (Fig. 14.11).

Serum sickness used to be solely a consequence of treatment with animal-derived antisera. Before the advent of antibiotics, sera from immunized animals were often administered to human patients to ameliorate infection or the effects of bacterial toxins, such as diphtheria toxin. Horses were commonly immunized with heat-inactivated toxin (called a toxoid). Intravenously administered horse antiserum is very efficient at neutralizing the harmful effects of bacterial toxins. Horse serum proteins persist in the patient's circulation and, unfortunately, are very good immunogens in humans. After 7 to 10 days, patients may develop symptoms of immune complex disease, corresponding to the advent of a primary antibody response to horse serum proteins. Serum sickness is a self-limiting disease, because the foreign antigen (antiserum) is cleared from the body.

CLINICAL APPLICATION
Drug-induced immune complex disease

An 18-year-old female presents in the emergency room with a two-day history of fever (39°C), cough, and labored breathing. A diagnosis of lobar pneumonia is made. She is admitted to the hospital, and because a Gram-negative organism is suspected, a 10-day course of oral penicillin G is prescribed. Within 48 hours, her temperature is 37.4°C (37°C is normal), and by 96 hours, her respiration has improved and she feels remarkably better. Sputum cultures grow penicillin-sensitive *Streptococcus pneumonia*, confirming the initial diagnosis. On the eighth day of treatment, she develops edematous eyelids and hives (urticaria) on her abdomen. Penicillin is immediately discontinued, and antihistamine is administered. Nevertheless, she develops tightness in the throat, swollen face, and widespread urticaria. Laboratory tests show an elevated leukocyte count with 67% lymphocytes (30% is normal), plasma cells are present in blood smears, and complement levels are decreased. She has developed a type III hypersensitivity response to penicillin. She is advised by her physician that she must avoid use of penicillin and penicillin derivatives in the future.

---

2. **Endogenous antigens:** These may also cause immune-complex disease. Unlike exogenous antigens, continually produced endogenous antigens are responsible for chronic antigen exposure, chronic immunization, and prolonged immune-complex disease. Autoimmune diseases are often accompanied by immune-complex disease. Each year, 50 new cases per million of the population of **systemic lupus erythematosis (SLE)** are diagnosed. This disease occurs approximately eight times more often in women than in men. SLE is a complex, multifaceted autoimmune disease. Individuals with SLE produce autoantibodies to a number of different self antigens. As a consequence, immune complexes are deposited in the vascular beds that activate complement and cause vasculitis.

CLINICAL APPLICATION
Acute rheumatic fever

"Strep" throat is an acute infection of the palatine tonsils often caused by *Streptococcus pyogenes*, making swallowing painful. For most individuals, streptococcal tonsillitis is a self-limiting illness. However, a small number of untreated individuals develop polyarthritis and complications arising from antibody responses to antigen (M protein) expressed in the cell wall of *S. pyogenes*. A minority of these individuals develop antibodies that cross-react with antigens expressed on heart valves, myocardial and smooth muscle sarcolemma, and myosin (anti-M antibodies), a disease known as **acute rheumatic fever (ARF)**. Because recurrent attacks of *S. pyogenes* result in increased severity of ARF, prophylactic measures are indicated. When *S. pyogenes* infection is confirmed by throat culture, antibiotic therapy (penicillin) is prescribed to help eliminate *S. pyogenes* and to minimize the development of a systemic antibody response.

V. TYPE IV HYPERSENSITIVITY

Type IV hypersensitivity reactions result from the interaction of T cell-initiated inflammation and do not involve antibody. Inflammatory responses result from the manner in which T cells encounter and respond to antigen. CD4$^+$ T cells may be sensitized and respond to topically applied antigen (**contact dermatitis, CD**, also called contact sensitivity), by antigen injected antigen [delayed (-type) hypersensitivity, DTH]. Alternatively, CD8$^+$ T cells may encounter cell-surface antigen and directly cause the lysis of that cell (CTL).

A. Contact dermatitis

Chemically reactive substances may be absorbed through the epidermis, where they bind to proteins. Potential **contact sensitizers** include synthetic chemicals, plant products, and certain metals (e.g., nickel). Generally, contact sensitizers are, by themselves, too small (<10,000 daltons) to be recognized by the immune system. Contact sensitizers interact with self proteins to form immunogenic **neoepitopes** or **neoantigens** on these proteins. Immunologists often refer to substances that are immunogenic only when bound to another molecule as **haptens**. First acute exposure to a contact sensitizer often occurs without apparent incident but serves to immunize the immune system. After seven or more days, reexposure or chronic exposure elicits a localized inflammation of the dermis. Clinical signs, like those seen for DTH, typically appear 24 to 72 hours after reexposure (Fig. 14.12).

CLINICAL APPLICATION
Poison ivy

Toxicondendron radicans, commonly known as poison ivy, is a woody vine that secretes a toxic oil known as urushiol. *T. diversiloba* (poison oak) and *T. vermix* (poison sumac) also secrete this compound. The name comes from *urushi*, a Japanese wood lacquer produced from the sap of *T. vermicifluum*. Minute amounts of urushiol (1 nanogram) are sufficient to elicit contact dermatitis in previously exposed individuals. Over 85% of individuals who contact urushiol will develop a type IV hypersensitivity to this compound.

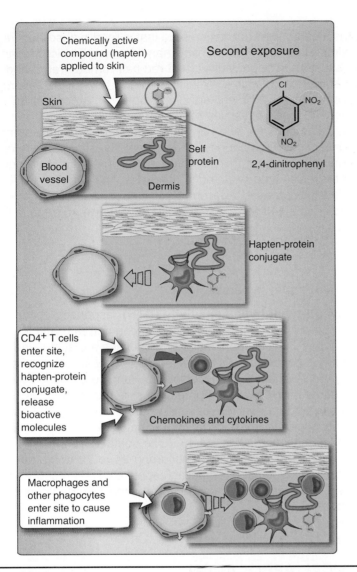

Figure 14.12
Contact dermatitis. Certain chemical compounds (e.g. 2,4-dinitrophenyl
or DNP) by themselves do not invoke an immune response (haptens).
However, they may penetrate the epidermis and covalently bind to self
proteins (hapten-protein conjugate). Following phagocytosis and presentation by resident dendritic cells in the context of MHC class II, CD4$^+$ T cells
entering the site may be activated and release chemokines to attract and
cytokines (e.g., IFN-γ) that induce type IV hypersensitivity.

CLINICAL APPLICATION
Canary girls and the munitions factory

As men fought in "the war to end all wars," World War I, Britain found
itself with severe shortages of war supplies and labor. The only way
to find sufficient labor for production needs was to hire young women
to manufacture and load trinitrotoluene (TNT) into explosive shells.

TNT is a pale yellow crystalline solid that is readily absorbed through the skin. Munitions workers who handled the chemical found that their skin turned bright yellow (and red hair turned green) and were nicknamed "canary girls." With time, many developed severe dermatitis, and over 100 workers died from TNT exposure. By themselves, TNT and derivatives of related compounds such as trinitrophenyl, dinitrophenyl, and nitrophenyl cannot stimulate an immune response. These compounds, termed haptens, penetrate the epidermis and readily bind to body proteins, where they may induce a hapten-specific type IV immune response. The plight of the canary girls led to increased awareness of industrial and environmental hazards and aided the cause that led to women's suffrage in Britain in 1918.

B. Delayed (-type) hypersensitivity

Delayed (-type) hypersensitivity (DTH) responses occur in sensitized individuals upon nontopical reencounter with antigen. In general, Type IV DTH hypersensitivity responses are stimulated by intracellular parasites such as bacteria (e.g., *Mycobacterium tuberculosis, M. leprae, Leishmania monocytogenes*), fungi (e.g., *Candida albicans*), and some viruses (e.g., mumps virus, a paramyxovirus). DTH responses occur upon reexposure to the stimulating antigen. Reexposure generally must occur more than one week after the initial antigenic encounter (Fig. 14.13). Like contact dermatitis responses, DTH responses are delayed, occurring 24 to 72 hours after restimulation. Unlike contact dermatitis responses, DTH responses are not limited to the dermis but can occur at almost any anatomical site in the body.

CLINICAL APPLICATION
Mantoux test

Tuberculosis (TB) is a potentially severe contagious disease caused by *Mycobacterium tuberculosis*. TB is spread from person to person through the air. More than 2 million people worldwide die from TB each year. Among people older than 5 years of age, TB disease is the leading cause of death due to infectious disease around the world.

The Mantoux skin test is a useful screening test to identify people who have been infected with TB. It involves injection of 5 TU (tuberculin units) of purified protein derivative (tuberculin), usually 0.1 mL, intradermally. Induration (swelling) is assessed at 48 to 72 hours. The induration is due to cell infiltration and occasionally vesiculation and necrosis. A positive response is an example of type IV hypersensitivity (DTH) and indicates that the subject has had prior exposure to *M. tuberculosis*.

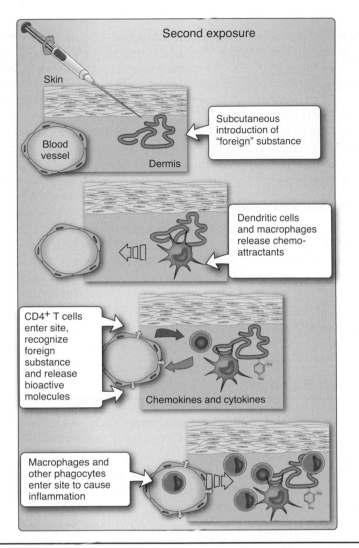

Figure 14.13
Delayed (-type) hypersensitivity. Proteins or intracellular organisms are phagocytosed and presented by resident dendritic cells in the context of MHC class II. CD4$^+$ T cells enter the site recognize the peptide-hapten conjugate and release chemokines to attract and cytokines (e.g. IFN-γ) to activate phagocytic cells to cause a type IV hypersensitivity.

CLINICAL APPLICATION
Hypersensitivity pneumonitis

John M., a previously healthy 46-year-old male with no prior history of immune-related illnesses presents with a persistent cough and shortness of breath associated with headache and malaise. Four weeks ago, his physician prescribed an antibiotic for some findings on his lung exam. The antibiotic did not alleviate his symptoms. At that time, his chest radiograph and screening spirometry were normal. For the last six months, he has worked in a new location.

Others at his workplace began to complain of similar symptoms, and an air quality analysis was performed, revealing fungal spore counts of more than 500 per cubic meter of air (reference: <200). Radiographs show diffuse patchy lung infiltrate consistent with the diagnosis of hypersensitivity pneumonitis, an example of type IV hypersensitivity mediated by CD4$^+$ T cells. John is prescribed a course of oral corticosteroids, and it is recommended that he find an alternative work location. John follows this advice, and his symptoms resolve quickly. He has remained symptom free since that time.

C. T cell-mediated cytotoxicity

In some instances, type IV hypersensitivity reactions are caused by CD8$^+$ T lymphocytes. These CTLs respond to reactive chemical agents (haptens) that pass through the cell membrane and bind to cytoplasmic proteins to produce neoantigens (Fig. 14.14). Peptides derived from haptenated cytoplasmic proteins (ubiquitin, proteasome, TAP pathway) are presented by MHC class I molecules to sensitize and elicit a CTL response.

Chapter Summary

- All four hypersensitivity responses occur upon second exposure or chronic exposure to antigen. Only type IV hypersensitivity reactions are antibody independent.
- Hypersensitivity reactions cause tissue injury by the release of chemical substances that attract and activate cells and molecules resulting in **inflammation.**
- Type I hypersensitivity reactions are rapid, occurring within minutes of exposure to an antigen, and always involve IgE-mediated degranulation of basophils or mast cells.
- **Anaphylaxis** ("against protection") is characterized by vascular smooth muscle constriction (**vasoconstriction**) combined with gap formation between adjacent capillary endothelial cells (**vasodilation**) that results in severe fluid loss and leads to **shock.**
- **Type II hypersensitivity** reactions are initiated by the binding of antibody to a cell membrane or to the extracellular matrix. Type II reactions are initiated by the interaction of antibody (IgM or IgG) with cell membranes or with the extracellular matrix. The antigens that are recognized may be intrinsic to the cell membrane or extracellular matrix, or they may be exogenous molecules such as a drug metabolite adsorbed onto the cell membrane or extracellular matrix.
- **Type III** hypersensitivity reactions involve the interaction of antibodies with soluble molecules to make soluble antigen-antibody complexes that become deposited in tissues. Circulating antigen-antibody complexes may lead to inflammation at their sites of deposition, often resulting in blood vessel inflammation (**vasculitis**). Immune complexes may cause injury resulting from the interaction with exogenous antigens (e.g., microbes, viruses, or chemically modified self proteins) or endogenous antigens (e.g., serum proteins).

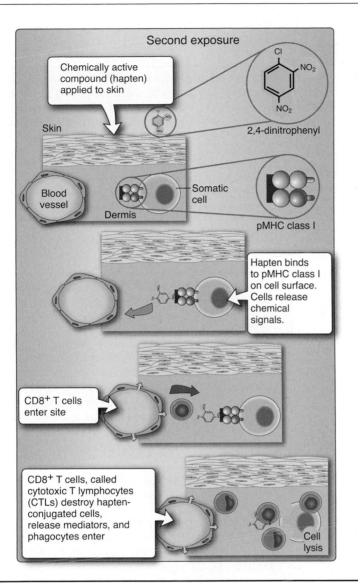

Figure 14.14
Type IV hypersensitivity mediated by cytotoxic CD8⁺ T lymphocytes. DNP that penetrates the epidermis may covalently bond to self proteins present on cell surfaces. CD8⁺ T cells enter the site, where they recognize and kill the hapten-modified cell and release substances that invoke an inflammatory response.

- **Type IV** hypersensitivity reactions involve direct attack of host cells by leukocytes in the absence of antibody. Included are contact dermatitis, delayed (-type) hypersensitivity (DTH), and, sometimes, cytotoxic T lymphocyte (CTL) responses. Type IV reactions result from T cell-initiated inflammation. Inflammatory responses result from the manner in which T cells encounter and respond to antigen. CD4⁺ T cells may be sensitized and respond to topically applied antigen (contact dermatitis), or they may be sensitized by injected antigen (DTH), or CD8⁺ T cells may encounter cell-surface antigen and directly cause cellular lysis (CTL).

Study Questions

14.1 A previously healthy 45-year-old male presents with rhinorrhea, nasal congestion, and persistent respiratory symptoms several months after returning to his home in New Orleans after Hurricane Katrina. He has noticed mold growing along the walls of his house. Skin testing for sensitivity to common mold spores gave positive results to several of them in less than 30 minutes. These findings indicate an example of:

A. contact dermatitis.
B. delayed (-type) hypersensitivity.
C. immediate hypersensitivity.
D. serum sickness.
E. type II hypersensitivity.

14.2 A 25-year-old female with a history of penicillin allergy unknown to her physician was given a single injection of penicillin for the treatment of syphilis. Within minutes, she developed diffuse urticaria (hives), tachycardia (rapid heart rate), and hypotension (decrease in blood pressure). This patient has experienced

A. anaphylaxis.
B. anergy.
C. antibody-mediated cytotoxicity.
D. asthma.
E. contact sensitivity

14.3 Which of the following is/are initiated by the interaction of host cell membranes with IgM or IgG antibody but never IgE antibody?

A. arthus reactions
B. serum sickness
C. type I hypersensitivity reactions
D. type II hypersensitivity reactions
E. type IV hypersensitivity reactions

14.4 An 8-year-old female with a known allergy to peanuts inadvertently ingests a cereal containing traces of peanuts. Within one hour, she develops diffuse erythema (redness of the skin) and urticaria associated with respiratory symptoms of shortness of breath and diffuse wheezing. These findings suggest which of the following events?

A. type I hypersensitivity reaction
B. arthus reaction
C. FcR-bearing cells binding to host cells coated with IgG
D. IgG binding to extracellular matrix of the respiratory passages
E. IgM-mediated interaction with cell membranes of lymphocytes

The correct answer is C. Type I (immediate) hypersensitivity is caused by the cross-linking of FcRε (also known as CD23) -bound IgE antibodies on cell surfaces, which triggers the release of vasoreactive amines from mast cell granules. Antigens (allergens) are often airborne and elicit type I reactions that cause respiratory distress. Neither contact dermatitis nor delayed (-type) hypersensitivity reactions involve antibody. Both serum sickness and type II hypersensitivity involve immune complexes.

The correct answer is A. This individual displays the hallmarks of a classical anaphylactic reaction to penicillin. Anergy is the impairment of effector immune responsiveness. Antibody-mediated cytotoxicity is most often localized to tissues bearing epitopes to which the antibody binds. Asthma causes respiratory distress due to the contraction of bronchiole-associated smooth muscle in response to the release of vasoactive mediators from mast cells. Contact sensitivity results from the epicutaneous application of a reactive antigen/hapten; in the present question, the antigen (penicillin) was administered intramuscularly.

The correct answer is D. Type II hypersensitivity reactions occur with host cell membranes or with the extracellular matrix. Arthus reactions and serum sickness are type III hypersensitivities that result from the interaction(s) of antibody with soluble antigen(s). IgE is not involved, thus ruling out type I hypersensitivity.

The correct answer is A. This individual has experienced an immediate or type I hypersensitivity. The clue here is that this reaction occurred within one hour of antigen (peanut) ingestion. Her presentation shows hallmarks of IgE-mediated anaphylactic reactions. Arthus reactions and those mediated by IgM and IgG do not cause mast cell degranulation; nor do they cause rapid respiratory distress.

14.5 The 8-year-old patient recovered from the event described in Study Question 14.4. The next day, she went to play with a friend who had recently returned from a family trip to Asia. The friend gave her a Japanese lacquered box as a gift. Two days later, she developed itchiness in her hands, and her mother noticed that they were bright red. Her mother also noticed clear fluid vesicles on her right forearm. These findings suggest which type of hypersensitivity?

A. type I, mediated by $CD4^+$ T cells
B. type I, mediated by $CD8^+$ T cells
C. type II, mediated by $CD8^+$ T cells
D. type III, mediated by $CD4^+$ T cells
E. type IV, mediated by $CD4^+$ T cells

The correct answer is E. Urushiol, common to poison ivy and poison oak, is a component of Japanese lacquer. The urticaria (itchiness) and fluid vesicles on her forearm are hallmarks of contact dermatitis, a type IV hypersensitivity mediated by $CD4^+$ T cells. Type I and type II hypersensitivities are mediated by antibodies; type IV is not.

14.6 A 45-year-old female with a history of hepatitis C viral infection presents with decreased renal function, hypertension (increased blood pressure), and anemia. Laboratory findings reveal decreased serum C3. Her urine sediment contains leukocytes, erythrocytes, and red blood cell casts (a proteinaceous mold of the renal tubules that includes erythrocytes). Her renal biopsy is consistent with glomerulonephritis. These findings suggest which type of hypersensitivity?

A. type I, mediated by $CD4^+$ T cells
B. type II, mediated by IgM antibodies
C. type III, mediated by IgG antibodies
D. type IV, mediated by $CD4^+$ T cells
E. type IV, mediated by IgG (and sometimes IgM) antibodies

The correct answer is C. Glomerulonephritis is often associated with immune complex deposition, a type III hypersensitivity. Red blood cell casts are indicative of glomerulonephritis, and reduced C3 levels indicate a high level of cleavage and activation of C3. Type I hypersensitivity is mediated by IgE, not by $CD4^+$ T cells. Type II hypersensitivity responses usually involve IgG. Type IV hypersensitivities do not involve antibodies.

14.7 A 35-year-old male presents with headache, fatigue, light-headedness, dyspnea (difficulty in breathing), and tachycardia (rapid heart rate). Laboratory findings reveal decreased hemoglobin and a positive direct Coombs' test (presence of antibodies on erythrocyte surfaces). The patient is currently taking an antibiotic for symptoms of upper respiratory infection. These findings suggest which type of hypersensitivity?

A. Type I, mediated by IgG antibodies
B. Type II, mediated by IgG antibodies
C. Type III, mediated by IgG antibodies
D. Type III, mediated by IgG or IgM antibodies
E. Type IV, mediated by $CD4^+$ T cells

The correct answer is B. Type II reactions involve antibodies directed against self cells (such as erythrocytes) or membranes. Certain drugs react with erythrocytes to form neoantigens. Type I responses are against foreign antigens (e.g., allergens), cause IgE responses, and do not invoke a Coomb's reaction. Type III reactions involve soluble antigen-antibody complexes, and type IV reactions do not involve antibody.

Immune Deficiency

15

I. OVERVIEW

It sometimes seems as if the immune system is so complicated that it cannot possibly work. Failure seems almost assured, and indeed, small deficits in the generation of T and B cell receptors are common (see Chapter 8). Because redundancy is built in, failure in one component of the immune system may sometimes be covered by another component with a similar or overlapping function. In other cases, failures in immune function become overt and may have a severe clinical impact.

Overt failures of the immune system leave the affected individual with a reduced ability to resist infection. **Immune deficiencies** or **immunodeficiencies** due to defects in various components of the immune system are infrequent, though not insignificant, and occur in two different ways. **Primary immune deficiencies** are those caused by intrinsic or congenital defects. These deficiencies usually are genetic in nature, but they may sometimes appear as the result of randomly occurring errors in development. Over 100 primary immune deficiency diseases are known in humans, and for many of these diseases, the specific defective genes have been identified.

Primary immunodeficiency diseases were once considered rare, but many are actually more common than was previously thought. Selective IgA deficiency has a frequency of about two individuals per thousand, compared with numerous others that occur with frequencies of one to ten per hundred thousand. However, because there are so many different primary immunodeficiency diseases, they become a significant health problem when considered collectively. Most primary immune deficiencies become apparent at about 6 months of age, when the maternally derived antibodies that entered the fetal circulation in utero begin to disappear and the infant becomes dependent upon his or her own immune system.

Secondary immune deficiencies are caused by environmental causes such as infection, therapeutic treatments, cancer, and malnutrition. These deficiencies may occur at any time of life, depending upon when the exposure to the causative factor(s) occurs. As with primary immune deficiencies, affected individuals are more susceptible to infection.

Immune deficiencies are characterized by several features. Some features occur in most forms of immunodeficiency, and some occur with a more limited set of deficiencies. Still others are associated only with specific diseases. These disease-specific features are often useful in diagnosis of a particular individual's disease.

Characteristics seen in many immune deficiency diseases include the following:

- recurrent or chronic infections
- inability to clear infectious agents after standard antibiotic therapy
- unusual infectious agents

Characteristics seen in a limited set of immune deficiency diseases include the following:

- failure of infants to gain weight normally, known as *failure to thrive* [severe combined immune deficiency disease (SCID), interferon γ receptor deficiency, bare lymphocyte syndrome]
- hepatosplenomegaly [common variable immune deficiency (CVID), interferon-γ receptor deficiency, Chediak-Higashi syndrome]
- skin rashes [SCID, Wiskott-Aldrich syndrome (WAS), X-linked agammaglobulinemia]
- diarrhea (associated with gastrointestinal infection) [CVID, WAS, X-linked agammaglobulinemia, bare lymphocyte syndrome, SCID, chronic granulomatous disease (CGD)]
- recurrent abscesses [CGD, leukocyte adhesion molecule defects]

Nonimmunologic characteristics that occur in specific immune deficiency diseases include the following:

- platelet deficiency (thrombocytopenia) [Wiskott-Aldrich syndrome]
- loss of balance (ataxia) and widened blood capillaries (telangiectasia) [immunodeficiency with ataxia-telangiectasia]
- partial or complete albinism [Chediak-Higashi syndrome]

II. PRIMARY (CONGENITAL) IMMUNE DEFICIENCIES

Defects causing primary immune deficiencies may occur in different cell lineages: the combined lymphoid cell lineage, T or B cell lineages separately, lineages producing phagocytic cells and natural killer (NK) cells, and even cells producing complement components. Additionally, defects in cells of one lineage may affect the development of other lineages that are intrinsically normal. For example, abnormalities in T cells may prevent the activation of B cells that are otherwise normal. And the interactions between cells from different lineages may result in a single defect inhibiting multiple types of immune responses.

Autosomal gene defects (whether recessive or dominant) affect both sexes equally. However, defective X-linked genes (usually recessive) affect males far more frequently than females. Unlike females, males cannot compensate for a defective X-linked gene with a normal counterpart of that gene on the other X chromosome.

A. Defects in stem cells

The **pluripotent stem cells** that ultimately generate the granulocytic, erythrocytic, monocytic, thrombocytic, and lymphocytic lineages of the hematopoietic system are initially found in the aorta-gonad-mesonephros of the developing embryo. These cells undergo two

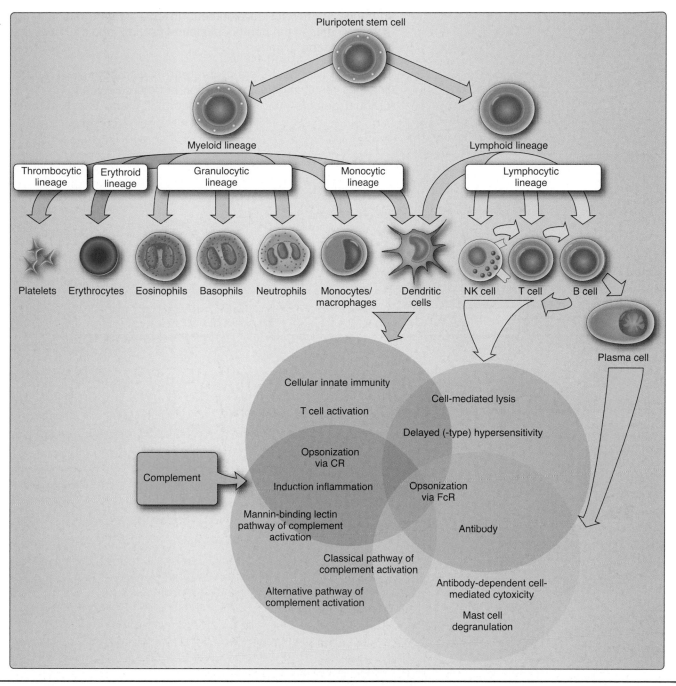

Figure 15.1
Hematopoietic stem cells and lineages. Pluripotent stem cells in the bone marrow give rise to all five hematopoietic cell lineages: lymphocytes, thrombocytes, monocytes, granulocytes, and erythrocytes. Note that both the lymphocytic and monocytic lineages produce dendritic cells.

migrations. During embryonic and fetal development, they migrate to the fetal liver. Later, before birth, they migrate again, this time to the bone marrow, where they remain for life. Some of the pluripotent stem cells differentiate into slightly differentiated stem cells that give rise to each of the five hematopoietic lineages (Fig. 15.1). Lymphoid stem cells generate both B cells (B-1 and B-2) and T cells ($\alpha\beta$ and $\gamma\delta$). Recall from Chapter 7 that the B-2 cell lineage remains within the bone marrow for development, the B-1 lineage relocates to and self-replicates in the peritoneal/pleural tissues, and the T cell lineage migrates to the thymus.

Defects in lymphoid stem cells giving rise to both the T and B cell lineages result in defective function of both cell types (Fig. 15.2). Individual defects may result in abnormal T and B cell numbers or

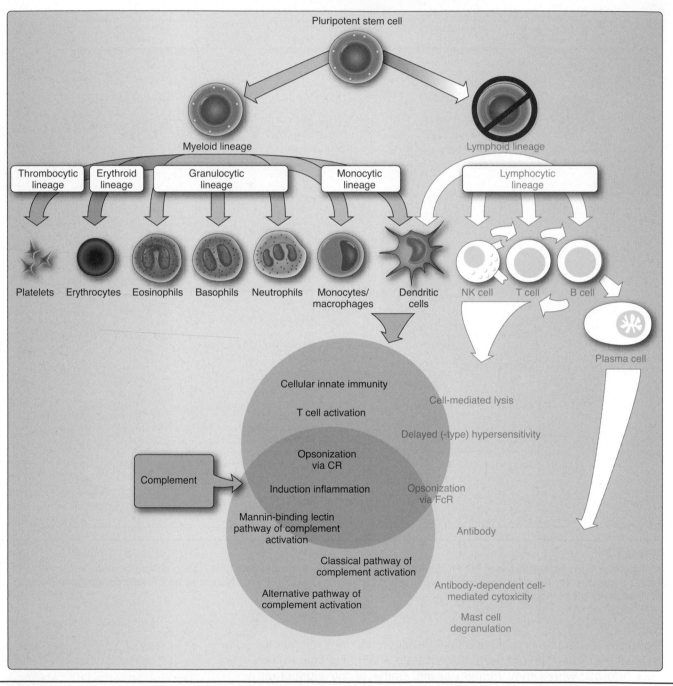

Figure 15.2
Effects of lymphoid cell lineage deficiencies. Defects in the lineage producing both T and B lymphocytes impair the development and/or functionality of both types of lymphocytes.

functions or both. Cell-mediated responses (e.g., cell-mediated lysis and delayed type hypersensitivity) are usually reduced, as is immunoglobulin production. The relative impacts of individual defects, however, are not always equal in T and B cells, nor do they always have equally severe consequences among affected individuals.

Severe combined immunodeficiency (SCID) is the classic example of defects in the combined lymphocyte lineage. SCID is not a single disease; it is a group of diseases caused by different defects in individual genes that have similar functional consequences (Table 15.1). SCID-related defects may occur in the genes that encode enzymes

Table 15.1
PRIMARY IMMUNE DEFICIENCY DISEASES ATTRIBUTABLE TO STEM CELL DEFECTS

Disease	Inheritance	Gene	Chromosome	Consequences
Adenosine deaminase (ADA) deficiency	Autosomal-recessive	*ADA* (adenosine deaminase)	20	Very susceptible to infection; impaired purine metabolism; T and B cells numbers and functions decreased due to toxic metabolites; immunoglobulin levels decreased
Immuno-deficiency with ataxia-telangiec-tasia	Autosomal-recessive	*ATM* (ataxia telangiec-tasia mutated)	11	Increased susceptibility to infection; frequent sinopulmonary infections; DNA repair affected and variable signs, including ataxia and telangiectasia (problems with balance and widened small capillaries); occurs at varying ages and in varying functions; T cell numbers and functions and immunoglobulin levels (especially IgG, IgA, and IgE) may decrease; B cell numbers may be normal; autoantibodies and chromosomal abnormalities are frequently found
Purine nucleoside phospho-rylase deficiency	Autosomal-recessive	*NP* (nucleo-side phos-phorylase)	14	Increased susceptibility to infection; impaired purine metabolism; declining T cell numbers over time (more susceptible than B cells to accumulated toxic metabolites); declining immunoglobulin levels due to decreased T cell help
Severe combined immune deficiency (SCID)	Autosomal-recessive	*RAG1* and/or *RAG2* (recombi-nation-activating genes)	11	High susceptibility to infection; unable to rearrange DNA to form variable regions of immunoglobulins and T cell receptors; T and B lymphocyte numbers/functions reduced or absent; immunoglobulin levels reduced or absent
	X-linked-recessive	*IL2RG* (common cytokine receptor γ chain, a component of the receptor complexes for IL-2, IL-4, IL-7, IL-9, and IL-15)	X	Multiple effects because common γ chain is a component of receptors for several cytokines; increased susceptibility to infection; T cell numbers and immunoglobulin levels decreased; B cell numbers normal or increased
	Autosomal-recessive	*JAK3* (janus kinase 3)	19	Increased susceptibility to infection; defective intracellular signaling; T cell numbers and immunoglobulin levels decreased; B cell numbers normal or increased
Wiskott-Aldrich syndrome	X-linked-recessive	*WAS* (Wiskott-Aldrich syndrome)	X	Increased susceptibility to infection, especially by *S. aureus*, develops during infancy and early childhood; T and B cell numbers and functions reduced, as are immunoglobulin levels; platelets abnormal and reduced in number

(RAG-1, RAG-2) responsible for the rearrangements of DNA that produce the variable regions of immunoglobulins and T-cell receptors. Other examples include defects in cytokine receptors and in molecules involved in cell-to-cell interaction for the activation of lymphocytes. Defective production of **purine nucleoside phosphorylase** provides an example of a genetic defect that affects both T and B cells but with differing intensity. The accumulated toxic metabolites resulting from this defect impair the functions of T cells far more severely than those of B cells.

CLINICAL APPLICATION
X-linked SCID

Timmy K., a 4-month-old male, presents with severe diarrhea and failure to thrive. Over the past two months, he has had two episodes of ear infections requiring antibiotic therapy. Examination reveals a poorly nourished child with minimal tonsillar tissue and the presence of oral thrush. Blood tests reveal lymphocyte counts significantly below normal with an absence of T cells (CD3$^+$) and NK cells (CD16$^+$, CD56$^+$) and significantly reduced numbers of B cells (CD19$^+$). A further workup by an immunology consultant results in a diagnosis of X-linked SCID. The hematology/immunology transplant team is notified, and the patient receives a bone marrow transplant.

B. Defects in T cells

Primary immune deficiencies intrinsic to T cells result in abnormal T cell numbers and/or functions. However, because T cell "help" is critical to the activation of naïve and memory B cells, many T cell defects also cause abnormalities in B cell numbers and immunoglobulin production (Fig. 15.3). Several representative diseases resulting from T cell defects are given in Table 15.2. Some are common to both CD4$^+$ and CD8$^+$ T cells; some affect only one T cell type or the other. Because the DTH response is largely responsible for clearance of fungi, frequent or recurrent fungal infections are suggestive of defects in T cell function.

A second category of T cell defects comprises those in which the responsible mutation(s) are not limited to T cells but may occur in cells that are critical to the development or activation of T cells. Some T cell defects arise from mutations in other cells that influence the development or activation of T cells. For example, **TAP-2 deficiency** (also known as **bare lymphocyte syndrome I**) is caused by defects in the transporter associated with the antigen presentation (TAP; either TAP1 or TAP2) system. These defects ultimately impair the loading of peptide fragments into nascent MHC class I molecules in all nucleated cells and reduce the number of MHC class I molecules that successfully reach the cell surface. This reduced MHC I expression decreases the number of functional CD8$^+$ T cells and can also affect the functions of NK cells monitoring MHC class I expression on body cells (although the NK cells appear not to attack uninfected

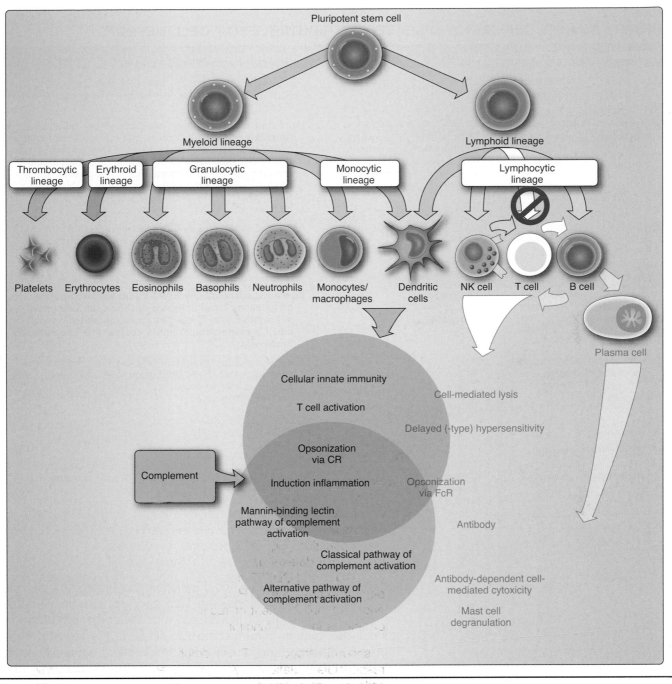

Figure 15.3
Effects of T lymphocyte deficiencies. Defective T cells not only reduce cell-mediated immune responsiveness, but also often reduce B cell functions because of the regulatory role for T cells in B cell activation.

host cells). Likewise, defects inhibiting expression of MHC class II molecules reduce the number of functional CD4$^+$ T cells. An additional example is **DiGeorge syndrome** (see Table 15.2), in which defects in thymic development arising from abnormal embryonic changes in the third and fourth pharyngeal pouches may inhibit or prevent development and thymic education of T cells. The severity of effects of DiGeorge syndrome is variable. In addition to abnormal

Table 15.2
PRIMARY IMMUNE DEFICIENCY DISEASES ATTRIBUTABLE TO T CELL DEFECTS

Disease	Inheritance	Gene	Chromosome	Consequences
CD3 deficiency	Autosomal-recessive	*CD3G* or *CD3E*	11	Increased susceptibility to infection; defects in CD3γ (CD3G) or CD3ε (CD3E) proteins; variable effects on T cell functions
DiGeorge syndrome	Autosomal-dominant or sponta-neous	Unknown Defects in embryonic thymic de-velopment	22 (when genetic)	Increased susceptibility to infections; T cell numbers and functions intrinsically normal but reduced and variable owing to abnormal development of thymus from third and fourth brachial arches; variable immunoglobulin levels; deletions in chromosome 22 frequently seen; often accompanied by other defects (e.g., facial fea-tures, palate, aorta, and parathyroid glands and cal-cium metabolism)
MHC class II deficiencies (bare lym-phocyte syndrome)	Autosomal-recessive	*CIITA* or *RFX5*	16 or 1	Increased susceptibility to infection; defective intra-cellular signaling; CD4$^+$ T cell numbers reduced; immunoglobulin levels decreased owing to defective T cell help
Purine nucleoside phospho-rylase deficiency	Autosomal-recessive	*NP* (nucleo-side phos-phorylase)	14	Increased susceptibility to infection; impaired purine metabolism; T cell numbers decline over time (more susceptible than B cells to accumulated toxic metabo-lites); immunoglobulin levels decline due to decreased T cell help
Transporter associated with anti-gen pre-sentation (TAP) -1 or -2 deficiency	Autosomal-recessive	*TAP1* or *TAP2*	6	Increased susceptibility to viral infections and to some intracellular bacteria; decreased MHC I expression and antigen presentation; CD8$^+$ T cell numbers and functions decreased
ZAP-70 deficiency	Autosomal-recessive	*ZAP70* (ζ chain associated protein kinase)		Recurrent severe infections; defective signaling from TCR; CD8$^+$ T cells absent; CD4$^+$ T cells present in normal numbers but nonfunctional

development of the pharyngeal pouches, the syndrome may include malformations of the aorta, the face and jaw, and the parathyroid glands. The majority of individuals with DiGeorge syndrome carry small deletions in chromosome 22, although the relevant gene or genes and their functions are still unidentified. These associated features allow early detection and treatment of DiGeorge syndrome at birth.

C. Defects in B cells

Several inherited genetic defects are intrinsic to B cells (Fig. 15.4). These B cell defects are responsible for the majority (more than 80%) of human immunodeficiency diseases (Table 15.3). Immunoglob-ulin levels are typically affected, but not necessarily B cell numbers. Some B cell deficiencies are characterized by abnormal production of all immunoglobulin isotypes, while others affect only one or a few. T cell numbers and functions are typically normal. The following examples illustrate the range of effects seen.

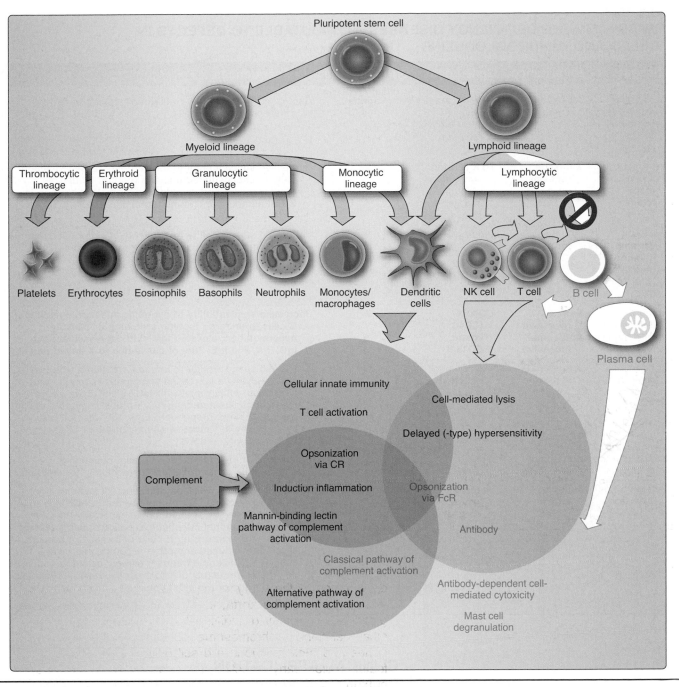

Figure 15.4
Effects of B lymphocyte deficiencies. Defective B cells affect humoral responses by altering B cell numbers and/or functions, including immunoglobulin production. T cells functions are usually unaffected.

Table 15.3
PRIMARY IMMUNE DEFICIENCY DISEASES ATTRIBUTABLE TO DEFECTS IN B CELLS AND IMMUNOGLOBULINS

Disease	Inheritance	Gene Locus	Chromosome	Consequences
Autosomal-recessive agamma-globu-linemia	Autosomal-recessive	Various genes involved in early differ-entiation	Various	Increased susceptibility to infection; failure in early differentiation of B cells
Bruton's agamma-globu-linemia	X-linked-recessive	*BTK* (Bruton agamma-globuline-mia tyro-sine kinase)	X	Increased susceptibility to infection; increased suscepti-bility to encapsulated bacteria (e.g., *H. influenzae*, *staphylococci*, and *streptococci*); drastic decrease in B cell numbers and immunoglobulin levels
Common variable immuno-deficiency (CVI or CVID)	Multiple forms	Unknown	?	Increased susceptibility to pyogenic infection; variable symptoms; varying isotypes (or combinations of isotypes) reduced or absent
Immuno-deficiency with hyper-IgM	X-linked-recessive Autosomal-recessive	*CD40LG* (CD40 ligand, CD154)	X	Increased susceptibility to pyogenic infection; inability of B cells to undergo isotype switching or somatic hypermutation; elevated IgM with decreased/absent IgG, IgA, and IgE; 70% of cases due to X-linked defect
Ig heavy chain gene deletions	Autosomal-recessive	Heavy chain constant genes	14	Increased susceptibility to infection (patients with IgG1 deficiency have increased susceptibility to pyogenic infections, while those with IgG2 or IgG3 are suscepti-ble to encapsulated bacteria); various immunoglobulin isotypes absent (dependent upon the affected heavy chain gene); IgG most frequently affected; B cell num-bers frequently reduced
Kappa chain deficiency	Autosomal-recessive	κ chain genes	2	Decreased or absent immunoglobulin containing κ chains; little or no effect on susceptibility to infection
Selective IgA deficiency	Multiple forms	Multiple genes	Various	Although patients with this deficiency display no increase in infections, an increased susceptibility to infections may be seen in some, especially recurrent pyogenic bacterial infections in patients also deficient in IgG2; IgA-expressing B cells decreased or absent; serum IgA reduced and often accompanied by IgG subclass deficiency; frequent allergic or autoimmune disorders; frequency of 1 to 2 per thousand individuals makes it one of the most common immune deficiency diseases

CLINICAL APPLICATION
Bruton's X-linked agammaglobulinemia

Bruton's X-linked agammaglobulinemia was named after an American pediatrician, Dr. Ogden Carr Bruton. In 1952, Dr. Bruton described the clinical case of an 8-year-boy who had recurrent bacterial infec-tions, including many episodes of pneumococcal sepsis. Dr. Bruton vaccinated the boy, but even then the patient did not produce any antibodies to *Pneumococcus*. In fact, the boy did not produce anti-bodies to any antigen and had undetectable levels of serum im-munoglobulins. Dr. Bruton treated this patient with monthly injec-tions of exogenous gamma globulin. The boy did not have any occurrences of sepsis over the 14 months during which he received injections. Because this condition was observed only in male patients, it was determined to be X-linked.

Bruton's agammaglobulinemia, a recessive X-linked disorder, is one of the best-known B cell immunodeficiencies, resulting from a defect in the gene (*BTK*) that encodes Bruton tyrosine kinase, an enzyme that is crucial to the early development of B cells. Consequently, in this disorder, B cells are few in number, and all immunoglobulin isotypes are diminished. Defects in several autosomal genes also lead to aberrant B cell development and similar agammaglobulinemias.

CLINICAL APPLICATION
Common variable immunodeficiency

Martha D., a 40-year-old woman, presents with recurrent sinusitis requiring antibiotic treatment. She has had two hospitalizations within the past two or three years for bacterial pneumonia. She also reports symptoms of chronic diarrhea, abdominal pain, weight loss, and fatigue. Laboratory tests reveal evidence of malabsorption due to infection with *Giardia lamblia*. Serum immunoglobulin assessments reveal a significantly decreased level of IgG and a mildly decreased level of IgA, consistent with common variable immunoglobulin deficiency. She is treated with passive immunoglobulin therapy, and her IgG level increases to within normal range. She continues to receive immunoglobulin therapy and remains free of significant infection or diarrhea for several years thereafter.

Selective IgA deficiency is the single most common immune deficiency disease, with a frequency estimated at one to two per thousand individuals. Multiple gene defects produce it, and there is evidence that some forms of the disease may involve defective isotype switch signaling from T cells. Individuals with selective IgA deficiency have normal levels of other isotypes and often display additional immunologic disorders (e.g., allergy or autoimmunity).

B cell activation is dependent in part on interaction with helper CD4$^+$ T cells. Some of this interaction involves the binding of CD40 on T cells to CD154 (CD40-ligand) on B cells. **Immune deficiency with hyper-IgM** results from a defect in the gene encoding the CD40 ligand. As a result, the isotype switch does not occur normally, and individuals with this defect produce high levels of IgM but are deficient in B cells that produce IgG, IgA, or IgE.

D. Defects in phagocytes and natural killer cells

Immune deficiency may also result from defects in nonlymphocytic cells such as phagocytes, neutrophils, and NK cells (Fig. 15.5, Table 15.4). Defects in phagocytic cells are significant because of their key

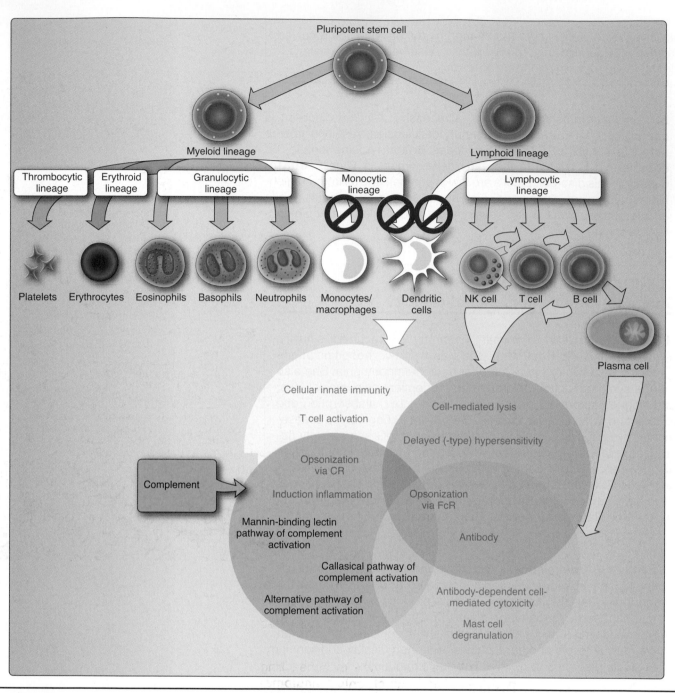

Figure 15.5
Effects of phagocytic cell and natural killer cell deficiencies. Defects in phagocytic cells reduce the ability to ingest and degrade microbes and to engage in antigen presentation to T cells. Defective NK cells have the ability to kill virally infected cells and participate in development of Th1 immune responses.

Table 15.4
PRIMARY IMMUNE DEFICIENCY DISEASES ATTRIBUTABLE TO DEFECTS IN ACCESSORY CELLS

Disease	Inheritance	Gene Locus	Chromosome	Consequences
Chediak-Higashi syndrome	Autosomal-recessive	*LYST* (lysosomal trafficking regulator; also called CHS1)	1	Increased susceptibility to infection by pyogenic bacteria; defective fusion of lysosomes and phagosomes due to defect in organelle membranes; reduced ability to kill ingested microbes; decreased NK and T cell functions; frequent albinism of eyes and skin and other defects of organelle membranes; giant granules in neutrophils and other cells
Chronic granulomatous disease (CGD)	X-linked-recessive	*CYBB* (β chain of cytochrome b; also called gp91phox)	X	Increased susceptibility to infection, especially *Staphylococcus aureus*, *Salmonella enteric*, *Typhimurium*, *Serratia marcescens*; macrophages and neutrophils affected; unable to produce superoxide metabolites
	Autosomal-recessive	*NCF1* (p47phox)	7	Increased susceptibility to infection; unable to produce superoxide metabolites for killing of ingested microbes; macrophages and neutrophils affected; NCF1 and NCF2 encode components of the NADPH oxidase complex; CYBA encodes the α chain of cytochrome b
		NCF2 (p67phox)	1	
		CYBA (p22phox)	16	
IFN-γ receptor deficiency	Autosomal-recessive	*IFNGR1* (IFN-γ receptor)	6	High susceptibility to mycobacterial infections; macrophages, neutrophils, NK cells, and Th1 cells are affected
Leukocyte adhesion defect 1 (LAD-1)	Autosomal-recessive	*ITGB2* (also known as CD18)	21	Increased susceptibility to recurrent infection by bacteria; frequent nonresolving abscesses; defective chemotaxis and adherence to endothelial surfaces by macrophages, neutrophils and NK cells
Leukocyte adhesion defect 2 (LAD-2)	Autosomal-recessive	*GDP-fucose transporter1*	11	Increased susceptibility to recurrent infection by bacteria and nonresolving abscesses; impaired synthesis of CD15s, a carbohydrate adhesion molecule; defects in ability of leukocytes to adhere to endothelial surfaces; reduced ability of leukocytes to move from vasculature into tissues; also causes Bombay blood group phenotype

roles in both innate and adaptive immune responses. The defects affect two major functions of these cells: their ability to kill microbes and their interactions with other cell types.

Several defects can interfere with the phagocyte's microbe-killing function. Defects in the genes associated with **chronic granulomatous disease** (**CGD**) result in defective enzymes and other microcidal molecules (e.g., toxic oxygen metabolites) involved in destruction and degradation of ingested microbes. In contrast, individuals with **Chediak-Higashi syndrome** have normal levels of these enzymes and microcidal molecules, but a defect in organelle membranes inhibits the normal fusion of lysosomes (carrying the enzymes and microcidal molecules) with phagosomes (containing the ingested microbes). Consequently, the phagocytes fail to destroy ingested microbes. Defects in receptors (e.g., pattern recognition receptors, IFN-γ receptors) used by phagocytic cells to respond to external activation signals can also leave the affected individuals susceptible to bacterial infections.

A second group of defects (e.g., **leukocyte adhesion defect 1 (LAD-1)** and **LAD-2** deficiencies) inhibit accessory cell function, including the ability of these cells to migrate and interact with other types of cells. For example, some leukocytes must interact with vascular endothelium to move from the vasculature into the tissues. Leukocytes of affected individuals may be unable to migrate to the organs in which lymphocyte activation occurs and to sites of infections, where they are needed to destroy and clear the infectious agents.

E. Defects in the complement system

Deficiencies in the complement system can affect both innate and adaptive immune responses (Fig. 15.6, Table 15.5). Numerous gene defects involving complement components and regulatory molecules increase susceptibility to infection and sometimes to the risk

Table 15.5

PRIMARY IMMUNE DEFICIENCY DISEASES ATTRIBUTABLE TO DEFECTS IN THE COMPLEMENT SYSTEM

Disease	Inheritance	Gene Locus	Chromosome	Consequences
C1q, C1r deficiency	Autosomal-recessive	*C1QA, C1QB, C1QC* (A, B, and C chains of C1q)	1	Increased incidence of infections; systemic lupus erythematosus (SLE) -like syndromes (type III hyper-sensitivities; see Chapter 8); impaired removal of immune complexes
		C1R or *C1S* (C1r and C1s)	12	
C2 deficiency	Autosomal-recessive	*C2*	6	SLE-like syndromes; vasculitis; impaired removal of immune complexes
C3 deficiency	Autosomal-recessive	*C3*	19	Recurrent pyogenic infections; impaired opsonization
C4 deficiency	Autosomal-recessive	*C4*	6	Increased incidence of infections; SLE-like syndromes; impaired removal of immune complexes
C5, C6, C7 deficiency	Autosomal-recessive	*C5, C6* or *C7*	9, 5, or 5	Increased susceptibility to *Neisseria*; unable to form membrane attack complex; SLE-like syndromes
C8 deficiency	Autosomal-recessive	*C8A* or *C8B* (α, β CD8 chains)	2	Increased susceptibility to *Neisseria*; unable to form membrane attack complex; SLE-like syndromes
C9 deficiency	Autosomal-recessive	*C9*	5	Increased susceptibility to *Neisseria*; unable to form membrane attack complex
Factor H deficiency	Autosomal-recessive	*CFH (Factor H gene)*	1	Recurrent pyogenic infections; increased activation of alternative pathway
Factor P (Properdin) deficiency	X-linked recessive	*PFC* (properdin factor, complement)	X	Increased susceptibility to infection, particularly by *Neisseria* ssp.; impaired alternative pathway; reduced stability of C3bBb convertase on microbial surfaces
Hereditary angio-edema	Autosomal-dominant	*SERPING1* (C1 inhibitor)	11	Excessive spontaneous activation of classical complement pathway (especially C2) causing local inflammation; swelling of tracheal and bronchial passages that can be life-threatening
Paroxysmal nocturnal hemoglo-binuria	X-linked-recessive	*PIGA* (phos phatidyl-inositol glycan)	X	Impaired synthesis of phosphatidylinositol glycan (PIG); absence of PIG prevents fixation of DAF and CD59 to the host cell membrane; unable to break down complement complexes on the host cell; excessive lysis of erythrocytes

of autoimmune disorders as well. In general, defects in the alternative pathway and mannan-binding lectin (MBL) pathways lead to increased susceptibility to infection. Defects in the classical pathway (except for C3) are not associated with significantly increased susceptibility to infection except for those caused by encapsulated bacteria. In these infections, antibodies, complement, and neutrophils are all required

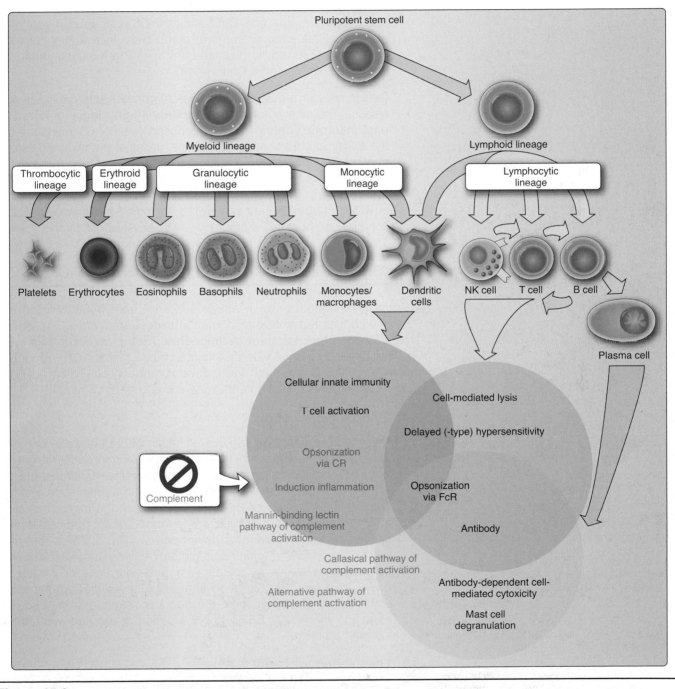

Figure 15.6

Effects of complement system deficiencies. Defective complement components can impair opsonization, lytic killing of microbes (via the membrane attack complex), and the ability to induce inflammation. Defects in regulatory components can lead to uncontrolled episodes of inflammation.

simultaneously to opsonize and kill these bacteria. **C3 deficiency** results in severe problems with recurrent infection and with immune-complex-mediated disease because of the central position of C3 in all three of the complement activation pathways.

The MBL and alternative pathways are able to generate sufficient complement-mediated protection against infection, even in the absence of the classical pathway. Deficiencies in the components of the alternative pathway (e.g., C3, B, D) are associated with increased susceptibility to infection. Deficiencies in C1, C2, and C4 can lead to inefficient clearance of immune complexes, increasing the risk of type III hypersensitivity diseases and injury to kidneys, joints, skin, and blood vessels (see Chapter 14).

Deficiencies in regulatory complement components can also cause disease. The most common is **hereditary angioedema** (or **hereditary angioneurotic edema**), in which reduced levels of C1 inhibitor reduce the ability to control activation of the classical pathway. As a result, uncontrolled inflammatory episodes occur that can become serious when the vascular system, respiratory tract, and GI tract are affected. Deficiencies in **decay accelerating factor** (DAF) or **CD59** allow accumulation of complement complexes, including the membrane attack complex, on host cell membranes with ensuing cell injury.

III. SECONDARY (ACQUIRED) IMMUNE DEFICIENCIES

Some immunodeficiency diseases arise not from genetic or developmental causes but from environmental exposures. These diseases are called **secondary immune deficiencies**. They may occur at any time of life, depending upon when exposure occurs (Table 15.6). Among the environmental factors that can induce immune deficiencies are therapeutic treatments, infections, malignancy, and general health.

A. Physiologic sequelae

Many factors that affect the overall health of the body can impair immune function. Stress, for example, has been associated not only with reduced general health, but also with impaired immune function. Among the most investigated of these environmental factors is nutrition. Malnutrition has been shown to diminish the immune system's ability to protect against infection. In some cases, reduced levels of specific dietary components have been shown to play a role in immunodeficiency. The amino acid glutamine, for example, is critical for normal levels of energy metabolism, and shortages of certain minerals and vitamins have been implicated in reduced immune function. Various reports indicate that reduced levels of iron, zinc, selenium and vitamins A, B6, C, and E are also associated with impaired immune function.

B. Therapeutic treatment

A normal individual's immune system may become suppressed, either intentionally or as a side effect of medical treatment (see Chapter 18). Transplant recipients usually undergo treatment to inhibit their immune responsiveness, at least for a period of time (see Table

Table 15.6
SOURCES OF SECONDARY IMMUNE DEFICIENCY

Cause	Examples	Mechanisms
Physiologic sequelae	General malnutrition	High impact on functions with high energy requirements
	Energy metabolism	Deficiencies of amino acids crucial for energy metabolism
	Trace metal deficiencies	Deficiencies of critical cofactors
	Vitamin deficiencies	Deficiencies of critical cofactors
Therapeutic treatment	Ionizing radiation	Damages replicating cells; induces oxidative stress
	Cytotoxic drugs (including many used for cancer treatment)	Damage/kill replicating cells
	Anti-inflammatory drugs (e.g., corticosteroids)	Interfere with production of some cytokines
	Immunosuppressive drugs (e.g., cyclosporine, tacrolimus, rapamycin)	Interfere with production of some cytokines
Infection	Human immunodeficiency virus (HIV)	Kills CD4$^+$ T cells, monocytes, and even CD8$^+$ T cells; the viral *nef* gene product also redirects pMHC I molecules from the cell surface and into lysosomes where they are degraded
	Epstein-Barr virus	Produces analog of interleukin-10
	Schistosoma	Secretes enzymes capable of cleaving immunoglobulins
	Herpesvirus	Inhibits MHC class I maturation within the endoplasmic reticulum
	Human cytomegalovirus (HCMV)	Interferes with transport of peptides into ER through TAP; redirects MHC class I molecules into cytoplasm rather than to cell surface
	Chlamydia	Interferes with phagocytic function by preventing fusion of phagosomes and lysosomes
	Staphylococcus	Produces toxin that kills phagocytic cells; produces protein that interferes with FcR-driven opsonization
	Yersinia	Produces toxin that kills phagocytes
	Streptococcus	Produces toxin that kills phagocytes
	Mycobacterium	Produces toxin that kills phagocytes; inhibits acidification within phagosomes by preventing fusion with lysosomes; inhibits oxidative degradation within phagosomes
	Salmonella	Inhibits oxidative degradation within phagosomes
	Leishmania	Inhibits oxidative degradation within phagosomes
Cancer	Multiple myeloma	Increasingly oligoclonal immune response
	Burkitt's lymphoma	Epstein-Barr virus (causative agent) produces an analog of IL-10
	Waldenström's macroglobulinemia	Excessive production of immunoglobulins; increased blood viscosity
	Chronic lymphocytic leukemia (CLL)	Reduced production of immunoglobulins
	Small lymphocytic lymphoma (SLL)	Reduced production of immunoglobulins

15.6), to heighten the chances of survival for the grafted tissue. During this treatment (and sometimes afterward), transplant recipients have a heightened susceptibility to **opportunistic infection** and must be monitored and treated to avoid the onset of overwhelming infection.

Similarly, individuals with autoimmune diseases (see Chapters 16 and 18) may be treated with agents that diminish the immune responses that are causing their problems, but again such treatment often leaves them more susceptible to opportunistic infection. Treatments aimed at other medical problems, such as cancer therapy, also injure the immune system, as they are directed at cells undergoing rapid division.

C. Infection

As was discussed in Chapter 13, many infectious organisms circumvent or evade immune responses generated against them. In many cases, these evasive tactics leave the host more susceptible to other infectious agents as well. For example, some bacteria secrete enzymes that destroy local immunoglobulins and complement components. Some bacteria and viruses protect themselves after ingestion by phagocytes by inhibition of several key phagocyte activities: fusion of phagosomes with lysosomes, synthesis and release of microcidal molecules, and presentation of peptides by MHC class I molecules. Yet other microbes (e.g., *Plasmodium*) evade the immune system by living within cells such as erythrocytes that express neither MHC class I nor II molecules on their surfaces. As a result, T cells cannot detect whether such cells are infected or not. Finally, some infectious organisms influence the entry of naïve T cells into either the Th1 or Th2 pathway, whichever is least effective for clearance of those particular microbes.

HIV (human immunodeficiency virus) destroys CD4$^+$ T cells, leading to **acquired immune deficiency syndrome (AIDS)**. HIV can also infect and kill monocytes and even CD8$^+$ T cells as the infection progresses. Because CD4$^+$ T cells are so central to the development of numerous immune responses, their progressive loss produces a gradual decline in humoral and cellular responses and an increasing susceptibility to opportunistic infection that eventually becomes fatal.

CLINICAL APPLICATION
HIV Infection and AIDS

AIDS (acquired immune deficiency) is caused by HIV (human immunodeficiency virus). HIV is a retrovirus that damages the cells of the body's immune system. People with HIV may develop opportunistic infections and various forms of cancer. The criteria for a diagnosis of AIDS are a CD4$^+$ T cell count less than 200 cells/mm^3 and the presence of at least one of the 26 different opportunistic infections, such as *Pneumocystis carinii* pneumonia, candida esophagitis, toxoplasmosis, cryptococcal meningitis, and tuberculosis caused by *Mycobacterium tuberculosis*.

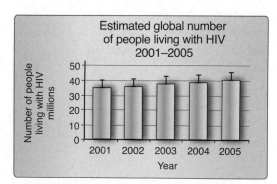

Figure 15.7
Impact of HIV/AIDS worldwide. The number of worldwide cases of HIV/AIDS has been steadily increasing. *(Data taken from: AIDS Epidemic Update. December 2005. World Health Organization and Joint United Nations Programme on HIV/AIDS).*

In 2005, it was estimated that 40 million people were living with HIV/AIDS worldwide (Fig. 15.7), with most of the HIV-infected people living in sub-Saharan Africa. Over 27 million people worldwide have died of AIDS since the first case was identified in 1980. However, since the early 1990s, the number of new cases of AIDS and HIV related to deaths has decreased significantly owing to effective antiviral therapies. These decreases have been most evident

unless the repaired cells are stem cells, the procedure constitutes passive therapy and will have to be repeated as the injected cells die. Second, once injected, the engineered cells must be able to migrate properly to the sites where they can grow and develop normally. Third, the "repaired" genes must be appropriately regulated and expressed, and the engineered cells must respond appropriately to signals affecting the expression and secretion of the new gene products. Finally, one must consider the risk that the engineering might lead to a malignant transformation or some other aberrant behavior in the engineered cell population.

Several successful attempts to treat immune deficiencies have been performed at the National Institutes of Health involving patients suffering from ADA deficiency, and in some cases, the engineering involved stem cells. While many of these patients have received considerable benefit, full functional replacement of sufficient numbers of stem cells has not yet been achieved, and the patients continue to receive periodic passive administration of engineered cells. It is hoped that continued research will improve the efficacy of these procedures.

Chapter Summary

- **Primary immune deficiencies** are caused by intrinsic genetic or congenital defects. Over 100 primary immunodeficiency diseases are known in humans, and the specific defective genes are known for many of them. Defects causing primary immune deficiencies occur in various cell lineages, affecting different sets of cells/molecules.

- **Secondary immune deficiencies** are caused by environmental factors such as infection, therapeutic treatments, cancer, and malnutrition. They may occur at any time of life, depending upon when the exposure to the causative factor(s) occurs.

- **Severe combined immunodeficiency (SCID)** is caused by defects in the combined lymphocyte lineage that impair T and B cell functions. SCID is a actually group of diseases caused by different individual genetic defects (autosomal and X-linked) that have similar functional consequences.

- **TAP deficiency** is a condition in which defects in the transporter associated with the antigen presentation (TAP) system impair the loading of peptide fragments into nascent MHC class I molecules in all nucleated cells. As a result, the number of MHC class I molecules that successfully reach the cell surface is reduced.

- **DiGeorge syndrome** results from defects in thymic development that prevent normal development and thymic education of T cells. DiGeorge syndrome varies in the severity of effects and may be accompanied by abnormalities due to abnormal development of embryologically related tissues: the aorta, the face and jaw, and the parathyroid glands.

- **Bruton's agammaglobulinemia** is a recessive X-linked disorder resulting from a defective gene (*BTK*) that encodes Bruton tyrosine kinase, an enzyme crucial to the early development of B cells. B cells are reduced in number or absent.

- **Selective IgA deficiency** is the single most common immune deficiency disease, with a frequency estimated at one to two per thousand individuals.

- **Immune deficiency with hyper-IgM** results from a defect in the gene encoding the CD40 ligand (CD154). As a result, the isotype switch does not occur normally, and individuals with this defect produce high levels of IgM but are deficient in B cells that produce IgG, IgA, or IgE.

- Defects in several different genes causing **chronic granulomatous disease** (**CGD**) encode defective enzymes and other microcidal molecules (e.g., toxic oxygen metabolites) involved in destruction and degradation of ingested microbes.

- **Chediak-Higashi syndrome** results from an inability to fuse lysosomes (carrying enzymes and microcidal molecules) with phagosomes (containing ingested microbes).

- Some immunodeficiencies (e.g., **leukocyte adhesion defect 1** (**LAD-1**) and **LAD-2** deficiencies) arise from defects in molecules needed for leukocytes to migrate and interact with each other or other cell types.

- **Hereditary angioedema**, caused by reduced levels of C1 inhibitor, reduces the ability to control activation of the classical pathway.

- **HIV** (**human immunodeficiency virus**) destroys $CD4^+$ T cells, leading to **acquired immune deficiency syndrome** (**AIDS**).

- Injection of **intravenous immunoglobulin** provides exogenous antibodies that boost insufficient intrinsic immunoglobulin levels.

- For long-term or permanent deficiencies, replacement of an immunodeficient patient's bone marrow with marrow from a normal donor may provide a permanent restoration of immune function. The requisite stem cells for lymphocytes, phagocytes, neutrophils, eosinophils, mast cells, and basophils are all present in the donated bone marrow.

Study Questions

15.1 A 2-month-old male infant presents with persistent diarrhea, signs and symptoms of *Pneumocystis carinii* pneumonia, and an oral fungal infection with *Candida albicans*. His weight is in the tenth percentile. Test results for HIV are negative by polymerase chain reaction. The most likely cause of these findings is

   A. grossly reduced levels of B cells.
   B. an X-linked inheritance of HLA genes.
   C. defective isotype switching.
   D. defective T cell function.
   E. selective IgA deficiency.

The correct answer is D. The fungal infection is highly suggestive of a T cell defect. Choices A, C, and E do not of themselves imply a deficiency in T cell function. HLA genes are autosomal, not X-linked.

15.2 A 5-year-old girl has a small deletion in chromosome 22. She has impaired thymus development with a significant deficiency in the number of functional T cells. The most likely etiology for these findings is

A. adenosine deaminase (ADA) deficiency.
B. Chediak-Higashi syndrome.
C. DiGeorge syndrome.
D. hereditary angioedema.
E. severe combined immunodeficiency (SCID).

The correct answer is C. Impaired thymic development leading to T cell dysfunction and small deletions in chromosome 22 are characteristic of DiGeorge syndrome. Thymic development is normal in all of the other choices.

15.3 A 3-year-old boy with an X-linked defect in the Bruton tyrosine kinase (BTK) gene is impaired in which of the following mechanisms?

A. antibody-mediated bacterial clearance
B. formation of the membrane attack complex
C. delayed (-type) hypersensitivity (DTH) responses
D. IFN-γ secretion by $CD4^+$ T cells
E. T cell precursor migration to the thymus

The correct answer is A. Bruton's agammaglobulinemia results in a near or total absence of B cells and immunoglobulins; hence antibody-mediated responses to microbes are severely impaired. Even in the absence of antibodies and the classical pathway of complement activation, the membrane attack complex can be generated through the MBL and alternative pathways. Antibodies are not involved in the other choices.

15.4 A 6-month-old male infant has diarrhea, extensive fungal infections, and skin rashes and has failed to gain weight. He is deficient in both T and B cell function. The thymus is of normal size. The most likely prospect for permanent restoration of normal immunity for this patient would be

A. an antibiotic "cocktail" given at regular intervals.
B. bone marrow transplantation.
C. exogenous immunoglobulins administered periodically.
D. isolation to an antiseptic environment.
E. thymic hormones given throughout his life.

The correct answer is B. The signs suggest a defect in the lymphocytic lineage. This could potentially be permanently alleviated by replacement of defective stem cells through bone marrow transplantation. Isolation is beneficial but is a severe imposition on the quality of life and constitutes protection rather than restoration of function. The remaining choices require constant repetitive application but not permanent restoration of function.

15.5 A female neonate has a malformed jaw, cardiac abnormalities, and hypocalcemia, in addition to diminished cell-mediated and B cell responses. Which of the following immune deficiencies should be included in the differential diagnosis of this patient?

A. adenosine deaminase (ADA) deficiency
B. DiGeorge syndrome
C. hereditary angioedema
D. severe combine immunodeficiency disease (SCID)
E. Wiskott-Aldrich syndrome

The correct answer is B. The defects in jaw and cardiac structure and the defective calcium metabolism (due to abnormal parathyroid development) point to aberrant development of structures derived from the third and fourth pharyngeal pouches. None of the other diseases given are associated with these accompanying features. This individual is likely to also include the thymus, and this patient is likely to have an underdeveloped thymus, which is a hallmark of DiGeorge syndrome.

15.6 A 21-year-old woman has a history since childhood of recurrent episodes of swelling of the submucosal and subcutaneous tissue of the gastrointestinal and respiratory tracts. Her C1 inhibitor level is less than 5% of the reference value. These findings support a diagnosis of

A. DiGeorge syndrome.
B. hereditary angioedema.
C. nutrition-based immune deficiency.
D. paroxysmal nocturnal hemoglobinuria.
E. Wiskott-Aldrich syndrome

The correct answer is B. Hereditary angioedema is caused by deficient levels of C1 inhibitor. DiGeorge syndrome is caused by aberrant development of the thymus. Nutrition-based immunodeficiencies are not characteristically identified by severely reduced levels of specific cell types or related molecules. Paroxysmal nocturnal hemoglobinuria is caused by a deficiency of CD59, and Wiskott-Aldrich syndrome is caused by a deficiency of the Wiskott-Aldrich syndrome protein.

15.7 A 3-month-old male infant has recurrent infections and is found to have an impaired ability to kill microbes by the nitroblue tetrazolium test (which evaluates effectiveness of degradative enzymes). Which of the following conditions is most likely responsible for the findings in this patient?

A. Chediak-Higashi syndrome
B. chronic granulomatous disease
C. hereditary angioedema
D. HIV/AIDS
E. Waldenström's macroglobulinemia

15.8 A 24-year-old male presents with fever, cough, and night sweats. Examination reveals an elevated temperature, increased respiratory rate, oral thrush (fungal infection), and decreased breath sounds in the right midlung field. Laboratory testing reveals a CD4 count of 60/μL (reference range: 400/μL). On the basis of these findings, the most likely underlying process is

A. autoimmune disease with pneumonia.
B. bacterial pneumonia.
C. HIV/AIDS with possible mycobacterium tuberculosis.
D. hypersensitivity pneumonitis.
E. *Mycobacterium tuberculosis* infection only.

The correct answer is B. Chronic granulomatous disease is caused by defects in a variety of degradative enzymes or other molecules involved in the oxidative burst. Chediak-Higashi syndrome is caused by an inability to fuse lysosomes with phagosomes. HIV/AIDS results from progressive destruction of CD4+ T cells. Although HIV can infect macrophages and dendritic cells, they remain capable of normal phagolysosome function. Hereditary angioedema results from a deficiency in C1 inhibitor, and Waldenström's macroglobulinemia is caused by excessive production of IgM.

The correct answer is C. The key feature is the extreme deficiency of CD4+ T cells that is characteristic of HIV/AIDS. None of the other choices would be associated with this finding. Respiratory difficulties due to *Mycobacterium tuberculosis* infection are frequently seen in HIV/AIDS patients.

Autoimmunity

16

I. OVERVIEW

The innate immune system relies upon a set of "hard-wired" genetically encoded receptors that have evolved to distinguish self from nonself. The adaptive immune system faces a much greater challenge in making such distinctions. The B cell receptors (BCRs) and T cell receptors (TCRs) of the adaptive immune system are randomly generated within each individual, without "preknowledge" of the epitopes that may be encountered. As a result, some BCRs and TCRs recognize nonself and others recognize self. Several mechanisms are utilized to identify and control or eliminate cells that are potentially self-reactive. The failure of these mechanisms to inactivate or eliminate self-reactive cells leads to **autoimmunity**.

Rheumatoid arthritis, some forms of diabetes, multiple sclerosis, psoriasis, and systemic lupus erythematosus, to name only a few, are autoimmune diseases. Autoimmunity is complex. It may arise by different mechanisms, and its risk is affected by a variety of environmental and genetic factors, many of which are as yet unidentified. Together, however, these various influences contribute to a breakdown in self tolerance, that is, the ability of the immune system to effectively distinguish self from nonself and to refrain from attacking self.

II. SELF TOLERANCE

Tolerance is the failure of the immune system to respond to an epitope in an aggressive way. Most **self-tolerance** results from the deliberate inactivation or destruction of lymphocytes bearing BCRs or TCRs that recognize and binds self epitopes. Inactivation or destruction may occur during early development (central tolerance) or may be imposed on lymphocytes in the periphery (peripheral tolerance). An understanding of how the immune system naturally imposes self-tolerance can provide critical clues for the development of therapeutic strategies for autoimmune diseases caused by the loss of self-tolerance.

A. Central tolerance

Central tolerance occurs during the early differentiation of B cells in the bone marrow and T cells in the thymus. Normally, both B and T cells that bind self-epitopes at distinct early stages of development meet an apoptotic death, thus eliminating large numbers of potentially self-reactive cells before they enter the circulation (see Chapter 9).

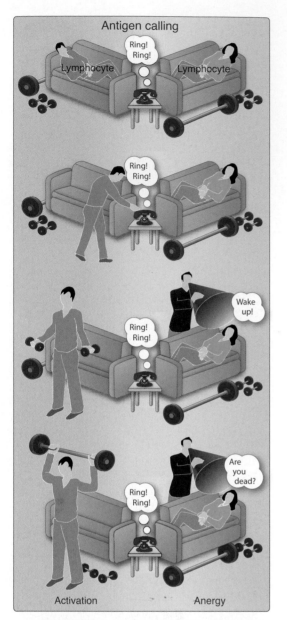

Figure 16.1
Anergy. Binding of antigen (for B cells) or pMHC (for T cells) can initiate either activation or anergy in lymphocytes.

B cells express surface IgM as their BCRs. Epitope recognition by BCRs of developing B cells within the bone marrow triggers their apoptotic death, a process known as **negative selection**. Likewise, the binding of peptide-MHC complex (pMHC I or pMHC II) by TCRs of single positive (CD4⁺CD8⁻ or CD4⁻CD8⁺) thymocytes causes them to undergo apoptotic death. This process removes many potentially autoreactive B and T cells before they enter the periphery (see Fig. 9.1). A major caveat imposed on central tolerance is that not all self-epitopes are to be found in the primary lymphoid organs, especially those self-epitopes that arise after lymphogenesis, such as those that arise during puberty. Other means are needed to prevent the autoreactive cells among them from inflicting damage on the body.

B. Peripheral tolerance

Several additional mechanisms, collectively called **peripheral tolerance,** control or eliminate autoreactive B and T cells after they exit the bone marrow or thymus. One such mechanism is the induction of **anergy**, a state of nonresponsiveness in lymphocytes after their receptors bind antigen (B cell) or pMHC (T cell) (Fig. 16.1 provides a whimsical view of anergy). Another mechanism is **suppression**, whereby regulatory cells inhibit the activity of other cells.

1. **Anergy:** Binding of TCRs to an appropriate pMHC I or pMHC II on the surface of antigen-presenting cells (APCs) provides the first signal for activation of T cells, but T cells must also receive second signals from the APCs (cytokines, etc.) for activation to proceed (see Chapter 5). Naïve CD8⁺ T cells may recognize and bind to self pMHC I on non-APCs as well as on APCs. In binding to non-APCs, engagement of their TCRs with pMHC I provides the first signal, but no second signals. Receipt of the first signal in the absence of second signals causes naïve T cells to enter a state of inactivity known as **anergy** (Fig. 16.2). So profound is this state that anergized CD8⁺ T cells usually cannot be activated by subsequent encounters with both first and second signals. There are, however, circumstances in which anergy can be broken and self-reactive CD8⁺ T cells can become activated, resulting in some autoimmune diseases. It is unclear whether CD4⁺ T cells can or cannot be anergized by comparable mechanisms because almost all binding by TCRs of CD4⁺ T cells occurs with pMHC II complexes on APCs.

    B cells can also undergo anergy. Some naïve autoreactive B cells leave the bone marrow. Their subsequent activation in the lymph nodes requires interaction with T cells, providing the necessary soluble signals and surface ligands. Like naïve CD8⁺ T cells, naïve B cells can be anergized if their surface immunoglobulins bind to self antigens in the absence of the additional necessary T cell signals.

2. **Suppression:** Tolerance to self-epitopes can also be induced by regulatory cells (Fig. 16.3). The molecular bases for these regulatory actions are still unclear, but in most cases, the regulatory cells are T cells. Examples include the following:

    •   CD4⁺CD25⁺ T cells diminish the activity of T cells stimulated by a variety of epitopes. They have been shown to have important roles in preventing development of inflammatory diseases (e.g., inflammatory bowel disease).

- Some CD8$^+$ T cells are able to inhibit the activation and proliferation of CD4$^+$ T cells, including some that mediate autoreactive type IV hypersensitivity (DTH) responses.
- CD8$^+$ and CD4$^+$ T cell subpopulations have been demonstrated, in various models, to inhibit antibody production.

Autoimmune responses vary in the pathologies they induce, and this sometimes depends upon the **Th1/Th2** balance in the responses (see Chapter 5) to a particular self antigen. For example, a Th2 response to a particular self-epitope may produce little or no pathology, but a Th1 response may produce an injurious cell-mediated inflammatory response such as DTH. As a result, the overt autoimmune disease may be determined by the relative balance in Th1 and Th2 responses generated against the epitope, and factors that influence that balance may alter the risk. Such a situation exists in the intestinal mucosal immune system of the gut-associated lymphoid tissues (see Chapter 13). Here, intestinal epithelial cells and some intraepithelial lymphocytes produce anti-inflammatory Th2 cytokines (IL-4, IL-10, and TGF-β) that create a microenvironment promoting production of IgA antibodies and inhibiting inflammatory cellular responses. Changes that favor development of Th1-like cell-mediated inflammatory responses, perhaps triggered by pathogenic bacteria, may be the basis for autoimmune **inflammatory bowel diseases** such as **Crohn's disease** and **ulcerative colitis**.

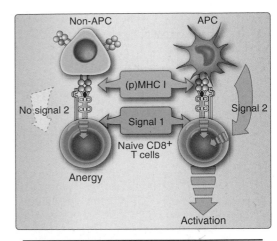

Figure 16.2
Induction of T cell anergy by binding to non-APCs. Engagement of TCRs on naïve CD8$^+$ T cells by binding to pMHC I on non-APCs provides the first signal for activation. T cells receiving signal 1 in the absence of signal 2 are anergized.

III. LOSS OF SELF-TOLERANCE

Despite the various mechanisms that are in place to prevent responses to self epitopes, autoimmunity still occurs occasionally. How does this happen? What types of situations provide opportunities for self-reactive immune cells to escape the traps set for them and become free to attack the body's cells and tissues? There are, in fact, several different situations that make this possible.

A. Molecular mimicry

Infection is frequently associated with development of autoimmunity. Experimental evidence in vitro has shown that under certain circumstances, the addition of high levels of exogenous cytokines can cause the activation of naïve T cells in the absence of interactions with APCs, and in some cases, even anergized T cells can be activated. Inflammation at sites of infection, originating with activated phagocytes responding to the presence of infectious agents, can generate elevated levels of pro-inflammatory cytokines that may mimic the effects seen in vitro. Within this setting, T cells recognizing self-epitopes may receive sufficient stimulation to become activated, even if they are not directly interacting with APCs (Fig. 16.4). While this mechanism has yet to be definitively demonstrated in vivo, the tendency for the development of autoimmune diseases to follow episodes of infection is suggestive.

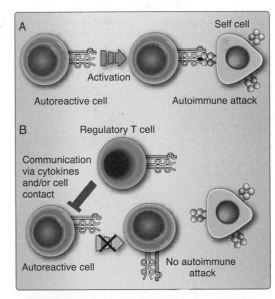

Figure 16.3
Regulatory cell inhibition. Regulatory cells (usually T cells) can prevent some responses by other lymphocytes. **A.** Autoreactive T cells that become activated can bind and attack host cells. **B.** Regulatory cells inhibit the activation of autoreactive cells and sometimes even of activated ones.

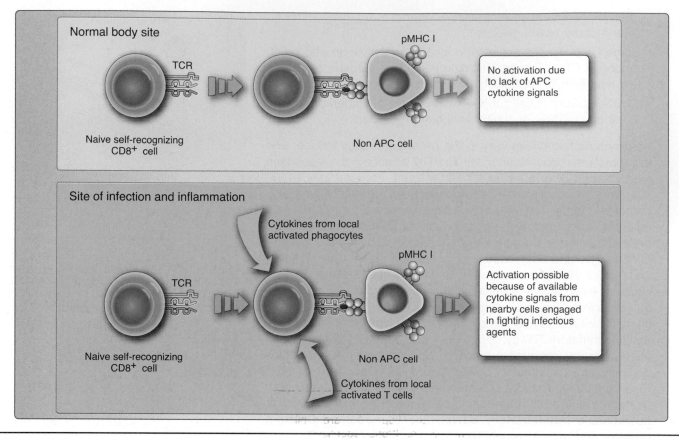

Figure 16.4
Inflammation and autoimmunity Under normal circumstances, autoreactive cells in the body are not activated by contact with self-molecules. Unless they are interacting with APCs, they are not also receiving cytokine signals necessary for activation. However, in inflammatory sites, local cytokine levels may be sufficient to activate autoreactive T cells when they are binding to self-epitopes on non-APCs.

Molecular mimicry is a process in which infection by particular microbes is associated with the subsequent development of specific autoimmune diseases. The antigenic molecules on some infectious agents are similar enough to some host self molecules that B and T cell responses generated against the microbial antigens can result in damage to host cells bearing similar molecules (Fig. 16.5). The best-understood example of this process is the cardiac damage resulting from rheumatic fever after infection by *Streptococcus pyogenes* ("strep," the causative agent of strep throat) (Fig. 16.6). Group A β-hemolytic strains of *S. pyogenes* express high levels of an antigen known as the M protein, a molecule that shares some structural similarities with molecules found on the valves and membranes of the heart. If the levels of IgM and IgG generated against the M protein during infection reach sufficient levels, there may be sufficient binding to host cells to induce damage and reduced cardiac function. In addition to cardiac sites, antibodies against the M protein can also cross-react to some degree with molecules on host cells in the joints and kidneys. The accumulated damage to cardiac and other tissues may be fatal. It is therefore important that patients who present with sore throats be tested to determine whether strep is present and, if

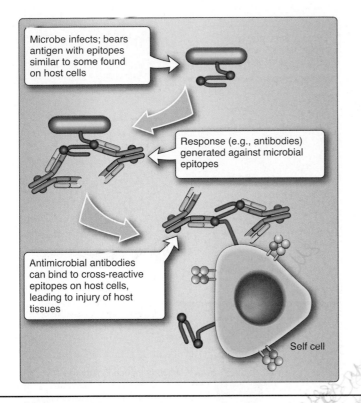

Figure 16.5
Molecular mimicry. Some microbial antigens bear epitopes that are similar to or identical to some epitopes on host molecules. Strong responses against the microbial epitopes can result in sufficient binding of host epitopes to produce immune-mediated injury.

so, to begin antibiotic therapy to clear the infection before vigorous antibody responses against strep antigens can develop.

Molecular mimicry appears to be involved in several autoimmune diseases, including diabetes. Certain peptide fragments from Coxsackie virus and cytomegalovirus cross-react with glutamate decarboxylase, a major target of autoreactive T cells found in patients with type 1 diabetes. In addition, peptides from other several viruses (e.g., cytomegalovirus, measles, hepatitis C virus) are cross-reactive with phosphatase IA-2, an enzyme produced by the pancreatic β cells, and may provide the basis for some cases of diabetes.

An association with infectious organisms has been demonstrated for several autoimmune diseases. A group of inflammatory arthritic diseases known as **reactive arthritis** occur more frequently in individuals who have had food poisoning. Two of these diseases, **ankylosing spondylitis** (usually involving the lower spine) and **Reiter's disease** (affecting the joints of the lower limbs and the gastrointestinal/genital/urinary tracts), have increased frequencies in individuals who carry the HLA-B27 gene and have been infected by *Klebsiella*. In fact, some structural similarities have been noted between the HLA-B27 molecule itself and certain proteins expressed by *Klebsiella*, suggesting a possible role for molecular mimicry. In addition,

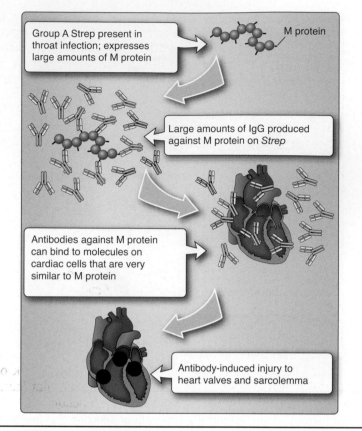

Group A Strep present in throat infection; expresses large amounts of M protein

M protein

Large amounts of IgG produced against M protein on *Strep*

Antibodies against M protein can bind to molecules on cardiac cells that are very similar to M protein

Antibody-induced injury to heart valves and sarcolemma

Figure 16.6

Association of cardiac damage and rheumatic fever. Rheumatic fever results from infection (usually of the throat) by Group A strep. High levels of antibodies can be generated against the bacterial M protein. IgG against M protein can cross-react with molecules on cardiac tissues that are highly cross-reactive with M protein. As a result, antibody-induced injury, especially to the valves and sarcolemma, can produce serious cardiac disease. Other tissues may also be affected.

the acetylcholine receptor, the self molecule that is targeted in autoimmune **myasthenia gravis**, shares some structural similarities with certain poliovirus proteins. As a whole, these data suggest that molecular mimicry could be an important factor in the generation of some autoimmune diseases.

B. Epitope spreading

Another phenomenon that may contribute to the influence of infectious organisms on autoimmunity is **epitope spreading.** The epitope that initiates a response leading to autoimmunity might not be the epitope that is targeted by immune responses that develop later during the pathogenesis of the disease. For example, initial responses against an infectious agent may result in damage that exposes self-epitopes in ways that subsequently trigger true autoimmune responses. In some animal models of human multiple sclerosis, responses to particular viral epitopes regularly precede the development of responses to specific epitopes associated with the myelin sheath that protects neuronal axons.

Additionally, the dominant self-epitope targeted by an autoimmune response does not necessarily remain constant over the course of the disease. In some experimental models of autoimmune diseases, in which a relapsing-remitting course of clinical signs may occur, these patterns may actually result from a series of independent responses generated against different self-epitopes rather than from alternating increased and decreased responses to a single epitope (Fig. 16.7). The possibility that the epitopes that initiate an autoimmune disease are different from those involved in the pathogenesis complicates attempts to devise therapies. Epitope spreading is suspected to play a role in several autoimmune diseases, including systemic lupus erythematosus, inflammatory bowel disease (Crohn's disease and ulcerative colitis), multiple sclerosis, pemphigus vulgaris, and some forms of diabetes.

C. Loss of suppression

Suppressor cells of various types serve to maintain peripheral tolerance. Evidence suggests that the numbers of these suppressor cells decline with age, increasing the risk that previously suppressed autoreactive lymphocytes can become active. A pattern of increasing risk with increasing age is indeed seen in some autoimmune diseases, such as **systemic lupus erythematosus (SLE)**. However, it can be difficult to differentiate between an increase in risk due to changes that result from aging and the simple fact that increased age provides more opportunity for a disease to occur.

D. Sequestered antigens

Some self-molecules are "sequestered" and are normally never exposed to the immune system for various reasons. As a result, if they do become exposed, as a result of injury for example, the immune system may view them as foreign and attack them. Among the best-understood examples of sequestered antigens are those associated with spermatogonia and developing sperm within the lumen of testicular tubules. The tubules are sealed off early in embryonic development, prior to development of the immune system, by enclosure within a sheath of tightly joined Sertoli cells. Immune cells do not penetrate the barrier presented by the Sertoli cells and therefore are never exposed to self-molecules that are unique to the testicular tubule lumen. If these are exposed by injury (or by procedures such as surgery or vasectomy), immune responses may occur against the self (but seemingly foreign) molecules. It is believed that some cases of male sterility are caused by this mechanism.

Collectively, sites in the body that are associated with some degree of isolation from the immune system are called **immunologically privileged sites**. In addition to the lumen of the testicular tubule, these sites include the cornea and the anterior chamber of the eye, the brain, and the uterine environment during pregnancy. The reduced vasculature of the cornea and the fluid-filled chamber of the anterior chamber of the eye, together with other immunosuppressive mechanisms, may help to protect the delicate structures of the eye from the damage and permanent injury that could follow strong inflammatory responses. For example, the fluid in the anterior chamber of the eye contains many anti-inflammatory molecules. In addition, cells in

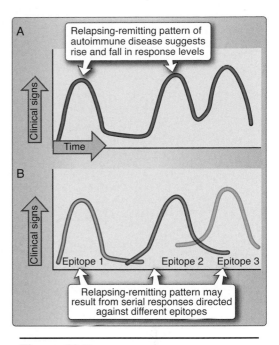

Figure 16.7
Association of autoimmune diseases with serial responses to different epitopes.
A. Some autoimmune diseases have alternating periods of exacerbation and remission of clinical signs (relapsing-remitting pattern). **B.** In some models of human autoimmune disease, the relapsing phases of exacerbation have been shown to be due to a series of newly generated responses to different epitopes.

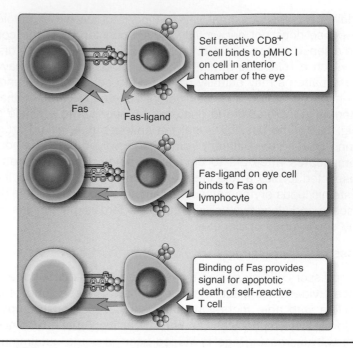

Figure 16.8

Role of Fas-ligand in protection of cells within immunologically privileged sites. Fas-ligand is widely expressed on cells in the anterior chamber of the eye. When autoimmune T cells attempt to bind to cells of the anterior chamber, Fas-ligand binds to Fas molecules expressed by T cells. This binding induces apoptotic death of the Fas-bearing cell (in this case, the T cell), and immune-mediated damage to the cells of the anterior chamber is avoided.

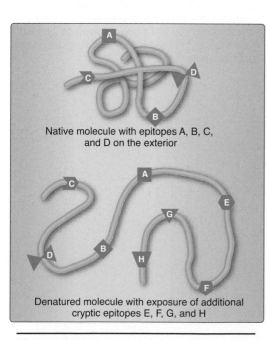

Figure 16.9

Cryptic epitopes. Some epitopes may not be readily available to the immune system because they are protected within the three dimensional structure of a molecule. A structural change in the molecule, such as cleavage or denaturation, may make these cryptic epitopes more accessible to antibodies.

the anterior of the eye widely express the **Fas-ligand** molecule (CD178) on their surface. When Fas-ligand binds to **Fas** (CD95) on activated T cells, those T cells undergo an apoptotic death (Fig. 16.8). Thus cells in the anterior chamber can protect themselves by killing autoreactive T cells that bind to them. Another mechanism helps to protect the brain. The **blood-brain barrier** consists of dense, tightly packed vascular endothelium that limits the flow of cells and large molecules from the vasculature into the brain, thus decreasing the ability of the immune system to infiltrate the brain. Again, the blood-brain barrier is thought to be beneficial because strong inflammatory responses could easily inflict irreparable damage upon the brain.

Molecules may also sometimes possess a type of immunologically privileged site. The three-dimensional configurations of some molecules may shelter epitopes in the interior from contact with the immune system. If the molecule is altered by denaturation or cleavage, however, the "hidden" internal epitopes may become exposed and available for recognition and binding by antibodies (Fig. 16.9). These are termed **cryptic epitopes**. The presence of rheumatoid factor, associated with inflammatory rheumatoid diseases, provides an example of this phenomenon (Fig. 16.10). The binding of IgG molecules trigger conformational changes in their Fc regions that expose "hidden" sites, some of which facilitate the binding of complement or Fc

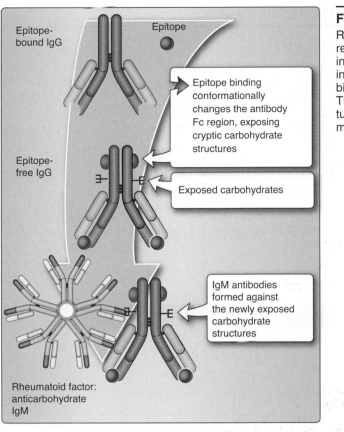

Figure 16.10

Rheumatoid factor. Rheumatoid factor (IgM produced against IgG) results from recognition of cryptic epitopes. Binding of antibodies, including IgG, to their epitopes produce a conformational change in the Fc region, exposing sites that become available for the binding of complement and recognition by cellular Fc receptors. The exposed sites include previously cryptic carbohydrate structures that, once available, can be recognized and bound by IgM molecules.

Epitope-bound IgG

Epitope

Epitope binding contormationally changes the antibody Fc region, exposing cryptic carbohydrate structures

Epitope-free IgG

Exposed carbohydrates

IgM antibodies formed against the newly exposed carbohydrate structures

Rheumatoid factor: anticarbohydrate IgM

receptors and some of which expose cryptic carbohydrate structures that can be recognized and bound by IgM antibodies. IgM antibodies directed at the cryptic carbohydrate structures on antigen-bound IgG molecules are called **rheumatoid factors**. The binding of IgM to IgG augments the formation of immune complexes and the activation of complement (see Chapter 14). The presence of rheumatoid factor is associated with several inflammatory autoimmune diseases.

E. Neoantigens

Responses to neoantigens may mimic autoimmune responses. **Neoantigens** are self antigens that have been modified by some extrinsic factor (e.g., binding of a reactive chemical) so that they appear foreign to the immune system. Thus they are not true autoantigens, and the reactions against them are not truly autoimmune. However, the effects of responses to neoantigens can be nearly identical to those against autoantigens. Some responses that are currently classified as autoimmune may in fact be due to neoantigens created by some unknown environmental agent. One feature that distinguishes responses against neoantigens from true autoimmune responses is that responses to neoantigens should cease if the agent responsible for creation of the neoantigens is removed. True autoantigens, by contrast, persist for the individual's lifetime and continue to stimulate autoimmune responses unless they are destroyed and eliminated.

IV. AUTOIMMUNE DISEASES

Table 16.1 lists several human autoimmune diseases. These diseases involve numerous different molecules, cells, and tissues that are targeted by the autoimmune responses. Some autoimmune diseases are systemic or diffuse, because of the distribution of the target antigens. For example, SLE and rheumatoid arthritis affect a variety of joints and other body tissues. Other diseases affect specific organs and tissues. Examples include:

- Crohn's disease (intestine)
- Goodpasture's disease (kidney and lung)
- Hashimoto's thyroiditis (thyroid gland)
- Insulin-dependent diabetes mellitus type I (β cells of the pancreas)

Table 16.1
AUTOIMMUNE DISEASES

Affected Tissue	Disease	Target Antigen
Anterior parts of the eye	Uveitis (anterior)	Beta B1-crystalin, other proteins of the ciliary body epithelium
Connective tissue	Scleroderma	Scl-70, PM-Scl antigens
Erythrocytes	Autoimmune hemolytic anemia	Erythrocyte surface molecules
Heart valves and sarcolemmal membranes	Rheumatic fever	Streptococcal M protein, cardiac muscle antigens
Joints of lower extremities; sometimes eyes and genital, urinary, or GI systems	Reiter's disease (reactive arthritis)	Possible association with infectious agents
Kidneys, lungs	Goodpasture's syndrome	Type IV collagen of basement membranes
Large intestine	Ulcerative colitis	Unknown
Lower spine	Ankylosing spondylitis	Unknown
Myelin of the central nervous system	Multiple sclerosis	Myelin proteins (several)
Pancreatic islet β cells	Type I insulin-dependent diabetes mellitus (IDDM)	Glutamate decarboxylase, preproinsulin, other β cell products
Platelets	Thrombocytic purpura	Platelet integrin molecules
Skeletal muscle	Myasthenia gravis	Acetylcholine receptor
Skeletal muscle	Polymyositis	Jo-1, PM-Scl antigens
Skin	Pemphigus vulgaris	Desmoglein-3
Skin	Psoriasis	Unknown, but there is some association with streptococcal infections
Skin, vasculature, muscle, joints, kidney	Systemic lupus erythematosus (SLE)	Nucleic acids, chromosomal proteins
Small intestine	Crohn's disease	Unknown
Spermatogonia, sperm	Male sterility (??)	Unknown
Synovial membranes, joints	Rheumatoid arthritis	Unknown
Tear ducts	Sjögren's syndrome	Ro/SS-A antigens
Thyroid gland	Graves' disease	TSH receptor
Thyroid gland	Hashimoto's thyroiditis	Thyroglobulin

- Multiple sclerosis (white matter of the brain and spinal cord)
- Sjögren's syndrome (tear ducts)

Autoimmune diseases can result from damage inflicted on cells and tissues by humoral responses, cell-mediated immune responses, or both. It should be noted that the assignment of humoral or cell-mediated damage is sometimes based on data from experimental models.

A. Humoral-associated autoimmune diseases

Some autoimmune diseases result from the binding of self-reactive antibodies, leading to Type II and Type III hypersensitivity responses. The antibodies responsible for initiating the diseases are usually of the IgG isotype, although IgM antibodies can contribute as well. The activation of complement and the opsonization of injured cells promote inflammatory responses that increase the damage inflicted on the targeted cells and tissues. Autoreactive T cells are typically present as well, but their role is primarily the activation of the autoreactive B cells rather than directly attacking host cells. Examples of these autoimmune diseases include:

- Autoimmune hemolytic anemia: type II hypersensitivity
- Goodpasture's syndrome: type II hypersensitivity
- Hashimoto's thyroiditis: type II hypersensitivity
- Rheumatic fever: type II hypersensitivity
- Rheumatoid arthritis: type III hypersensitivity
- Systemic lupus erythematosus: type II and type III hypersensitivity

B. Cell-mediated autoimmune diseases

Type IV hypersensitivity responses involve cell-mediated injury leading to autoimmune disease. These may include cytotoxic T cell responses or macrophages driven by DTH responses. The inflammation that is generated can eventually involve numerous simultaneously ongoing responses. In some diseases, particular antibodies may also be characteristically present, but they have not been demonstrated to contribute to the disease pathologies. The following are examples of autoimmune diseases involving type IV hypersensitivity responses. Rheumatoid arthritis provides an example of an autoimmune disease that involves both humoral and cell-mediated injury.

- Insulin-dependent diabetes mellitus (type 1)
- Multiple sclerosis
- Reactive arthritis
- Rheumatoid arthritis

V. HLA ASSOCIATION WITH AUTOIMMUNE DISEASES

The risks for many autoimmune diseases appear to be associated with the presence of particular HLA genes (Table 16.2). In some cases (e.g., HLA-B27 and HLA-DR3), a single HLA gene is associated with increased risk for multiple autoimmune diseases. The molecular

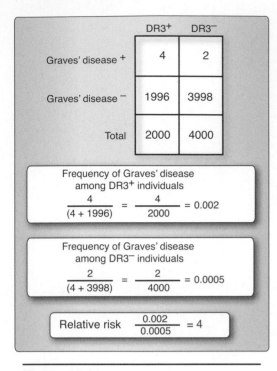

Figure 16.11
Relative risk. The statistical association between an autoimmune disease and a specific HLA gene is expressed as the relative risk. Relative risk is the ratio between the incidence of the disease among carriers of the gene in question and the incidence among noncarriers.

mechanisms underlying these statistical associations are still uncertain but presumably involve some influence on processing and presentation of self epitopes to self-reactive T cells.

The strength of the statistical association between a particular HLA gene and a particular autoimmune disease is expressed as the **relative risk.** The relative risk compares the frequency of the particular disease among carriers of a particular HLA gene with the frequency among non-carriers (Fig. 16.11). For example, the relative risk of 6 for the association of SLE with HLA-DR3 means that SLE occurs approximately three times more frequently among DR3$^+$ individuals than among DR3$^-$ individuals. Relative risk calculations are made within defined populations, and results may vary among groups of different ethnic or geographic origin.

Because genetics is only one of several possible factors contributing to the risk of a particular autoimmune disease, most relative risks are modest, in the range of 2 to 5. However, some HLA genes display much higher associations. For example, HLA-B27 and ankylosing spondylitis have relative risks around 100, and over 90% of individuals with ankylosing spondylitis are B27$^+$. The impact of relative risk should also be considered in the context of actual frequency. A disease occurring at a rate of 3 per million in one group and 1 per million in the other has a relative risk of 3, but the practical impact is diluted by the rarity of the condition.

Table 16.2
MHC ASSOCIATIONS WITH AUTOIMMUNE DISEASES

Disease	HLA Gene[a]	Relative Risk[b]
Acute uveitis	B27	10
Ankylosing spondylitis	B27	100
Goodpasture's syndrome	DR2	15
Graves' disease	DR3	4
Hashimoto's thyroiditis	DR5	3
Type I insulin-dependent diabetes mellitus	DR3/DR4 heterozygote	20–25
Multiple sclerosis	DR2	5
	DR3	10
Myasthenia gravis	DR3	3
	B8	3
Pemphigus vulgaris	DR4	15
Psoriasis vulgaris	Cw6	5–13
Reiter's disease	B27	35
Rheumatoid arthritis	DR4	4
Systemic lupus erythematosus	DR3	6

[a]Studies done in different populations may implicate different genes.
[b]Relative risks can vary among different studies. Values given are typical.

Chapter Summary

- **Tolerance** is the failure to respond in an aggressive way against an epitope recognized by the immune system.

- **Autoimmunity** results from a loss of **self-tolerance** through the failure to inactivate or eliminate self-reactive cells.

- **Central tolerance** occurs in the primary lymphoid organs (bone marrow and thymus) during the early development of B and T cells.

- **Peripheral tolerance** results from mechanisms that inactivate or eliminate B and T cells that are in circulation.

- **Anergy** (inactivation) of B and T cells occurs when naïve lymphocytes bind via their BCR or TCR ("first signal") but fail to receive the second signals provided by T cells (for B cells) and APCs (for T cells) that are necessary for activation.

- Suppressor T cells inhibit responses by other immune cells.

- Loss of self tolerance may occur through molecular mimicry, epitope spreading, loss of suppression, or the exposure of sequestered antigens.

- **Molecular mimicry** involves the generation of responses to microbial epitopes that may cross-react with host epitopes that are structurally very similar to the microbial ones.

- **Epitope spreading** occurs when a response to an epitope leads to the generation of responses to one or more other epitopes.

- Suppressor T cell numbers may decline with age, permitting other self-reactive cells to escape regulation and initiate autoimmune diseases.

- Sequestered antigens are located in anatomical sites that are normally sheltered from the immune system by specialized anatomic structures or other mechanisms.

- **Neoantigens** are not self-antigens but may lead to conditions that mimic autoimmunity. If the condition creating the neoantigens is removed, the condition should be resolved. Responses to true self-antigens, on the other hand, should be permanent as a rule.

- Numerous autoimmune diseases have been identified. Their effects are determined largely by the localization of the self-epitope. Some diseases, such as systemic lupus erythematosus and rheumatoid arthritis, are systemic and affect several body sites simultaneously. Others, such as Hashimoto's thyroiditis and Sjögren's syndrome, affect specific tissues or organs.

- Autoimmune pathology may result from antibody-initiated damage (hypersensitivity types II and III), cell-mediated responses (type IV hypersensitivity), or both.

- Some autoimmune diseases have elevated frequencies in individuals carrying certain HLA genes. The statistical association between the disease and the HLA gene is expressed as the **relative risk**.

Study Questions

16.1 The failure to inactivate or eliminate self-reactive cells results in

    A. autoimmunity.
    B. positive selection.
    C. negative selection.
    D. suppression.
    E. tolerance.

> The correct answer is A. Autoimmunity results from the failure to inactivate or eliminate self-reactive immune cells. Positive selection is the promotion of lymphocytes that can function within the body. Suppression, negative selection, and tolerance are various mechanisms by which the immune system produces tolerance.

16.2 Failure of the immune system to respond against an epitope in an aggressive way is termed

    A. autoimmunity.
    B. positive selection.
    C. negative selection.
    D. suppression.
    E. tolerance.

> The correct answer is E. Tolerance is the failure to generate a destructive response against an epitope that the immune system recognizes.

16.3 Deliberate inactivation or destruction of lymphocytes bearing BCRs or TCRs capable of recognizing and binding specific self-epitopes results in

    A. hypersensitivity.
    B. autoimmunity.
    C. molecular mimicry.
    D. positive selection.
    E. self tolerance.

> The correct choice is E. The inactivation or destruction of lymphocytes bearing particular antigen receptors is one of the mechanisms producing tolerance. Hypersensitivity responses are heightened and destructive. Autoimmunity results from the absence of self tolerance. Mimicry is a means of breaking tolerance. Positive selection is the promotion of lymphocytes that bear receptors capable of particular self-molecules.

16.4 Lymphocytes expressing both the CD4 and CD25 markers on their surfaces function as

    A. antigen-presenting cells.
    B. autoantibody-secreting B cells.
    C. cytotoxic T cells.
    D. natural killer-like T cells.
    E. T regulatory cells

> The correct answer is E. $CD4^+CD25^+$ T cells are a regulatory subset of T cells. They do not act as antigen-presenting cells, nor do they secrete antibodies. Cytotoxic T cells are $CD8^+$. They do not belong to the natural killer-like T cell subset of T cells.

16.5 During an infection with *Streptococcus pyogenes*, an individual generated sufficiently high levels of IgM and IgG antibodies against a *S. pyogenes* antigen with structural similarity with molecules on the heart that cardiac damage was caused. In this example, the microbe contributed to autoimmunity via a process known as

    A. anergy.
    B. central tolerance.
    C. epitope spreading.
    D. loss of suppression.
    E. molecular mimicry.

> The correct answer is E. Molecular mimicry contributes to autoimmunity by triggering responses with microbial molecules that are cross-reactive with host molecules. Anergy and central tolerance are mechanisms for preventing autoimmunity. Epitope spreading involves the generation of responses to a series of different antigens, not to cross-reactive ones. The loss of suppression is a different mechanism by which tolerance can be broken.

16.6 A previously healthy 12-year-old female lost eight pounds over the past several weeks without dieting. Her parents are concerned about this weight loss and believe that she has an eating disorder. The patient's history reveals polydipsia (excessive thirst), polyuria (excessive urination), and nocturia over the last several weeks. A fasting blood glucose of 460 mg/dl is obtained (reference range: 70 to 100 mg/dl). The patient is diagnosed with an autoimmune disease. On the basis of these findings, which of the following conditions was most likely diagnosed in this patient?

A. anorexia nervosa
B. hyperthyroidism
C. nephrolithiasis (kidney stones)
D. type 1 diabetes mellitus
E. urinary tract infection

The correct answer is D. Type I diabetes mellitus is the autoimmune disease, among those listed, that impairs regulation of blood glucose levels. Some forms of hyperthyroidism can result from autoimmune diseases attacking thyroid receptors. Anorexia nervosa, nephrolithiasis, and urinary tract infections are not autoimmune diseases.

16.7 In Question 16.6, a defect or deficiency in which of the following is associated with the patient's condition?

A. adipose tissue
B. kidney tubules
C. pancreatic β cells
D. thyroid gland
E. skeletal muscle

The correct answer is C. Destruction of pancreatic β cells reduces insulin production. The other tissues listed are not targets of the autoimmune attack, although they may incur later secondary damage if the primary disease is not sufficiently treated and controlled.

16.8 A previously healthy 65-year-old female presents with complaints of frequent bowel movements, weight loss, and nervousness. Her physical examination was remarkable for slight exophthalmos (protrusion of the eyeball) and atrial fibrillation (abnormal heart rhythm). Laboratory findings supported a diagnosis of Graves' disease. Which of the following tissues/organs will be most affected by the ensuing immune reactions?

A. connective tissue
B. joints of lower extremities
C. heart valves
D. kidneys
E. thyroid gland

The correct answer is E. Graves' disease results from autoimmune responses targeting the thyroid gland. The other tissues and organs listed are not targets of the autoimmune responses producing Graves' disease.

16.9 Graves' disease is an example of which of the following immunologic processes?

A. autoimmune disease associated with HLA gene B27
B. autoimmune disease associated with HLA gene DR3
C. immune deficiency associated with HLA gene DR2
D. immune deficiency associated with HLA gene DR4
E. type III hypersensitivity associated with HLA gene Cw6

The correct answer is B. Graves' disease is an autoimmune disease that is associated with the presence of the HLA-DR3 gene. It is not associated with HLA-B27, -DR2, -DR4, or -Cw6. It does not result from immunodeficiency.

16.10 A 35-year-old male presents with symptoms of fatigue, paresthesia (numbness and tingling) of his arms and legs, and occasional blurred vision of two months' duration. Tests reveal several areas of demyelination within the central nervous system. Diagnosis of which of the following conditions is supported by these findings?

A. ankylosing spondylitis
B. Hashimoto thyroiditis
C. multiple sclerosis
D. reactive arthritis
E. systemic lupus erythematosus

The correct answer is C. Multiple sclerosis is an autoimmune disease that results in demyelination within the central nervous system. Ankylosing spondylitis and reactive arthritis involve joints, Hashimoto's thyroiditis involves the thyroid gland, and systemic lupus erythematosus is a systemic disease with primary effects on joints, muscles, skin, and kidneys.

16.11 Which of the following is the underlying immunological process in ankylosing spondylitis?

A. autoimmune disease associated with HLA gene B27
B. development of autoantibodies against nucleic acids
C. immune mediated destruction of neurons
D. immune deficiency associated with HLA gene DR4
E. molecular mimicry of the acetylcholine receptor

The correct answer is A. Ankylosing spondylitis is an autoimmune disease in which over 90% of people with the disease carry the HLA-B27 gene. The autoimmune response does not target nucleic acids or acetylcholine receptors. It is not an immune deficiency disease.

16.12 A 30-year-old female presents with fatigue, weight loss, arthritis of her hands, and a malar ("butterfly") rash. Blood tests reveal decreased hemoglobin and the presence of antinuclear antibodies. These findings support which of the following diagnoses paired with its underlying immunologic process?

A. Graves' disease: autoantibodies to thyroid stimulating hormone receptor
B. myasthenia gravis: autoimmunity associated with HLA gene DR3
C. Reiter syndrome: immune-mediated destruction associated with HLA gene B27
D. rheumatoid arthritis: immune deficiency associated with HLA gene DR4
E. systemic lupus erythematosus; autoantibodies to chromosomal proteins

The correct answer is E. Systemic lupus erythematosus results from the generation of autoimmune antibodies against chromosomal proteins (and nucleic acids). It is associated with the presence of HLA-DR3, but not -B27 or -DR4. Myasthenia gravis results from autoantibodies against acetylcholine receptors on muscle cells. Reiter's syndrome and rheumatoid arthritis target joints. The thyroid gland is not a target of the antinuclear antibodies.

16.13 A 55-year-old female presents with complaints of pain and stiffness in her hands and wrists that occurs mainly in the morning. Examination reveals tenderness and swelling in both wrists and hands. Testing reveals the presence of rheumatoid factor. The patient is diagnosed with rheumatoid arthritis. Resulting injury that will likely occur in this patient will result from

A. both cell mediated and humoral immunity.
B. both type II and type III hypersensitivity.
C. IgE-mediated immune responses only.
D. self tolerance.
E. type II hypersensitivity only.

The correct answer is A. Rheumatoid arthritis involves damage inflicted by both antibody-driven type III hypersensitivity responses and cellular type IV hypersensitivity responses. It does not involve type II hypersensitivity responses or IgE mediated (type I) responses. It results from the loss of self-tolerance.

16.14 A 47-year-old-male has a history of end-stage renal failure and required a kidney transplant. Approximately four weeks after receiving his transplanted kidney, he developed oliguria (decreased production of urine), fever, hypertension, and pain or tenderness over the allograft. On the basis of these findings, the most likely underlying immunological process is

A. autoimmunity.
B. acute rejection.
C. chronic rejection.
D. hyperacute rejection.
E. peripheral tolerance.

The correct answer is B. The time span is appropriate for acute rejection of the transplanted organ but not for chronic or hyperacute rejection. There is no information suggesting autoimmunity. Peripheral tolerance is a mechanism for preventing responses to self-antigens.

16.15 A 20-year-old woman presents with right lower abdominal cramp-type pain associated with diarrhea and weight loss . Blood tests reveal a low hemoglobin level and high white blood cell counts. She is diagnosed with Crohn's disease. The tissue that is most affected in this autoimmune disease is

A. connective tissue.
B. erythrocytes.
C. pancreatic β cells.
D. the small intestine.
E. the thyroid.

The correct answer is D. Crohn's disease targets the small intestine. It is not directed at connective tissue, erythrocytes, pancreatic β cells, or the thyroid gland.

Transplantation

17

I. OVERVIEW

The ability to replace or restore damaged tissues, or even whole body parts, has long been a dream of the healing professions. The broad application of transplantation in human medicine has been available only for the past five or six decades. Among the obstacles that had to be overcome were infection control, the genetic matching of donors with hosts, an understanding of the immunologic processes involved, and the development of agents that could inhibit the immune system. The development of antiseptic techniques coupled with antibiotics reduced the risk of infection, while tissue typing and immunosuppressive drugs increased the probability of transplant success.

II. GENETIC BASIS OF TRANSPLANTATION

The genetic basis for transplantation was recognized in the early twentieth century by pioneers such as Loeb, Tyzzer, and Little. The genetic match (similarity/disparity) between the donor and the host is perhaps the most important factor determining the likelihood of a successful transplant. The recipient's immune system looks for certain genetically encoded molecules (**histocompatibility antigens**) on the surfaces of the donor cells. Thus the response against transplanted cells and tissues has parallels to the body's response to foreign infectious organisms.

A. Histocompatibility genes and antigens

Histocompatibility genes encode histocompatibility antigens. It is estimated that there are several scores of such loci, probably more than a hundred. Among these are the MHC class I and II molecules encoded within the **major histocompatibility complex** (**MHC**). With the possible exception of a few loci whose expression is not understood, the products of histocompatibility genes are codominantly expressed. **Codominance** means that they are expressed whether present as a single copy (heterozygous or hemizygous) or two copies (homozygous). Thus an individual heterozygous at a particular histocompatibility locus (e.g., $H1^a/H^b$) would simultaneously express both $H1^a$ and $H1^b$ molecules on the same surface cell surface (Fig. 17.1). The same would be true for other histocompatibility loci (e.g., $H2^a/H2^b, H3^a/H3$).

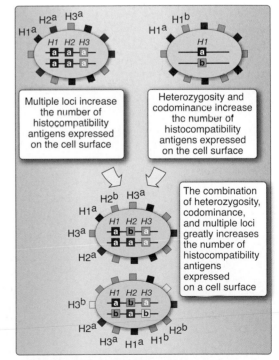

Figure 17.1
Histocompatibility antigens.

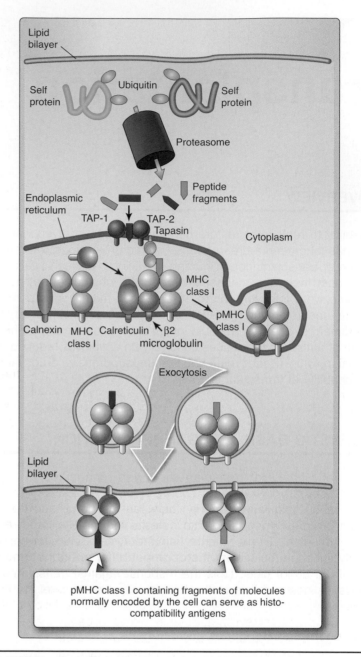

Figure 17.2
Display of histocompatibility antigens. Peptide fragments that result from proteasome degradation of cytoplasmic molecules and their subsequent loading onto MHC I molecules in the endoplasmic reticulum are present on the surface of all nucleated cells.

The structures and functions are known for only a very few of these molecules, namely, the MHC class I and II molecules. Little is known about the other non-MHC histocompatibility antigens except that they include molecules encoded by a large number of genes scattered among all of the chromosomes (including X and Y). In principle, any peptide fragment brought to the cell surface and presented by either MHC class I or II molecules could serve as a histocompatibility antigen (Fig. 17.2). Such fragments could be derived from cytosolic proteins or from cell debris ingested and degraded by phagocytic cells. The important distinction is that the molecules are encoded within the transplanted donor cells and not derived from infectious agents.

B. Types of grafts

Transplants may be categorized by location or by the genetic relationship between the recipient and the donor. With respect to location, tissues or organs that are placed in their normal anatomic location are called **orthotopic** grafts. However, many transplanted tissues or organs can function quite well in other sites as well. Grafts that are placed into a site other than their normal one are called **heterotopic** grafts. Heterotopic grafts are especially useful in cases in which orthotopic placement may be technically difficult.

Classification of grafts by the donor-recipient genetic relationship (Fig. 17.3) is more complex. **Autografts** are those transferred from one part of an individual to another location on that same individual. **Syngeneic** grafts are those transferred between different individuals who are genetically identical or nearly so (e.g., identical twins or members of an inbred strain). **Allogeneic** grafts (or **allografts**) are transferred between two genetically disparate individuals of the same species (e.g., brother and sister, parent and child, or totally unrelated individuals). Finally, **xenogeneic** grafts (or **xenografts**) are those exchanged between members of different species (e.g., the placement of primate hearts into human recipients).

C. The laws of transplantation

The **laws of transplantation** were originally established in experimental studies, particularly in mice, but are applicable to human transplantation as well. Genetic diversity in humans virtually ensures that no two individuals are genetically identical (identical twins are an exception). The histocompatibility antigens of concern in transplantation vary from one case to another, depending upon what specific genetic differences are present in each donor-recipient combination (Fig. 17.4). Experimental animals and plants can be deliberately bred to reduce their genetic heterogeneity so that genetic variability becomes a controlled variable rather than an uncontrolled one. This process, called **inbreeding**, is accomplished by mating of closely related individuals. When laboratory mice are subjected to brother-sister matings for 20 or more consecutive generations, **inbred strains** are produced. The animals within a given inbred strain are hypothetically homozygous for more than 99% of their genetic loci and, for practical purposes, are all genetically identical.

Transplants between members of the same inbred strains and between members of different inbred strains were used to deduce the laws of transplantation, which can be summarized as *a host can recognize as foreign, and mount a response against, any histocompatibility antigen not encoded within its own cells* (Fig. 17.5). Grafts exchanged between individuals of the same species who are completely different (homozygous for different alleles) at a histocompatibility locus can potentially be rejected. Such differences do not necessarily

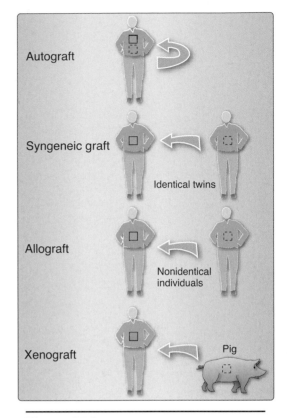

Figure 17.3
Classification of grafts by donor-recipient genetic relationship.

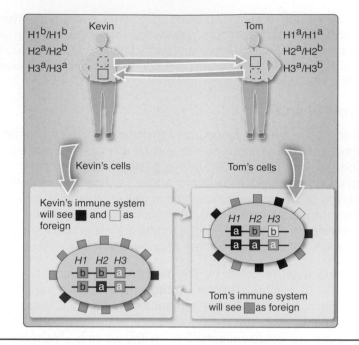

Figure 17.4

Histocompatibility differences vary among donor-recipient combinations. Which donor antigens stimulate the recipient immune response depends upon the specific combination of donor and recipient histocompatibility genes involved.

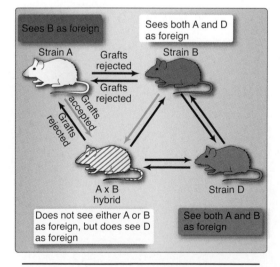

Figure 17.5

Laws of transplantation.

cause rejection on every occasion, for a variety of reasons, but the potential is always present. Each member in the exchange will recognize the allelic form of the histocompatibility antigen expressed by the other as foreign. Heterozygous recipients, on the other hand, will see nothing foreign on grafts received from homozygous parental donors. Heterozygous grafts placed onto either type of homozygous parental type recipients will be rejected, as they express histocompatibility antigens that are foreign to one or the other parental recipient.

The utility of inbred strains can be extended by further subjecting them to programs of selection and breeding that utilize normal genetic recombination for the transfer of small chromosomal segments from one inbred strain to another. These new sets of inbred animals are called **coisogenic strains,** and they permit comparisons among organisms that differ from one another by only a small section of a chromosome or, conversely, that have only a small chromosomal segment in common (Fig. 17.6). Comparisons among coisogenic strains allow the mapping and analysis of individual histocompatibility genes within the transferred segment.

The most thoroughly characterized histocompatibility genes are those encoding the MHC class I and II molecules. As was discussed in Chapter 6, the MHC class I and II molecules are normally quite polymorphic within populations. As a result, MHC class I and II

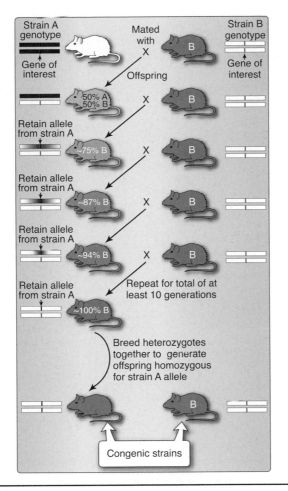

Figure 17.6
Congenic strains. Congenic strains, attained by systemic breeding and selection, differ only by small chromosomal regions.

molecules (or, more precisely, fragments of different MHC I and II molecules being presented on intact and normally functioning MHC class I and II molecules) that differ between a host and a donor are readily recognized as foreign and trigger host immune responses directed against the donor cells (Figs. 17.7A and 17.7B). Foreign MHC molecules (especially the class I molecules) present a strong barrier to transplant survival, and it has been estimated that 5% to 10% of an individual's $CD8^+$ T cells can recognize and bind fragments of foreign MHC class I.

A number of different characteristics have been noted that distinguish the effects on transplantation of differences between host and donor at MHC I and II loci from those of differences at non-MHC (or minor) histocompatibility loci (Table 17.1). While exceptions can often be found, there are valid generalizations that can be made.

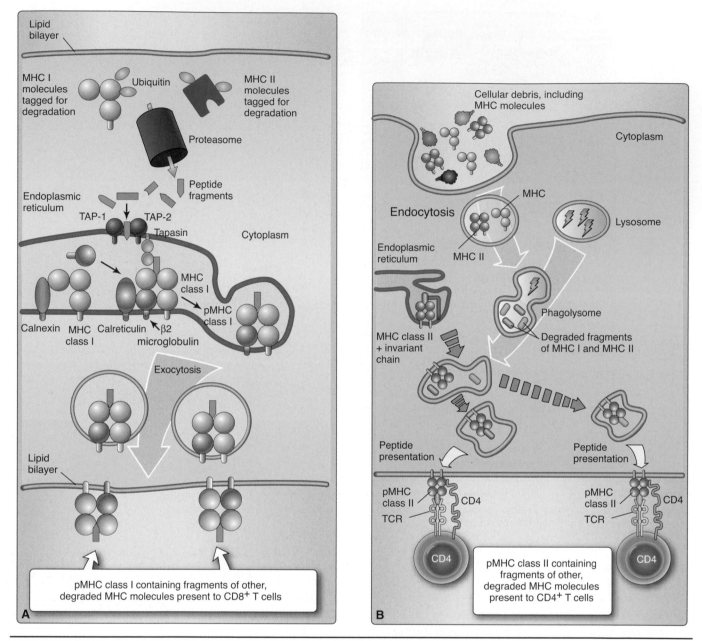

Figure 17.7
Fragments of MHC I and II molecules can be presented as histocompatibility antigens by intact MHC I and MHC II molecules. **A.** Erroneously translated, misfolded or otherwise damaged cytoplasmically synthesized MHC class I and II molecules may be ubiquinated and degraded by proteasomes. The resulting fragments can be transported into the endoplasmic reticulum by TAP and loaded onto nascent MHC I molecules for eventual presentation to CD8+ T cells. **B.** Ingested MHC class I and II molecules may be degraded and loaded onto MHC II molecules for presentation.

Table 17.1
HISTOCOMPATIBILITY GENES AND ANTIGENS

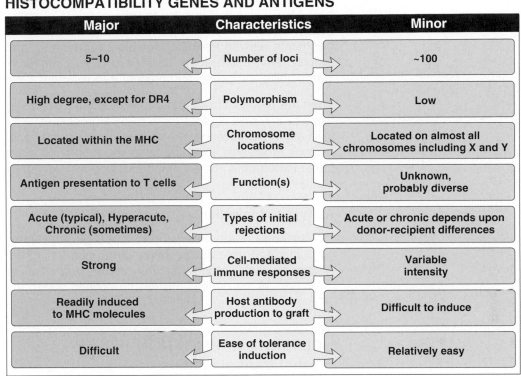

Major	Characteristics	Minor
5–10	Number of loci	~100
High degree, except for DR4	Polymorphism	Low
Located within the MHC	Chromosome locations	Located on almost all chromosomes including X and Y
Antigen presentation to T cells	Function(s)	Unknown, probably diverse
Acute (typical), Hyperacute, Chronic (sometimes)	Types of initial rejections	Acute or chronic depends upon donor-recipient differences
Strong	Cell-mediated immune responses	Variable intensity
Readily induced to MHC molecules	Host antibody production to graft	Difficult to induce
Difficult	Ease of tolerance induction	Relatively easy

III. TISSUE REJECTION

The recipient immune system recognizes peptide fragments presented by MHC class I or II molecules, whether those fragments are derived from infectious organisms or from the degradation of self molecules encoded by host genes (see Figs. 10.6 and 10.7). In the case of transplanted tissues, the genes of the engrafted cells may encode nonself molecules that also can be detected by the recipient immune system and function as histocompatibility antigens. T cells can detect and be activated against histocompatibility antigens through two different pathways of recognition: direct or indirect (Fig. 17.8). Direct recognition involves antigen presentation by donor antigen-presenting cells (APCs) to recipient T cells, while indirect recognition involves antigen presentation by recipient APCs to recipient T cells.

Direct recognition can occur only when some of the MHC class I or II molecules on the donor cells are identical to those on recipient cells. Like other cytosolic proteins, MHC class I and II molecules can be degraded by proteasomes and the resulting fragments presented on the cell surface by intact MHC class I molecules. If the donor and recipient have MHC class I molecules in common, APCs of donor origin may be able to present those peptide fragments directly to the TCRs of recipient $CD8^+$ T cells. Because the MHC class I molecules on the donor cells are the same as those present in the host thymus during thymic education, the recipient TCRs are able to recognize and bind the pMHC

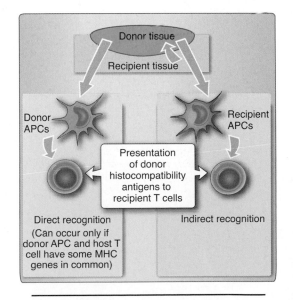

Figure 17.8
Direct recognition and indirect recognition.

I molecules on the donor cells. Direct recognition may also occur if donor APCs ingest cellular debris of donor origin and process/present it via MHC class II molecules to recipient CD4$^+$ T cells. **Indirect recognition** occurs when recipient APCs process and present peptide fragments derived from the ingestion, processing, and presentation of cellular debris from donor cells—debris that contains the donor histocompatibility antigens—and present it to recipient T cells.

Thus the recognition of foreign histocompatibility antigens and the activation of T cells against them involve processes very similar to those involved in the initiation of responses against antigens derived from infectious organisms. Indeed, the recipient immune system may view the transplanted cells as just another batch of infected cells—infected by nonself genes.

A. Types of rejection

Rejection responses fall into three general categories—chronic, acute, and hyperacute—depending upon timing and intensity. Each type involves particular sets of immune responses and is determined in part by the genetic mismatch between donor and recipient.

CLINICAL APPLICATION
Renal transplantation

Doug, a 42-year-old male, presented initially three years ago with weakness. He developed type 1 diabetes at age 18 and hypertension at age 32. He had been taking insulin and an antihypertensive medication. Blood tests revealed low hemoglobin and decreased renal function. He was diagnosed with anemia associated with chronic kidney disease. He was referred to a nephrologist, who managed the patient's hypertension with an angiotensin-converting enzyme inhibitor, erythropoietin for anemia, dietary protein restriction, and vitamin D supplementation. Now, three years later, he has developed end-stage renal disease with worsening renal function requiring replacement therapy. The patient is advised to undergo dialysis or renal transplantation. He is advised that renal transplantation provides a good quality of life and is less expensive overall than chronic hemodialysis.

Fortunately, his brother has volunteered to be a kidney donor and is found to be an appropriate genetic match. The patient received his brother's healthy kidney together with immunosuppressive therapy. The kidney is functioning satisfactorily as he recovers from surgery.

B. Immune responses involved in rejection

Chronic rejections are the slowest and the least vigorous type of rejection. The transplanted tissues or organs establish a vascular connection and proceed to function for weeks, months, and even years before signs of deterioration due to immune attack become evident.

Even after the first signs of rejection appear, the graft destruction proceeds slowly and gradually as the graft tissue is replaced by intracellular matrix and scar tissue. Chronic rejections are typical of situations in which the donor and recipient differ by only non-MHC histocompatibility gene differences, although there are exceptions.

Acute rejections occur much sooner after graft emplacement than do chronic rejections. The grafts establish vascular connections and function normally for a relatively short period of time (e.g., two to four weeks) before the first signs of rejection appear. Unlike chronic rejections, acute rejections proceed rapidly once underway. The grafts become edematous and inflamed, with an influx of blood and mononuclear cell infiltrates, and complete destruction and sloughing of the grafted tissues may take only a very few days following the first signs of deterioration. Acute rejections are commonly seen when the donor and recipient differ at MHC histocompatibility genes, especially those involving the MHC class I loci.

Hyperacute rejections are the most rapid type of rejection. They are initiated and completed within a few days of graft placement, usually before the grafted tissue or organs can establish connections with the recipient vasculature. The immune attack is typically directed at the vasculature of the graft and is mediated (in various situations) by complement, natural killer (NK) cells, and/or preexisting antibodies. Hyperacute rejections have also been called "white grafts" because in the case of skin, the failure to establish a vascular connection gives the engrafted skin a blanched appearance. The term can be misleading; it does not describe the comparable condition of other rejected tissues. A hyperacutely rejected kidney, for example, may be bluish in color owing to the large amount of deteriorating blood trapped within it.

Like responses to infectious organs, immune responses against transplanted tissues or organs can display memory. Attempts to repeat grafts that have previously been rejected usually result in an accelerated graft rejection, a phenomenon termed **second set rejection** (Fig. 17.9). Grafts that are rejected chronically on the initial occasion may be rejected acutely when repeated. During the initial rejection, activated T and B lymphocytes can generate populations of memory cells that provide the basis for accelerated and heightened secondary responses. Second set responses are therefore simply secondary immune responses directed against histocompatibility antigens.

While not every type of immune response is necessarily generated for every allograft or xenograft, almost every relevant type of immune response has been observed among various rejection episodes: antibodies, T cell responses, complement, and even NK cells.

Antibodies against graft antigens occur from two primary sources. **Natural antibodies** are preexisting antibodies that are present in the absence of known exposure or immunization. They provide, for example, the basis for transfusion reactions against ABO antigens on red blood cells, a topic that is discussed later in this chapter. Natural antibodies are produced, probably by B-1 B cells, following stimulation by antigenic molecules on the natural flora found in the body

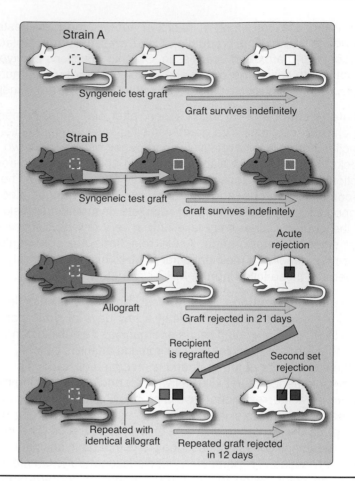

Figure 17.9

Second set rejections. Initial allografts between different inbred strains usually undergo acute rejection. If the rejected graft combination is repeated, the newly placed graft is rejected in an accelerated ("second set") manner.

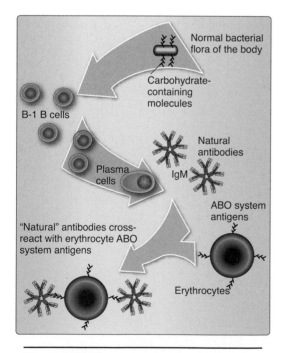

Figure 17.10

Naturally occurring antibodies. Naturally occurring antibodies against A and B antigens were so named because they were already present at the time of transfusion, prior to any known exposure or immunization.

(Fig. 17.10). They are of the IgM isotype and are directed against carbohydrate antigens. These antibodies are stimulated by microbial carbohydrate molecules but may cross-react with carbohydrate molecules on eukaryotic cells (e.g., human). Thus, for example, they can act immediately to damage erythrocytes in transfusions that are mismatched for carbohydrate ABO antigens. Similarly, in the case of xenografts, they can bind immediately to some carbohydrate molecules associated with the graft vasculature and initiate fatal damage to the graft.

The second source of antibodies involved in graft rejection occurs by the activation of B cells and generation of plasma cells synthesizing antibodies against histocompatibility antigens on graft tissue. Typically, sufficient amounts of antibodies to affect graft survival are generated only after prolonged or repeated exposures. Antibodies usually have little or no role in chronic or acute rejections unless they have been elevated by previous rejections of grafts bearing the same histocompatibility antigens. Acute rejection of first-time grafts is mediated by T cell responses. While it is relatively easy to generate significant levels of antibodies against MHC class I and II molecules by repeated exposures to allogeneic grafts (or injected cells), it has been difficult to demonstrate the consistent generation of antibodies against minor (non-MHC) histocompatibility antigens. Binding of antibodies to graft cells can initiate destructive actions such as complement activation, opsonization, and antibody-dependent cell-mediated cytotoxicity. The effects of these actions can vary, depending upon the nature of the targeted tissue.

Development of delayed (-type) hypersensitivity (DTH) and cytotoxic T lymphocyte (CTL) responses directed against histocompatibility antigens has been demonstrated in both acute and chronic rejections. The inflammatory nature of the DTH response, with the recruitment and activation of macrophages, suggests that it plays a significant role. While CTLs specifically directed against histocompatibility antigens are clearly generated, how much they contribute to a given rejection can be difficult to discern because their killing is directed against a single target cell at a time. Both DTH and CTL responses can be generated against MHC (class I and II) and non-MHC histocompatibility antigens.

Complement activation and the ensuing inflammation can inflict considerable injury and even death on grafted cells. As was mentioned, this inflammation can be targeted through the attachment of graft-specific IgG and IgM molecules. However, complement has also been found to have an important impact on xenografts that does not involve the classical pathway of activation. Host cells are protected from the potential threat of deposition of complement fragments (e.g., C3b and C4b) on host cell membranes by the presence of various cell receptors and membrane-associated enzymes that continuously break them down and remove them. These protective mechanisms, however, are species-specific. Thus, when a graft from a miniature swine is placed on a human recipient, the enzymes and receptors that effectively protect the pig cells from pig complement are not effective against human complement, and the graft cells can be rapidly attacked by fragments of human complement initiating opsonization and formation of the membrane attack complex. The rapid action of these preexisting complement components leads to hyperacute rejection of xenografts.

NK cells recognize molecules produced by damaged or stressed cells and prepare to kill those cells. They refrain from doing so, however, if they recognize sufficient levels of appropriate MHC class I molecules on the targeted cells. In the case of xenografts, host NK may recognize stress molecules on graft cells but will not find appropriate host MHC class I molecules on the graft cells to inhibit them. As a result, host NK cells can cause considerable injury to the graft and constitute another significant barrier to successful xenotransplantation.

C. Therapeutic intervention

The initial effort to minimize the risk of rejection is to genetically match the donor and recipient as closely as possible. However, some degree of mismatch is present in the vast majority of transplants. The next step that can be taken is to inhibit the ability of the recipient immune system to attack and damage the engrafted tissues. This inhibition is approached in two general ways:

- **Specific immune tolerance** involves a selective inhibiting of the responsiveness to a given antigen or set of antigens.
- **Immune suppression** (or **immunosuppression**) involves inhibiting general immune responsiveness without regard to the specificity.

While specific immune tolerance to foreign grafts can be induced in experimental systems, it usually requires some advance information about the precise genetic differences involved and sufficient lead time to prepare the recipient. These requirements have limited its use in humans so far. In addition, some of the techniques are ethically inappropriate in humans. Therefore immunotherapy for transplant patients still relies upon immunosuppression.

Immunosuppressive techniques such as whole-body irradiation or the use of toxic drugs effectively eliminate immune responses that could damage transplanted organs and tissues (Table 17.2). The treated recipients, however, are then open to opportunistic infections that can be fatal if not successfully monitored and controlled. Over the past few decades, additional drugs (e.g., cyclosporine, tacrolimus, and rapamycin) have been developed that have more restricted effects on the immune system. Their effects are targeted more closely on cells that react to graft antigens while leaving the remainder of the immune system relatively uninhibited in its ability to deal with infectious agents. They are not without risk, however. Patients must often receive the drugs for an extended period of time. If a significant infection occurs during this period, the immune cells respond-

Table 17.2

IMMUNOSUPPRESSIVE AGENTS RELEVANT TO TRANSPLANTATION (ALSO SEE CHAPTER 18)

Agent	Affected Cells	Mode of Action
Azathioprine	Multiple cell types	Inhibition of nucleotide synthesis
Corticosteroids (e.g., prednisone)	Multiple cell types	Inhibition of transcription for numerous cytokines and other products involved in inflammation
Cyclophosphamide	Multiple cell types	Inhibition of nucleotide synthesis
Cyclosporine	Lymphocytes	Inhibition of transcription for multiple cytokines (e.g., IL-2, IL-4)
Mycophenolate mofetil	Lymphocytes	Inhibition of lymphocyte nucleotide synthesis and proliferation
Sirolimus (rapamycin)	T cells	Inhibition of some signal transduction induced by cytokines (e.g., IL-2)
Tacrolimus (FK506)	T cells	Inhibition of gene transcription in lymphocytes, inactivation of calcineurin
Irradiation	Many cell types	Induction of DNA damage, especially in rapidly proliferating cells
Antibodies against lymphocytes or against T cells	Lymphocytes, T cells	Destruction or inhibition of lymphocytes or lymphocyte subsets
Anti-CD4 antibodies, anti-CD8 antibodies	$CD4^+$ T cells, $CD8^+$ T cells	Interference with TCR binding
Anti-MHC I/II antibodies	Antigen-presenting cells	Interference with antigen presentation and T cell activation by blockading

ing to the infectious agent could be inhibited in the same way as those responding to graft alloantigens. In addition, extended use of these drugs is sometimes associated with damage to organs such as the liver. These and other therapeutic drugs are discussed in greater detail in Chapter 18.

A second approach to inducing a less than global inhibition of the immune response has been the use of antibodies directed at molecules on the surface of the cells involved in immune responses, particularly lymphocytes and APCs. Antibodies against MHC class I or class II molecules can inhibit with T cell activation. Antibodies against CD4 or CD8 molecules, when administered during active rejection, have been shown to inhibit or destroy T cells and halt the rejection at least temporarily. However, antibodies against broad categories of T lymphocytes (e.g., anti-CD3 antibodies) have problems similar to those seen with immunosuppressive drugs, and their long-term use can reduce the body's ability to respond to infectious agents.

IV. TISSUE-SPECIFIC CONSIDERATIONS

Special problems may arise when particular tissues are transplanted. We will discuss two of these situations: those involving blood transfusions and the transfer of bone narrow.

A. Transfusion

Transfusion is essentially the transplantation of blood. Erythrocytes and white cells in the transfused blood bear hundreds of molecules that can vary among individuals and act as histocompatibility antigens on these cells. Erythrocytes alone are estimated to express over 400 such types of antigens. Fortunately, mismatches for the vast majority of these antigens seldom have clinical consequences, and those tend to be of minimal severity when they do occur. There are, however, two antigen systems that are of major clinical concern: the ABO and Rh systems.

1. **ABO:** The **ABO antigen system** is a set of carbohydrate structures on erythrocyte surfaces and on some endothelial and epithelial cells. They are synthesized by glycosyl transferases encoded by two loci: the H locus and the ABO locus (Fig. 17.11, Table 17.3). The H locus has two alleles: dominant H and recessive h. The recessive h allele encodes a nonfunctional product, but the H allele encodes a fucosyl transferase that attaches fucose to a precursor molecule normally present on erythrocyte surfaces to produce H substance. H substance is the precursor for the glycosyltransferases encoded by the alleles of the ABO locus that modify the H substance to produce A and B antigens (Fig. 17.11).

   A and B antigens are recognized and bound **by natural antibodies** (also called **naturally occurring antibodies**) present in the serum without any stimulation from prior transfusions or intentional immunizations. These natural antibodies, of the IgM isotype, are probably generated against carbohydrates on normal body flora, and their role in transfusion is probably due to cross-reaction with

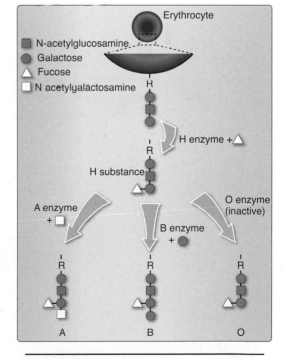

Figure 17.11
Synthesis of ABO blood group antigens.

Table 17.3
ABO ANTIGEN SYSTEM

Genotype of Individual		Phenotype of Individual	Natural Antibodies Present In Serum
H Locus	*ABO* Locus		
HH or *Hh*	*AA*	A	Anti-B
HH or *Hh*	*AO*	A	Anti-B
HH or *Hh*	*AB*	AB	None
HH or *Hh*	*BB*	B	Anti-A
HH or *Hh*	*BO*	B	Anti-A
HH or *Hh*	*OO*	O	Anti-A and anti-B
hh	*AA*	O	Anti-A and anti-B
hh	*AO*	O	Anti-A and anti-B
hh	*AB*	O	Anti-A and anti-B
hh	*BB*	O	Anti-A and anti-B
hh	*BO*	O	Anti-A and anti-B
hh	*OO*	O	Anti-A and anti-B

certain carbohydrates on erythrocytes that share structural similarities with those on the microbial flora. Individuals who have neither A nor B on their own erythrocytes generate IgM antibodies against both A and B. Individuals of blood type A, tolerant to their own A antigens, will produce only anti-B antibodies. Similarly, type B individuals are tolerant to their own B antigens and therefore generate only anti-A antibodies.

Mismatched transfusions (e.g., type A erythrocytes given to a type B recipient) can have serious consequences. The naturally occurring IgM antibodies react almost immediately with the transfused erythrocytes to initiate agglutination and complement-mediated lysis. It is the agglutination that produces the clumping seen in demonstrations of ABO typing commonly performed in laboratories (see Chapter 20). ABO mismatching can result in massive destruction of transfused red blood cells (**transfusion reaction**) and, if severe enough, can produce a type of transfusion reaction known as an **acute hemolytic reaction** within 24 hours of transfusion. This reaction is caused by widespread hemolysis within the vasculature from the binding of IgM to erythrocytes and the ensuing complement activation. Clinical signs include fever, chills, shortness of breath, and urticaria. If it is extensive enough, a potentially fatal condition known as disseminated intravascular coagulation can develop.

Such situations emphasize the necessity of correct typing and matching of donors and recipients. Type A individuals can safely be given blood of phenotypes A and O, while type B recipients can safely receive blood of phenotypes B or O (Table 17.3). Type O recipients should receive erythrocytes only from other type O donors. AB individuals are "universal recipients" and can safely

Table 17.4
PERMISSIBLE ABO HOST-DONOR COMBINATIONS

Recipient Phenotypes	Can Accept Erythrocytes from Donors of Phenotypes
A	A, O
B	B, O
AB[a]	AB, A, B, O
O	O[b]

[a]Because they can safely accept erythrocytes from all donor types, type AB individuals are called *universal recipients*.

[b]Because they can safely donate erythrocytes to all recipient types, type O individuals are called *universal donors*.

receive transfusions from donors of phenotypes A, B, O, or AB (Table 17.4).

CLINICAL APPLICATION
Blood transfusion reaction

Aileen, a 55-year-old female, has had breast cancer for several years requiring chemotherapy. She is hospitalized for chemotherapy-induced anemia requiring a blood transfusion.

Within minutes after beginning the blood transfusion, she develops fever, nausea, back pain, and hypotension. The blood transfusion is immediately stopped. She is given intravenous fluid and acetaminophen. The patient's blood type is retested, and the original typing is found to be erroneous, confirming that the reaction was caused by a transfusion reaction. Fortunately, her symptoms resolve without any complications, such as acute kidney failure.

---

2. **Rh:** The **Rh ("Rhesus") antigens** on erythrocyte surfaces are proteins. When an Rh-negative (Rh⁻) individual is exposed to Rh-positive (Rh⁺) erythrocytes, he or she can generate antibodies, some of which are of the IgG isotype. Rh antigens can be typed prior to transfusion, and Rh-related transfusion reactions can be avoided by avoiding the transfusion of Rh⁻ recipients with Rh⁺ blood. Rh incompatibility during pregnancy presents a special concern for an Rh⁻ mother who carries an Rh⁺ fetus. Fetal blood immunizes the mother's immune system to make IgG antibodies that may cross the placenta and destroy fetal erythrocytes in utero.

   Rh antigens are encoded by a series of closely linked loci (*D* and *CE*) with dominant alleles (e.g., *D*) and recessive alleles (e.g., *d*), the most important of which is *D*. *DD* or *Dd* individuals have the Rh⁺ phenotype, while those with *dd* are Rh⁻ (Table 17.5). When the father is Rh⁺, an Rh⁻ mother may carry an Rh⁺ fetus (Fig. 17.12). The maternal immune system is exposed to fetal blood as early as the first trimester of pregnancy and begins to generate anti-Rh

Table 17.5
Rh ANTIGEN SYSTEM

D locus (alleles *D* and *d*)	C locus + E locus (alleles *C* or *c* and *E* or *e*)	Rh phenotype of individual
DD	All combinations (*C* + *E*, *C* + *e*, *c* + *E*, or *c* + *e*)	Rh⁺ (positive)
Dd	All combinations (*C* + *E*, *C* + *e*, *c* + *E*, or *c* + *e*)	Rh⁺ (positive)
dd	All combinations (*C* + *E*, *C* + *e*, *c* + *E*, or *c* + *e*)	Rh⁻ (negative)

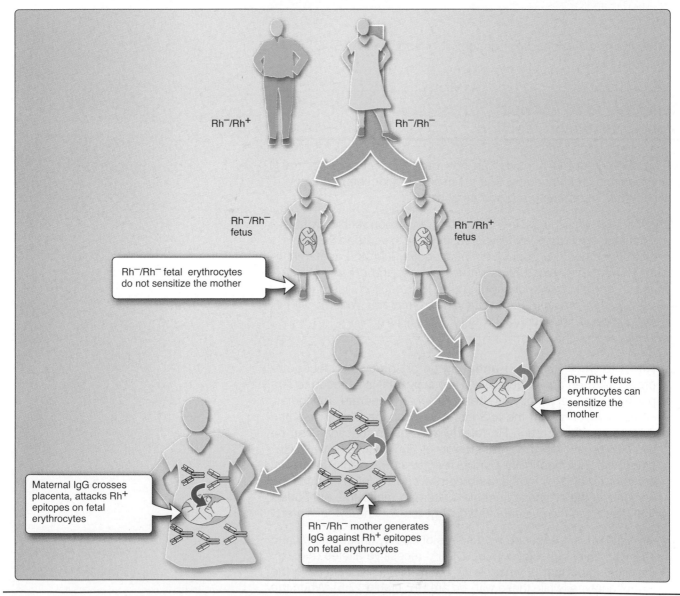

Figure 17.12
Hemolytic disease of the newborn. An Rh⁻ mother carrying an Rh⁺ fetus can be exposed to fetal erythrocytes during pregnancy and delivery. The maternal immune system can generate anti-Rh IgG antibodies that cross the placenta and bind to Rh⁺ fetal erythrocytes. Upon binding, these antibodies can induce destruction of fetal erythrocytes that may lead to anemia and other consequences.

IgG antibodies. The first Rh$^+$ fetus is rarely at risk because of the time needed for injurious levels of anti-Rh antibodies to develop. However, subsequent Rh$^+$ fetuses are at risk because maternal anti-Rh antibodies can increase rapidly and enter the fetus. Binding to fetal erythrocytes can lead to anemia and damage to other fetal organs. This is called **hemolytic disease of the newborn (HDN)** or sometimes **erythroblastosis fetalis**. The Rh antigen is a protein and elicits an IgG response. Every conception between an Rh$^+$ male and an Rh$^-$ female has the potential to produce an Rh-incompatible fetus. Aborted (spontaneous or induced) conceptions can also lead to the development of an IgG antibody response to Rh$_0$ (*D*).

In HDN, binding of anti-Rh antibodies to erythrocytes activates fetal complement, causing lysis of erythrocytes. The resulting anemia may become so severe that the fetus sustains severe damage or dies in utero. To compensate for the anemia, the fetal bone marrow releases immature erythrocytes (or erythroblasts). The abnormal presence of these erythroblasts in the fetal circulation is the hallmark of the disease (hence the term *erythroblastosis fetalis*).

Preventive therapy, especially the use of Rh$_0$ (*D*) immune globulin to minimize the risk of the mother becoming sensitized against Rh, is now routinely available for this situation. This involves the injection of a high-titer anti-Rh antibody preparation such as RhoGAM® or MICRhoGAM®. These preparations contain pooled anti-Rh antibodies, prepared from human serum obtained from mothers who have made antibodies to Rh antigens. Rh$_0$ (*D*) immune globulin should be administered after the twelfth gestational week for ongoing pregnancy was well as for spontaneous or induced abortion. Use of Rh$_0$ (*D*) immune globulin may also be appropriate after a blood transfusion of an Rh$^-$ female.

CLINICAL APPLICATION
Hemolytic disease of the newborn

Kim, a 30-year-old female is pregnant for the third time. Her first pregnancy resulted in a miscarriage, and she did not follow up with any additional testing. During her second pregnancy, the baby was jaundiced at birth and exhibited anemia and hepatosplenomegaly consistent with hemolytic disease of the newborn. Kim was found to be Rh$^-$, and the baby's father was Rh$^+$. Elevated levels of anti-Rh antibodies were found in Kim's blood.

During her third pregnancy, she has been very concerned. To prevent complications, she receives injections of RhoGAM, a high-titer anti-Rh antibody prepared from human serum from mothers who have made antibodies against Rh antigens. RhoGAM is given at 28 weeks of pregnancy and again within 72 hours of delivery if the baby is Rh$^+$. Kim delivers a healthy baby boy.

Although apparently healthy, the child should be followed to check for sequelae that may not be apparent at birth. Where appropriate prenatal care is observed, HDN has become rare. However, it is still a danger where appropriate prenatal care is avoided or unavailable.

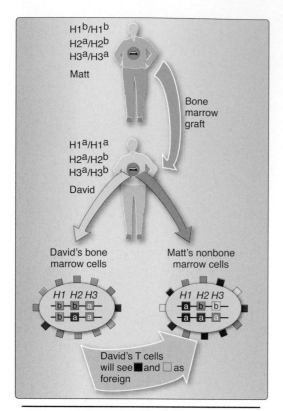

Figure 17.13
Bone marrow transplantation. Immunocompetent T cells in the donor bone marrow may recognize host antigens as foreign and initiate a graft-versus-host (GVH) response. The risk of GVH can be greatly reduced by removing mature T cells from the bone marrow inoculate prior to its introduction.

B. Bone marrow

The bone marrow carries stem cells for the entire hematopoietic system and (at least hypothetically) could be used to treat individuals in whom some or all of the these tissues are intrinsically defective or may have been damaged. Examples include those with immune deficiency diseases, some anemias, and the effects of cancer therapies. Indeed, transplantation of bone marrow can provide benefits to some of these patients, but it also carries unique risks. Bone marrow transplantation involves the placement of an immunocompetent tissue into a recipient who is usually immunodeficient for natural or therapeutic reasons. Even recipients with intact immune systems, however, undergo procedures that deliberately damage their immune systems to enable the transplanted bone marrow to establish itself in its new environment.

Under these circumstances, the immunocompetent cells in the transplanted bone marrow may recognize histocompatibility antigens on recipient cells as foreign and attack the host tissues (Fig. 7.13). This is a **graft-versus-host** (**GVH**) response, and the resulting damage is **graft-versus-host disease** (**GVHD**), which can be potentially fatal. GVHD can develop from two sources within the transplanted bone marrow: the stem cells and the mature T cells present in the implanted bone marrow. The most immediate and serious threat comes from the mature T cells because they are capable of generating rapid and severe GVH responses. These responses can be minimized by pretreatment of the bone marrow inoculate to remove the T cells prior to implantation. It is hoped that lymphocytes generated from the implanted stem cells will become tolerant to host histocompatibility antigens as they undergo positive and negative selection in the recipient thymus. However, this tolerance is sometimes imperfect, but when GVH responses do result from the activity of donor stem cell-derived lymphocytes, they are usually transient and less severe than the GVH responses initiated by mature T cells within the bone marrow inoculum.

Although genetic matching of donor and recipient can minimize the risk of GVHD, it is also important for another reason. T cells generated by implanted stem cells must undergo thymic education in the recipient thymus. Some degree of matching between the MHC class I and II genes of the host and donor is required for the positive and negative selection events of thymic education to proceed properly. Bone marrow recipients are also vulnerable to opportunistic infection while the new marrow becomes established and must be carefully monitored for infection and treated appropriately. Once established and functioning, the transplanted hematopoietic stem cells can often provide a normal or near-normal condition to recipients for the remainder of their lives.

C. Immune-privileged sites

Some anatomic sites are "permissive" in tolerating genetic mismatches between donor and recipient that would lead to prompt rejection in most parts of the body. Allogeneic and xenogeneic grafts that would be rapidly rejected at most sites in the body can often survive when placed into these areas. These sites are termed **immune-privileged**

sites, and each has features that limit the immune response to cells and molecules within them. The immune-privileged sites include the eye, the testicular tubules, the brain, and perhaps the placenta.

The eye has several features that make it a privileged site. The aqueous humor of the anterior chamber allows cells and molecules to exist without close contact with the vasculature, thus hiding them from the immune system to some extent. In addition, the immunologic processes that inhibit immune responses, such as the apoptotic death of lymphocytes attacking tissues in the eye, operate very rapidly, perhaps protecting the eye from damage from more extensive inflammation. This mechanism may also account, at least in part, for the ease with which corneas can be transplanted between individuals with genetic differences that would be difficult to overcome with other tissues.

The lumen of the testes also provides an immunologically privileged site. The testicular tubules are developed and closed prior to the development of the immune system. Because the Sertoli cells and other tubular elements prevent any subsequent passage of immune cells into the testicular tubules, the molecules and cells that are unique to that environment (e.g., spermatogonia and developing sperm) are never recognized as self by the immune system. As a result, if the testicular tubules are breached by infection, injury, or surgical intervention, the immune system can react against the seemingly foreign antigens that become exposed. It is estimated that a portion of male infertility cases may stem from immune responses against exposed testicular tubule elements.

The brain is sometimes cited as an immune-privileged site, because the blood-brain barrier can limit the exchange of cells and large molecules between the vasculature and the nervous system. The extent of this isolation is still somewhat unclear, as is the extent to which the cells of the immune system recirculate through nervous tissue. It appears that mechanisms that rapidly suppress potentially dangerous immune-mediated injury, similar to those seen in the eye, may also exist in the brain.

The placenta presents an interesting conundrum. The developing fetus typically expresses numerous histocompatibility antigens that are foreign to the mother. Therefore why does the maternal immune system not attach and destroy the fetus? While the basis for the sheltering of the fetus from the maternal immune system (aside from maternal IgG crossing the placenta to provide passive protection to the fetus) has yet to be clarified, several structural and biochemical features of the fetal/uterine environment have been suggested as contributing factors.

V. TISSUE SOURCES

Tissues available for transplantation can come from a variety of different sources. Traditionally, they have been harvested from voluntary living donors or from cadavers. In the case of cadaver donors, permission must usually be obtained through the documented permission of the donor given prior to death or through the agreement of family or guardians. Depending upon the nature of the tissue, donated cells can sometimes be expanded or modified in vitro prior to implantation. Increasing research into the use of stem cells, either from adult or embryonic sources, provides yet another potential source but has had limited use in humans to this point. Finally, the search for available organs has been extended to other species, and the use of primate and swine donors has provided some benefits, though it has been limited by other problems inherent in xenogeneic exchanges.

A. Human tissues and organs

The total number of transplants that have been performed now exceeds a half million worldwide. The increased efficacy of transplantation has been made possible by continual improvements in techniques, in the ability to genetically match donors and recipients, and in the ongoing development of immunosuppressive and antibiotic agents that can be used to manipulate the recipient immune system to permit graft survival without an accompanying overwhelming sepsis.

1. **Organ procurement and distribution:** A growing imbalance exists between the number of organs available for transplantation and the number of patients awaiting them, and the effective distribution of available organs has become increasingly complicated. In the United States, organ distribution is managed through the United Network for Organ Sharing (UNOS), the organization that administers the federally founded Organ Procurement and Transplantation Network. UNOS utilizes various factors, including the degree of genetic matching, potential benefit to the recipient, and geographical priorities to prioritize the assignment of donated organs as they become available. UNOS maintains a regularly updated web site available to the public that details the types of organs, number of transplants performed, success rates, waiting lists, and other criteria.

2. **Stem cell and fetal sources:** The ability to transfer healthy stem cells that are self-renewing and capable of generating new cells and/or tissues offers benefit to a variety of injuries (e.g., burn wounds, spinal cord injuries) and diseases (e.g., arthritis, diabetes, cardiovascular disease, and neurologic diseases such as Alzheimer's disease and Parkinson's disease). In some cases, these represent new forms of therapy; in other cases, they extend the effectiveness of previous therapies. For example, transplantation of pancreatic islet cells has been used to treat diabetes, but the transplanted cells have finite life spans. The transplantation of stem cells that are capable of generating these cells provides a potentially permanent replacement therapy.

Adult stem cells have already been used in a limited number of human cases, but their ability to generate a variety of new tissues is more limited. In addition, much has yet to be learned about how best to obtain and prepare them for use. Their primary application thus far has been the use of hematopoietic stem cells in bone marrow transplantation. **Embryonic stem cells** have a broader capacity for regeneration, as has been demonstrated in experimental animal models, but their use in humans has been restricted by practical and ethical considerations.

3. **Ethical considerations:** Transplantation involves decisions that sometimes create ethical difficulties for some individuals. In some cases, cultural or religious customs forbid individuals from participating as either donors or recipients of transplantation and even blood transfusion. Even when there are no such general limitations, individuals are often personally reluctant to offer themselves as potential donors. As a result, the need for donated organs greatly exceeds the supply, creating the need for a system such as UNOS that regulates their distribution to prevent availability from becoming dependent upon a potential recipient's wealth or social/political influence.

The potential use of embryonic stem cells faces social and religious opposition from some segments of the scientific, religious, and general communities. Currently, this opposition has imposed severe limitations on obtaining and using human embryonic stem cells for either research or therapeutic use.

B. Nonhuman (xeno-) tissues and organs

The shortage of available human organs has spurred research into the use of nonhuman alternatives. Numerous attempts have been made to utilize animal donors. Primates are an obvious donor choice because of their close genetic relationship to humans. Pigs have many physiologic similarities to humans, and some breeds have organs that are an appropriate size for use in human recipients. Pig skin has also been used on occasion for temporary coverage of damaged areas in human burn victims.

Xenotransplantation has not been very successful or widely used, however. Xenografts face significant immunologic obstacles. Concern also exists about the potential for introducing zoonotic infections (infections passed from one species to another) through xenotransplantation. Finally, some individuals oppose the use of xenografts on ethical grounds.

Naturally existing antibodies in human serum, such as those against ABO antigens on human erythrocytes, can react with xenogeneic tissues to produce hyperacute rejections. NK cells can detect stress molecules on xenograft cells and bind to them via their killer activation receptors. However, the absence of human MHC class I molecules on the xenografts prevents the NK cells from ceasing the killing response through binding of their killer inhibition receptors. Xenogeneic cells lack enzymes that protect them against the attachment of human complement components that lead to cell lysis. These various mechanisms often destroy xenografts before the T cell-mediated responses typically associated with allograft rejection are even generated. Attempts to resolve these problems have utilized genetic engineering of the animal donors to introduce various human genes. While there have been promising experimental advances, they have not yet significantly increased the clinical application of xenotransplantation.

Chapter Summary

- The genetic match (similarity/disparity) between the donor and the host is a very important factor in determining the likelihood of a successful transplant.

- **Histocompatibility genes** encode histocompatibility antigens. Among these are the MHC class I and II molecules encoded within the **major histocompatibility complex** (**MHC**).

- Grafts that are placed in their normal anatomic location are called **orthotopic** grafts. Grafts that are placed into a site other than their normal one are called **heterotopic** grafts.

- **Autografts** are those transferred from one part of an individual to another location on that same individual. **Syngeneic** grafts are those transferred between different individuals who are genetically identical or members of the same inbred strain of experimental animals. **Allogeneic** grafts (or **allografts**) are transferred between two genetically disparate individuals of the same species. **Xenogeneic** grafts (or **xenografts**) are those exchanged between members of different species..

- The **laws of transplantation** can be summarized as follows: *A host can recognize as foreign, and mount a response against, any histocompatibility antigen not encoded within its own cells.*

- The recipient immune system recognizes peptide fragments presented by MHC class I or II molecules. In the case of transplanted tissues, the genes of the engrafted cells may encode molecules that also can be detected by the recipient immune system and function as histocompatibility antigens. The recognition of foreign histocompatibility antigens and the activation of T cells against them involve processes that are very similar to those involved in the initiation of responses against antigens derived from infectious organisms.

- **Chronic rejections** are the slowest and the least vigorous type of rejection. Chronic rejections are typical of situations in which the donor and recipient differ by only non-MHC histocompatibility gene differences. **Acute rejections** occur much sooner after graft emplacement than do chronic rejections (e.g., two to four weeks). **Hyperacute rejections** are the most rapid type of rejection. They are initiated and completed within a very few days of graft placement, usually before the grafted tissue or organs can establish connections with the recipient vasculature. **Second set rejection are** grafts that are rejected more rapidly when repeated upon a recipient who rejected the same type of graft on a previous occasion

- Development of delayed (-type) hypersensitivity (DTH) and cytotoxic T lymphocyte (CTL) responses directed against histocompatibility antigens have been demonstrated in both acute and chronic rejections

- Steps can be taken to inhibit the ability of the recipient immune system to attack and damage the engrafted tissues. **Specific immune tolerance** involves a selective inhibition of the responsiveness to a given antigen or set of antigens. **Immune suppression** (or **immunosuppression**) is a broad and general inhibition of immune responsiveness without regard to specificity. A second approach to inducing a less than global inhibition of the immune response has been the use of antibodies directed at molecules on the surface of the cells involved in immune responses, particularly lymphocytes and antigen-presenting cells

- ABO mismatching can result in massive destruction of transfused red blood cells (**transfusion reaction**) and, if severe enough, can produce a type of transfusion reaction known as an **acute hemolytic reaction** within 24 hours of transfusion.

- When an Rh-negative (Rh⁻) individual is exposed to Rh-positive (Rh⁺) erythrocytes, he or she can generate antibodies, some of which are of the IgG isotype. In the case of an Rh⁻ mother carrying an Rh⁺ fetus, the maternal anti-Rh IgG antibodies can cross the placenta and bind to fetal erythrocytes. This can lead to **hemolytic disease of the newborn**.

- **Graft-versus-host disease** (**GVHD**) can develop from two sources within transplanted bone marrow: the stem cells and the mature T cells present in the implanted bone marrow. The latter present the most serious risk of developing GVHD, but the risk can be minimized by removing them from the bone marrow inoculate prior to its infusion

- Tissues available for transplantation can come from a variety of different sources. Traditionally, they have been harvested from voluntary living donors or from cadavers.

Study Questions

17.1 A 38-year-old female requires a kidney graft. Her HLA genotype is A3/A8, B1/B8, C4/C1. For each locus, the maternal allele is listed first and the paternal allele second. Several potential donors are available. Which of the following donors would be the best choice?

A. Donor A: A8/A27, B24/B8, C4/C9
B. Donor B: A3/A3, B27/B8, C1/C1
C. Donor C: A8/A6, B44/B8, C4/C1
D. Donor D: A6/A27, B1/B8, C4/C2
E. Donor E: A3/A8, B1/B27, C9/C4

The answer is B. The best donor will have the fewest mismatched HLA genes not present in the recipient. Donor B contains only HLA B27, which is not present in the recipient. Donor A has three mismatches, Donor C has two mismatches, Donor D has three mismatches, and Donor E has two mismatches.

17.2 After receiving a kidney transplant from the most appropriate available donor, a 38-year-old female is administered immunosuppressive drugs, including cyclosporine, in order to

A. decrease T cell production of IL-2.
B. destroy stem cells in her bone marrow.
C. induce involution of her thymus.
D. inhibit macrophage release of IFN-γ.
E. reduce plasma cell secretion of IgG antibodies.

The answer is A. Cyclosporine decreases T cell production of IL-2, resulting in decreased T cell proliferation. Cyclosporine treatment does not destroy bone marrow stem cells, nor does it induce thymic involution. Neither macrophage release of IFN-γ nor plasma cell secretion of IgG antibodies is affected by cyclosporine.

17.3 A 6-year-old male receives a bone marrow transplant from his father during treatment for acute myelogenous leukemia. Of primary concern will be the potential development of

A. acute rejection.
B. an allergic reaction.
C. autoimmune responses.
D. graft-versus-host disease.
E. immediate hypersensitivity.

The answer is D. Graft-versus-host (GVH) disease is a risk because bone marrow contains immunocompetent tissue. The GVH response is directed against host antigens that are not present in the donor bone marrow. Recipients of bone marrow transplants are immunocompromised or immunosuppressed, resulting in little risk for development of host-versus-graft responses such as acute rejection. Allergic reactions, also described as type I or immediate hypersensitivity reactions, do not occur in response to bone marrow transplantation. An autoimmune response is one directed by the immune system against self antigens.

17.4 With no therapeutic intervention, the most likely outcome for a transplanted skin graft obtained from an unrelated donor who is HLA identical to the recipient is

A. acute rejection.
B. chronic rejection.
C. graft-versus-host disease.
D. hyperacute rejection.
E. long-term success.

The answer is B. Chronic rejection is most likely to occur, over months to years, in such a situation. Unrelated HLA identical individuals will have numerous mismatches of minor histocompatibility genes. Because the major histocompatibility genes match, hyperacute and acute rejections are unlikely to occur. Skin does not contain immunocompetent tissue and cannot mount a graft versus host response. Even with identical major histocompatibility genes, long-term success of a transplanted skin graft will require immunosuppressive therapy.

17.5 What are the possible ABO blood types of children to the union of a man who has blood type AB and a woman who has blood type O?

A. A only
B. A and B only
C. A, B, and AB only
D. A, B, AB, and O
E. O only

The answer is B. Blood types A and B are both possible in children of parents with type AB and type O. The genders of the parents and of the children are inconsequential, since inheritance of ABO blood group is autosomal. A and B are codominant and are both dominant to O. In this example, children will inherit either the A or B allele from the father and the O allele from their mother and will have either blood type A or blood type B. Inheritance of both A and B or of O only is not possible, eliminating types AB and O as possible blood types among the children of this couple.

Immune
Pharmacotherapy

18

I. OVERVIEW

It is sometimes desirable to boost or supplement the normal immune response to maintain good health. However, on other occasions, as in the case of transplantation, the normal response of the immune system creates problems. And in other instances, such as allergy or autoimmunity, undesirable immune responses develop. In many of these situations, immune response can be enhanced, diminished, or altered by pharmacologic agents or other treatments, as described in this chapter.

II. MEASURES THAT ENHANCE THE IMMUNE RESPONSE

Immunotherapy is the application of therapeutic treatments for the purpose of increasing or augmenting immune function. Such treatments may include the use of agents (e.g., **adjuvants**) that enhance immune responses in a nonspecific way. More specifically targeted therapies include the application of cytokines that stimulate the activity of particular cell types or the administration of human serum immunoglobulin to supplement or replace suboptimal immunoglobulin levels or isotypes in patients with a variety of immune deficiencies.

A. Adjuvant therapy

In addition to the primary treatment, adjuvant therapy is administered to nonspecifically stimulate immune responses, either directly or indirectly. Adjuvants administered with vaccines can indirectly enhance the effect of the vaccine indirectly by attracting antigen-presenting cells and increasing their expression of costimulatory molecules. **Bacillus Calmette-Guérin** (**BCG**), prepared from an inactivated form of *Mycobacterium* and is commonly used around the world as a tuberculosis vaccine, can serve as an effective adjuvant for vaccination or immunization. However, it can also be used directly for postsurgical treatment of superficial bladder cancer. A BCG suspension is periodically instilled into the bladder over a period of six weeks; this promotes inflammation and, in doing so, stimulates antitumor immune responses.

Levamisole, a veterinary antihelminthic agent that provides immunostimulation with low toxicity, has been used in conjunction with other therapies to elevate cell-mediated immunity in a variety of infections. In combination with the cancer chemotherapeutic agent 5-fluorouracil, levamisole is used to treat colon cancer, in which it is thought to stimulate the production of antitumor cytokines and factors by macrophages and T cells.

B. Cytokine therapy

Innate and adaptive immune responses are regulated by a variety of influences, including cytokines. Cytokines affect the induction and intensity of cellular growth and differentiation, cell activation, tissue inflammation, and tissue repair. Both **type I (IFN-α/β)** and **type II (IFN-γ) interferons** have been used as immunotherapeutic agents to heighten immune responsiveness in patients with viral infections such as hepatitis B or hepatitis C virus. Both natural and engineered interferons are rapidly cleared from the circulation, but their availability can be prolonged by conjugation to **polyethylene glycol**. Chronic treatment with pegylated recombinant IFN-α decreases the risk of subsequent hepatocarcinoma in about 20% of individuals with chronic hepatitis C viral infection. Additionally, IFN-α2b combination therapy with ribavirin, an antiviral agent, can result in a sustained clinical response in approximately 50% of the cases. Interferons can also be effective in treating patients with immune deficiency diseases such as chronic granulomatous disease (CGD, a disease due to defective killing of microbes by phagocytes). The incidence of serious infection is greatly diminished in CGD patients treated with pro-inflammatory cytokines such as recombinant IFN-γ. The most common side effects of interferon therapies are flulike symptoms that can become severely debilitating.

Cytokine therapy has also been applied in the treatment of cancer. Immunotherapy against tumors has been traditionally unreliable, and only recently have more reliable treatment regimens been developed. These include the use of IFN-α for treatment of hairy-cell leukemia, IL-2 for treatment of some renal carcinomas and melanomas, and IFN-γ and TNF-α for treatment of ovarian tumors. IL-2 can activate NK cells, an important component for the destruction of tumor cells.

Tumors can sometimes outgrow the immune response. An attempt to increase antitumor immune responses has involved the isolation of T cells from excised tumors and their proliferation in vitro by adding IL-2 to the cultures. It is presumed that these T cells (tumor-infiltrating lymphocytes) will include many that are specifically directed against tumor antigens. Proliferation in vitro before reinfusion increases the probability that the cells will encounter their target tumor cells. Exogenous IL-2 may also be given to the patient to encourage continued proliferation of the antitumor T cells in vivo.

Another antitumor approach is the engineering of tumor cells to make them more immunogenic. Transfection with active cytokine genes, as well as genes producing constitutive expression of molecules such as CD80 and CD86, can convert tumor cells into a type of quasi-antigen-presenting cells that express tumor antigens. When returned to the patient, the engineered tumor cells may be able to interact with tumor antigen–specific T cells and facilitate their activation.

Finally, cytokines can even sometimes function to a degree as adjuvants. For example, immune responses to melanoma peptide vaccines appear to be enhanced when IL-12 is injected together with the vaccines.

C. Antibody replacement therapy

The administration of exogenous immunoglobulin (**human immune globulin**, or **HIg**) can be effective therapy for individuals with generalized antibody deficiencies (hypogammaglobulinemia or agammaglobulinemia). The immune globulin products are typically administered intravenously (**intravenous immune globulin**, or **IVIG**). HIg consists mostly of IgG with trace amounts of IgM and IgA. Because it is derived from pooled immune human sera, it can react against a broad range of epitopes. The benefit provided by HIg lasts for approximately one month (the serum half-life of IgG is about 23 days); therefore HIg injections must be repeated at monthly intervals to maintain sufficient antibody levels for protection. Since HIg is an immunomodulating agent that can modulate complement activation, alter antibody production, and suppress various inflammatory mediators, HIg can be beneficial in situations in which immune deficiency is not the underlying problem. It has been demonstrated to be beneficial in treatment of autoimmune idiopathic thrombocytopenic purpura, B cell chronic lymphocytic leukemia, and Kawasaki syndrome (a disease, usually affecting children, that involves inflammation of the blood vessels and other tissues such as heart muscles).

Antibody replacement therapy need not always involve broad-range HIg. People with selective antibody deficiencies, groups at high risk for certain infections (the elderly or infants), or those exposed to certain infectious diseases (e.g., health care workers or laboratory personnel) may benefit from intramuscular injections of a broad-spectrum immune globulin or preparations of immune globulins containing specific antibodies. Preparations of immune globulins containing specific antibodies (e.g., against tetanus, hepatitis B, rabies, cytomegalovirus, and varicella zoster virus) are available for those at high risk or high exposure. With the advent of **monoclonal antibody** technology, large quantities of antibodies against specific epitopes are available for other therapeutic uses as well. For example, monoclonal antibodies against the CD20 marker are particularly useful in treatment of B cell non-Hodgkin's lymphoma.

III. MEASURES THAT DIMINISH THE IMMUNE RESPONSE

The immune system can aggressively reject newly transplanted organs or activating immune cells and thus inducing autoimmune diseases. The immune response can be controlled by using drugs or other measures to prevent or to treat these conditions. Measures that diminish the immune response can be either specific or nonspecific.

A. Anti-inflammatory agents

Inflammation is a response to foreign substances, causing direct or indirect activation of the innate immune system. Inflammation is characterized by increased blood flow, increased capillary permeability, and leakage of plasma and blood components into the interstitial spaces and the migration of leukocytes into the inflamed site. Histamine, serotonin, prostaglandins, bradykinin, chemokines, and leukotrienes are chemical mediators of inflammation that are released from granulocytic cells such as mast cells, basophils, and eosinophils. Phagocytic cells such as neutrophils and macrophages can engulf foreign substances, triggering the release of inflammatory molecules. Anti-inflammatory drugs, such as corticosteroid and prednisone, and nonsteroidal anti-inflammatory drugs (NSAIDs), such as ibuprofen and aspirin, are used to control inflammation.

1. **Corticosteroids:** These drugs, specifically glucocorticoids, have broad and potent anti-inflammatory and immunosuppressive effects. Glucocorticoids have been used for the treatment of rheumatoid arthritis since 1949. This drug is currently widely used to nonspecifically treat many inflammatory diseases and conditions, including autoimmune disorders, allergic diseases, and asthma, and to prevent organ rejection.

Glucocorticoids are steroid hormones that bind to the cytosolic glucocorticoid receptor (Fig.18.1). This newly formed complex then enters into the cell nucleus and binds to the glucocorticoid response elements in the promoter region of the specific gene, causing an increase in expression of the target genes or prevents the expression of the target genes. Glucocorticoids are effective anti-inflammatory agents, although the specific mechanism of their anti-inflammatory effect is not completely understood. Known effects of corticosteroids include the following:

- Inhibition of translation of genes encoding cytokines IL-1, IL-2, IL-3, IL-4, IL-5, IL-6, IL-8, and TNF-α
- Diminished B cell clone expansion and decreased antibody synthesis
- Decreased IL-2 production, reducing T cell proliferation
- Decreased size and lymphoid content of the spleen and lymph nodes
- Functional modification of certain T cell subsets
- Increased synthesis of lipocortin-1, which inhibits the production of lipid mediators such as prostaglandin, and leukotrienes
- Decreased numbers of T cells, eosinophils, and mast cells in the lamina propria of the airways
- Inhibition of monocyte and neutrophil chemotaxis
- Changes in leukocyte distribution, causing lymphopenia (decreased numbers of lymphocyte) and neutrophilia (increased numbers of neutrophils)

Many conditions and diseases, such as inflammatory bowel disease, systemic lupus erythematosus, autoimmune hemolytic anemia, idiopathic thrombocytopenic purpura, and rheumatoid arthritis, respond to corticosteroids. Corticosteroids are currently available in many forms, such as oral, intravenous, intramuscular, inhalation, and topical administrations. Inhalation and intranasal

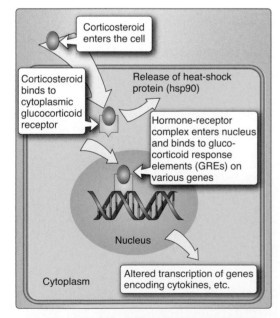

Figure 18.1
Glucocorticoid and the cytosolic glucocorticoid receptor.

corticosteroids are widely used in the treatment of asthma and rhinitis. Topical administration is effective in the treatment of atopic dermatitis and ocular allergy. To minimize immune responses against graft antigens, corticosteroids are useful in organ transplant rejection crises, particularly in cases of imperfectly matched grafts.

There are risks associated with corticosteroid usage. Clinically significant adverse effects due to corticosteroid usage are related to the dose, duration, and route of administration. Chronic high-dose systemic therapy can cause significant adverse effects. In children, for example, chronic administration of glucocorticoids can slow linear bone growth. Other clinically significant adverse effects include hypothalamic pituitary axis suppression, infection, hypertension, cataracts, hyperglycemia, and osteoporosis. Individuals using corticosteroids should be closely monitored for any adverse reactions.

2. **Nonsteroidal anti-inflammatory drugs (NSAIDs):** These drugs include aspirin and ibuprofen. NSAIDs have anti-inflammatory, antipyretic and analgesic effects (Fig. 18.2). In addition to providing clinical benefit in the treatment of anti-inflammatory diseases, aspirin is also used to treat conditions requiring inhibition of platelet aggregation. NSAIDs irreversibly block the prostaglandin synthase enzyme, which has two isoforms: cyclooxygenase-1 (COX-1) and cyclooxygenase-2 (COX-2). COX-1 is responsible for thromboxane synthesis, and COX-2 is responsible for

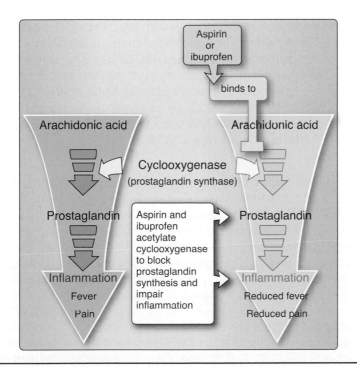

Figure 18.2
NSAIDs: aspirin and ibuprofen. Inhibition of prostaglandin synthesis diminishes inflammation by blocking cyclooxygenase.

prostaglandin synthesis. The inhibitory effects of prostaglandins include decreases in edema, leukocyte infiltration, pain, and fever. The inhibition of thromboxane production reduces platelet aggregation. The anti-inflammatory effect of NSAIDs is usually observed at high doses, while the analgesic (pain-relieving) effect is dose-responsive (Fig. 18.2).

The desirable effects of NSAIDs are thought to be due to the inhibition of COX-2, and the side effects are thought to be due to inhibition of COX-1. For this reason, COX-2-selective agents were developed. However, long-term treatments with COX-2-selective inhibitors have been shown to increase the risk of myocardial infarctions. As a result, some of these COX-2-selective inhibitors have been withdrawn from the market.

In general, NSAIDs are used clinically to treat mild to moderate pain and inflammatory conditions, such as rheumatoid arthritis. Aspirin's inhibition of platelet aggregation makes it clinically useful in the prevention of coronary artery thrombosis and transient ischemic attack. The main adverse effects of chronic NSAID use are gastric irritation, erosion, and hemorrhage. Other clinically significant effects include renal tubular necrosis and acute renal failure.

B. Immunosuppressive measures

Autoimmune diseases occur when adverse immune response develops against self epitopes. Autoimmune diseases can result from damage inflicted on cells and tissues by humoral or cell-mediated immune responses and sometimes by both. Suppressor cells of various types serve to maintain immune tolerance. When the numbers of these suppressor cells decline with age, the risk of autoimmune diseases is enhanced in aged individuals by allowing previously suppressed autoreactive lymphocytes to become active. Immune responses in autoimmune diseases such as rheumatoid arthritis, inflammatory bowel disease, and systemic lupus erythematosus can be diminished in some cases by pharmacologic agents. Immune suppressive measures are also used to diminish overt and often catastrophic effects of graft rejection or in the treatment of bronchial asthma.

1. **Rheumatoid arthritis therapy:** Rheumatoid arthritis (RA) is a chronic multisystem, inflammatory, autoimmune disease that affects the synovia and cartilages of small and large joints as well as other organ systems. It is a destructive disease that involves both cell-mediated and humoral immune responses (Fig. 18.3). The initial underlying cause of RA is still unknown. Cartilage damage is due to the $CD4^+$ T-cell recognition of antigen(s) within the joint that triggers the release of inflammatory cytokines that lead to the accumulation of neutrophils and macrophages. Within the inflamed synovia are B cells, plasma cells, $CD4^+$ T cells, and various types of inflammatory cytokines, such as tumor necrosis factor-α (TNF-α), IL-1, IL-8, and IFN-γ. **Rheumatoid factors** (IgM or IgG autoantibodies directed against the Fc region of circulating IgG) are formed that facilitate the formation of immune complexes. In advanced stages of RA, deposition and complement

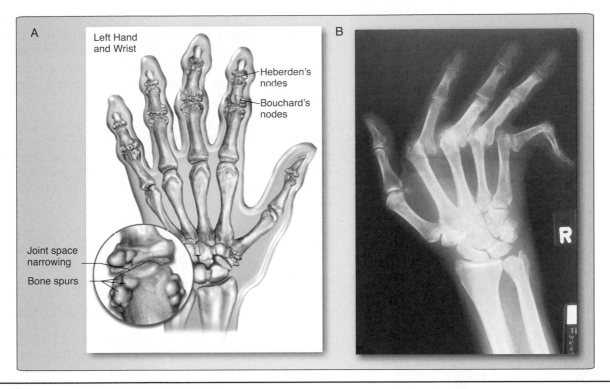

Figure 18.3
Rheumatoid arthritis. **A.** Rheumatoid arthritis–induced damage to joint cartilage is due to the CD4$^+$ T cell recognition of the initiating antigen within the joint, triggering the release of inflammatory cytokines. Production of IgG antibodies against the initiating antigen also contributes to the inflammation through the formation of immune complexes. **B.** X-ray of hand of patient with severe rheumatoid arthritis.

fixation of these immune complexes may contribute not only to joint destruction but also to vasculitis, carditis, and pleuritis.

In addition to glucocorticoids such as prednisone, therapies for RA include disease-modifying antirheumatic drugs (DMARDs), TNF-α inhibitors, IL-1 receptor inhibitors, and immunomodulators. NSAIDs that inhibit cyclooxygenase and blocking prostaglandin formation help to reduce the pain and inflammation associated with RA. DMARDs such as methotrexate, antimalarial drugs, gold salt therapy, and sulfasalazine can mitigate the disease process but usually do not lead to complete remission.

How DMARDs actually work is not fully understood, but it appears that they modify the immune system. DMARD treatment may take up to six to eight months to become fully effective. Although effective in treating RA, the side effects of DMARD treatment are often significant, and people taking the drug require frequent monitoring.

The most widely used DMARD as an immunosuppressive agent in the treatment of rheumatic disease is methotrexate. This drug inhibits DNA synthesis by inhibiting dihydrofolate reductase, an enzyme required for the conversion of folic acid into its active form, tetrahydrofolate (an enzyme that is involved in the synthesis of thymidine). Toxicity of methotrexate treatment is mainly associated with rapidly dividing cells. Therefore it can have significant adverse effects within the gastrointestinal mucosa and bone marrow, mainly suppression. Other clinically significant adverse effects include hepatic fibrosis and hypersensitivity pneumonitis. Because of the severe side effects, only low doses of methotrexate are used to treat RA.

Other DMARDs agents that are used in the treatment of RA are alkylating agents such as cyclophosphamide and purine analogs such as azathioprine. These agents inhibit cell proliferation. These immunosuppressive agents also have significant adverse effects, including hepatic toxicity, and are associated with an increased risk of cancer and infection.

Systemic inflammatory processes and local joint destruction in RA involves cytokines. The development of drugs that inhibit cytokines and cytokine function proved to be useful in treating patients with RA. TNF-α-neutralizing monoclonal antibodies, soluble recombinant TNF-α receptors, and IL-1 receptor–blocking proteins are several treatment options currently available for patients.

Using monoclonal antibodies to effectively bind TNF-α, a cytokine that is crucial to the disease process, is one way of treating RA. Another is to use a so-called **immunoadhesin** molecule, a fusion protein produced by recombinant DNA technology that combines the constant domain of an antibody molecule with the ligand-recognition domain of a cytokine receptor. A third way is by using a recombinant protein that mimics a naturally occurring IL-1 receptor antagonist, which would effectively block the IL-1 binding site.

TNF-α receptor inhibitors, such as adalimumab, etanercept, and infliximab, can effectively inactivate TNF-α. TNF-α inhibitors can decrease the signs and symptoms of RA and can reduce the progression of joint damage. In addition, their onset of action is faster than that of DMARDs. Adverse effects associated with cytokine inhibitors include infections, such as the reactivation of latent tuberculosis infections.

Anti-IL-1 receptor antagonist is yet another agent that is used in the treatment of RA. IL-1 is a protein found in increased amounts in joints of individuals with RA. Use of the antagonist reduces the binding of IL-1 to the IL-1 receptor (IL-1R). Serious side effects of this drug are an increase in infection and a decrease in the number of white blood cells and platelets.

2. **Asthma therapy: Asthma** is a common, chronic inflammatory respiratory disorder. The pathogenesis of asthma involves inflammatory cells such as mast cells, neutrophils, eosinophils, and CD4$^+$ Th2 cells. Inflammation of the bronchi causes bronchial constriction and airway hyperresponsiveness, leading to recurrent dyspnea and episodes of wheezing and coughing in susceptible individuals (Fig.18.4). Chronic asthma can develop into refractory inflammation of the airways, accompanied by increased bronchial edema, mucus production and bronchial obstruction. Airflow obstruction is often reversible, either spontaneously or following treatment. A predisposing factor in the development of bronchial

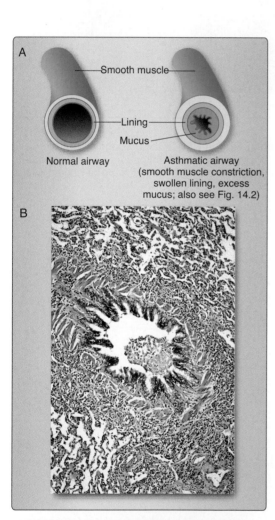

Figure 18.4
Bronchial asthma. **A.** A normal bronchus and the bronchus of a patient with asthma; bronchial inflammation associated with edema, mucus production, and obstruction. **B.** Histologic section of asthmatic bronchiole.

asthma is **atopy**, the genetic predisposition to develop IgE-mediated responses to common allergens such as mold. Other causes or common triggers of asthma include respiratory infections and animal dander (e.g., from cats).

Treatments for asthma include bronchodilatory agents such as β_2-adrenergic receptor agonists (albuterol), methylxanthines (theophylline), and anticholinergic agents (ipratropium bromide); anti-inflammatory agents, such as corticosteroids, inhibitors of mast cell degranulation (e.g., cromolyn), and leukotriene antagonists (zileuton, montelukast, and zafirlukast); and novel immunomodulatory agents, such as omalizumab, a monoclonal anti-IgE antibody.

3. **Transplantation:** Most transplants involve some degree of genetic mismatch between host and donor. Transplanted cells, tissues, and organs are susceptible to destruction by the host immune system (host versus graft), and in the case of bone marrow transplantation, it is the host tissues that are susceptible to attack from the immunocompetent cells of the graft (graft versus host). In either case, the successful coexistence of host and graft may depend upon the applications of therapy to diminish the destructive responses of the immune system, whether derived from host or donor.

One approach has been the use of immune suppression (or immunosuppression), which is treatment that imposes a broad and general inhibition of immune responsiveness, without regard to specificity. Over the past few decades, however, drugs such as cyclosporine, tacrolimus, and rapamycin have been developed that have more restricted effects on the immune system. Their effects are targeted more closely to those cells reacting to graft antigens while leaving the remainder of the immune system relatively uninhibited in its ability to deal with infectious agents. They are not without risk, however. Patients must often receive the drugs for an extended period of time. If a significant infection occurs during this period, the immune cells responding to the infectious agent could be inhibited in the same way as those responding to graft alloantigens. In addition, extended use of these drugs is sometimes associated with damage to organs such as the liver.

Cyclosporine is an essential immunosuppressive agent that was discovered in 1976. It has demonstrated significant efficacy in the treatment of graft-versus-host syndrome after transplantation of bone marrow and other organs and in treatment of some autoimmune diseases. Cyclosporine is a specific inhibitor of T cell–mediated immunity. In vitro studies have shown that it selectively alters the immune regulation activities of helper T cells. Specifically, cyclosporine inhibits calcineurin, which is necessary for the activation of T cells. Therefore, it suppresses the production of IL-2. Clinically significant adverse effects include nephrotoxicity, neurotoxicity, and hepatotoxicity.

Tacrolimus is a macrolide antibiotic derived from the bacterium *Streptomyces tsukubaensis* and is about 50 to 100 times more potent than cyclosporine. Its mechanism of action is similar to that

Table 18.1
TREATMENT OF AUTOIMMUNE AND INFLAMMATORY DISEASES

Disease	Affected Tissues/Organs	Common Signs And Symptoms	Immunosuppressive/ Anti-inflammatory Agents
Crohn's disease (Fig. 18.5)	Intestinal mucosa layers	Diarrhea, right lower quadrant abdominal pain with an inflammatory mass, fever, and weight loss	Sulfasalazine, corticosteroid, azathioprine, methotrexate, TNF-α inhibitors
Multiple sclerosis	White matter of brain and spinal cord	Sensory symptoms, optic neuritis, diplopia, limb weakness, ataxia, cognitive and affective abnormalities, fatigue, constipation, urinary urgency/ frequency, and sexual dysfunction	IFN-β-1a, IFN-β-1b, glatiramer acetate, mitoxantrone, natalizumab, corticosteroid
Systemic lupus erythematosus (Fig. 18.6)	Joints, muscle, vasculature, kidneys, skin, mucosa, central nervous system, blood, heart, and lungs	Arthritis, weight loss, fever, fatigue, rash, mouth sores, alopecia, and photosensitivity	Aspirin, NSAIDs, corticosteroid, hydroxychloroquine. cyclophosphamide, mycophenolate mofetil
Myasthenia gravis	Muscle motor end plate (neuromuscular junction)	Muscle weakness (ptosis, diplopia, and dysarthria)	Corticosteroids, cyclosporine, azathioprine
Dermatomyositis	Skin and muscle	Weight loss, fever, arthralgias, proximal muscle weakness, fatigue, rash, and photosensitivity	Corticosteroid, methotrexate, azathioprine, cyclophosphamide, mycophenolate mofetil
Ulcerative colitis	Colonic mucosa and submucosa	Diarrhea and hematoschezia	Sulfasalazine, corticosteroid, azathioprine, methotrexate, TNF-α inhibitors
Psoriasis	Skin	Inflamed, edematous skin lesions covered with a silvery white scale	Topical steroid and retinoids, TNF-α inhibitors
Psoriatic arthritis	Joints	Arthritis, arthralgia (oligoarticular joint inflammation)	NSAIDs, corticosteroid, methotrexate, sulfasalazine, TNF-α inhibitors
Ankylosing spondylitis	Axial skeletal and sacroiliac joints	Inflammatory back pain, and arthritis of the hips and knees	NSAIDs, sulfasalazine, methotrexate, TNF-α inhibitors

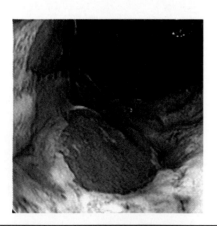

Figure 18.5
Crohn's disease. A segmental involvement of the intestine is seen, with discontinuous areas of inflammation. The inflammation involves all layers of the intestine.

of cyclosporine in that it also selectively alters the activities of helper T cells by inhibiting calcineurin and thus IL-2 synthesis and secretion. Clinically significant adverse effects of tacrolimus are similar to those for cyclosporine, including nephrotoxicity.

Sirolimus (rapamycin) is also a macrolide antibiotic, isolated from the fungus *S. hygroscopicus*, that is structurally similar to tacrolimus. However, rapamycin interferes with the immune response by blocking IL-2 receptor signaling and inhibiting protein synthesis. Clinically significant adverse effects of rapamycin include hyperlipidemia, leukopenia, and thrombocytopenia.

4. **Other autoimmune and inflammatory diseases:** Preferred treatments for several autoimmune diseases, some of which are discussed in Chapter 16, are given in Table 18.1. Some of these diseases are systemic (e.g., SLE), while others have more limited effects on specific organs and tissues. Autoimmune diseases can result from pathology initiated by humoral responses, cell-mediated immune responses, or both.

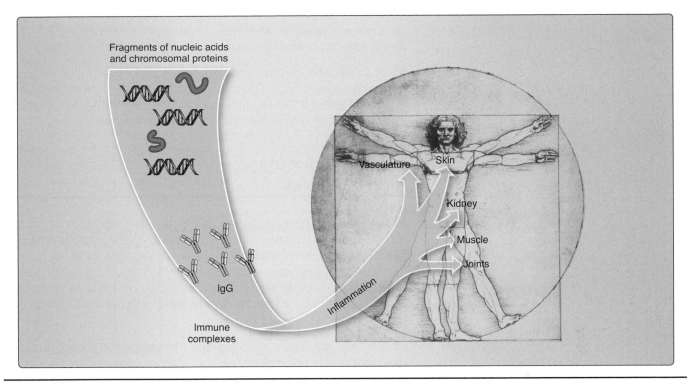

Figure 18.6
Systemic lupus erythematosus. This disorder is associated with autoantibodies against fragments of nucleic acids and chromosomal proteins, producing a systemic inflammation (type III hypersensitivity) that affects many organs and tissues of the body.

CLINICAL APPLICATION
Ankylosing spondylitis

Jeff, a 35-year-old-male, presents with low back pain that has persisted for more than three months. He describes pain mainly in the sacrum and in the buttocks area and occasionally radiating down the legs. The pain sometimes wakes the patient up at night, and in the morning, he feels that his back is stiff. Physical examination is remarkable for mild loss of lateral flexion of the lumbar spine. Laboratory examination reveals an increased in erythrocyte sedimentation rate and leukocytosis. The rheumatoid factor test is negative. This patient's human leukocyte antigen typing is positive for HLA-B27. Radiograph of the spine shows mild subchondral bony erosions on the iliac side of the bone calcification and ossification in the sacrum area.

This patient presents with symptoms and signs consistent with ankylosing spondylitis. The pathophysiology of **ankylosing spondylitis** is due to inflammation associated with cellular infiltration of lymphocytes, plasma cells, and leukocytes in the affected joints, particularly sacroiliac, spinal facet joints, and paravertebral soft tissues. The etiology is unknown. However, approximately 90% to 95% of patients are positive for human leukocyte antigen HLA-B27, and these patients commonly have a family history of the disease.

Initial treatments for this patient include a lifelong exercise program and analgesics such as NSAIDs. Other alternative anti-inflammatory agents (Table 18.1) may provide clinical benefit. As the disease progresses, spinal and hip surgery may be indicated.

CLINICAL APPLICATION
Ulcerative colitis

Rob, a 30-year-old-male, presents with frequent episodes of bloody diarrhea, abdominal pain, fecal urgency, and low grade fever for 1 week. Physical examination reveals a temperature of 38°C, tachycardia, abdominal pain, and bloody stool. Laboratory examination reveals mild anemia and leukocytosis. Colonoscopy examination reveals crypt abscesses and superficial inflammation from the rectum to the colon.

This patient presents with signs and symptoms suggesting **ulcerative colitis**. The findings on the colonoscopy confirm the diagnosis. The etiology of ulcerative colitis is unknown. Interestingly, the risk of developing ulcerative colitis is associated with nonsmokers and former smokers. Medical treatment options for ulcerative colitis are similar to those listed for Crohn's disease in Table 18.1. For patients with severe disease that is refractory to medical therapies, surgery may be indicated.

CLINICAL APPLICATION
Systemic lupus erythematosus

Joy, a 25-year-old-female presents, with a butterfly-shaped rash on her cheeks and mild joint pain. Physical examination reveals a temperature of 38°C and a fixed erythema on her cheeks. She also has mild tenderness, and swelling in the joints of both of her hands. Laboratory tests revealed mild anemia, leukocytosis, and positive tests for antinuclear antibody and anti-double-stranded DNA.

This patient has signs and symptoms consistent with **systemic lupus erythematosus (SLE)**, a disorder associated with autoantibodies against fragments of nucleic acids and chromosomal proteins, producing inflammation that affects many organs and tissues of the body.

For definitive diagnosis, a patient must have four of the following findings at any time: malar rash (butterfly rash, appearing on the face), discoid skin lesion, photosensitivity, oral ulcers, nonserosive arthritis, serositis, renal disorders, neurologic disorder, hematologic disorder, immunologic disorder, and antinuclear antibody. Medical treatment options for SLE are listed in Table 18.1.

IV. THERAPIES USED TO ALTER THE IMMUNE RESPONSE

Therapies are sometimes used to alter the immune response by prevention, stopping the immune response before it starts, or by redirecting it to less harmful immune responses. The management of allergic symptoms or severe and potentially fatal response such as anaphylaxis, on the other hand, provides an example in which redirecting the immune response to less harmful effects provides benefit.

A. Preemptive measures

Once an immune response begins, it is difficult to fully suppress the effect. A more successful approach is to use therapeutic measures before an immune response develops, but this requires that a possible adverse immune response is imminent. Antibiotic therapy is an example of preemptive measure.

1. **Antibiotic therapy:** Antibiotics are sometimes given to prevent a bacterial infection and limit the development of adaptive immune responses that may be potentially injurious. For example, in addition to causing structural heart disease, rheumatic heart fever was the leading cause of death in many children before 1960. With the development of preventive antibiotic treatment, the incidence of rheumatic fever has declined significantly. Rheumatic fever is associated with a prior group A streptococcal infection such as acute pharyngitis. Rheumatic fever is generally a self-limiting illness; symptoms spontaneously subside over a period of days in the large majority of patients. In some patients, complications develop that lead to the production of self-reactive antibodies that causes autoimmune acute rheumatic fever (ARF), a condition that can result in rheumatic heart disease. Inflammation of the heart, specifically valvular vegetations and mitral valve regurgitation are causes of long-term morbidity. Joints, central nervous system, skin, and subcutaneous tissues may also be affected. Rheumatic fever occurs because of cross-reactivity between streptococcal cell wall and heart tissues, and the use of penicillin or other antibiotics decreases the probability that sufficient antibody will be produced to cause heart disease.

B. Modification of ongoing disease

Therapeutic measures provide benefit by minimizing the course of the disease. Systemic administration of cytokines has been used clinically to alter the course of a number of diseases. Allergen immunotherapy administered to patients with allergic diseases is a way of redirecting the immune response to less harmful effects.

1. **Cytokines:** These protein molecules act as messengers between cells and affect their functions. Systemic administration of cytokines has been used clinically to alter the course of many diseases, including cancer. Clinical research studies support the use of IFNs as treatments for several malignancies as well as other diseases. IFN-α has been used to treat malignant, chronic myelogenous

leukemia; Kaposi's sarcoma; hairy cell leukemia; and hepatitis B and C. IFN-β has been used to treat the relapsing type of multiple sclerosis and IFN-γ to treat chronic granulomatous disease. In addition, IFN-γ has also been used to treat patients with severe atopic (IgE-mediated) dermatitis. IFN-γ downregulates IL-4 production and decreases the development of IgE responses. Although the interferons have therapeutic benefits, there are systemic side effects associated with this agent. The most commonly reported side effect is flulike symptoms.

HIV, the virus that causes AIDS, kills $CD4^+$ T cells and reduces the numbers of monocytes/macrophages. $CD8^+$ T cell numbers can also become reduced. Recently, deaths due to HIV infection in developed countries have declined dramatically owing to **highly active antiretroviral therapy (HAART)**. However, although the viral load is decreased with HAART, the virus is not eliminated. A number of cytokine therapies are currently being tested in clinical or preclinical trials with the objective of restoring the functional immune cells and preventing opportunistic infections, including the following:

- IL-2 to reverse $CD4^+$ T cell lymphopenia
- IL-12 to enhance HIV specific cell-mediated immunity
- IL-15 to enhance $CD8^+$ T cell function
- IFN-α/IFN-γ to enhance CTL responses
- GM-CSF to enhance monocyte/macrophage function
- G-CSF to increase myeloid cell precursors.

As with most other types of treatments, systemic cytokine therapy is accompanied by adverse side effects. For example, IL-2 supports the growth of T lymphocytes and NK cells but also increases apoptosis in T cell populations. IL-15 also simulates proliferation of both $CD8^+$ and $CD4^+$ T cell populations and appears to be anti-apoptotic.

2. **Allergen immunotherapy:** Allergen immunotherapy involves subcutaneous administration of an aqueous extract of the allergen repeatedly over a period of weeks to months in gradually increasing doses. The objective of allergen immunotherapy is to reduce responses to allergic triggers, decrease inflammatory responses, and prevent development of persistent disease.

With repeated immunization, antibody production is redirected from being predominantly IgE to being predominantly IgG. IgG antibodies bind and remove the allergen before it can interact with IgE antibodies bound to the surfaces of mast cells. This treatment is indicated for patients with allergic rhinitis, allergic asthma, or stinging insect hypersensitivity. These patients have symptoms that are not easily controlled by avoiding exposure to an allergen, or pharmacologic therapy for them has not proven to be effective. Allergen immunotherapy is normally safe. However, a serious adverse reaction—anaphylaxis—may develop. All patients receiving immunotherapy should be observed for at least 20 minutes following injection, and emergency treatments, including antihistamine and epinephrine, should be available if necessary.

Chapter Summary

- **Adjuvants** administered with vaccines can indirectly heighten the effect of the vaccine indirectly by attracting antigen-presenting cells and increasing their expression of costimulatory molecules.

- Cytokines affect the induction and intensity of cellular growth and differentiation, cell activation, tissue inflammation, and tissue repair. Both type I (IFN-α/β) and type II (IFN-γ) interferons have been used as immunotherapeutic agents to heighten immune responsiveness in patients with viral infections such as hepatitis B or hepatitis C.

- The administration of exogenous immunoglobulin (human immune globulin, or HIg) can be effective therapy for individuals with generalized antibody deficiencies.

- Glucocorticoids are anti-inflammatory steroid hormones that bind to cytosolic glucocorticoid receptors, forming complexes that can enter the nucleus and alter transcription of particular sets of genes. They are used to treat inflammatory bowel disease, systemic lupus erythematosus, autoimmune hemolytic anemia, idiopathic thrombocytopenic purpura, and rheumatoid arthritis.

- NSAIDs reduce inflammation by inhibiting prostaglandins and thromboxane synthesis through the inactivation of cyclooxygenase (prostaglandin synthase).

- Rheumatoid arthritis is a chronic multisystem, inflammatory, autoimmune disease that affects the synovia and cartilages of small joints, large joints, and other organ systems. Therapies include glucocorticoids disease-modifying antirheumatic drugs (DMARDs), TNF-α inhibitors, interleukin-1 receptor inhibitors, and immunomodulators.

- Bronchial asthma is a common, chronic inflammatory respiratory disorder. The pathogenesis of asthma involves inflammatory cells such as mast cells, neutrophils, eosinophils, and CD4$^+$ Th2 cells.

- Cyclosporine inhibits calcineurin, suppressing the production of IL-2. Tacrolimus has a mechanism of action similar to that of cyclosporine in selectively inhibiting calcineurin and inhibiting IL-2 synthesis and secretion. Rapamycin blocks the response by blocking IL-2 receptor signaling and inhibiting protein synthesis.

Study Questions

18.1 Which of the following describes a common use of an adjuvant?

A. to diminish B cell clone expansion and antibody synthesis
B. to enhance the effect of a vaccine
C. to improve antibody deficiencies
D. to inhibit translation of genes encoding numerous cytokines
E. to treat inflammatory diseases including autoimmune disorders

The correct answer is B. Adjuvants are commonly used to enhance the effect of a vaccine. Adjuvant therapy is given in addition to a primary treatment to nonspecifically stimulate immune responses, either directly or indirectly. Antibody deficiencies are sometimes treated with human immune globulin (HIg). Anti-inflammatory agents such as glucocorticoids can diminish B cell clone expansion and antibody synthesis and can also inhibit translation of cytokine genes. Glucocorticoids are also used to treat inflammatory diseases.

18.2 An individual is given therapy with human immune globulin (HIg). Which of the following conditions would be appropriate for this type of therapy?

A. agammaglobulinanemia
B. allergy
C. rheumatoid arthritis
D. superficial bladder cancer
E. systemic lupus erythematosus

The correct answer is A. HIg is used to treat agammaglobulinemia, a generalized antibody deficiency that may be improved by administering HIg. Consisting primarily of IgG, HIg is obtained from pooled immune human sera and can provide reactivity against a broad range of epitopes. Anti-inflammatory agents, such as glucocorticoids, are often used to treat allergic disease and rheumatoid arthritis. Superficial bladder cancer is sometimes treated with the direct administration of the Bacillus Calmette-Guérin (BCG) adjuvant. HIg does not have antiviral properties; type I interferons have been used to heighten immune responsiveness in patients with hepatitis B or hepatitis C viruses.

18.3 Glucocorticoids exert immunosuppressive effects by

A. binding to intracellular receptors and influencing gene transcription.
B. impairing the ability of platelets to aggregate.
C. inhibiting cyclooxygenase and thromboxane production.
D. stimulating IL-2 production and T cell proliferation.
E. upregulating cell-surface receptors for cytokines.

The correct answer is A. Glucocorticoids bind to intracellular receptors located in the cytosol and then influence (inducing or inhibiting) the transcription of responsive genes. NSAIDs inhibit cyclooxygenase and therefore inhibit the production of prostaglandins, resulting in reduction in edema, leukocyte infiltration, pain, and fever. The NSAID aspirin impairs platelet aggregation by irreversibly inhibiting the cyclooxygenase enzyme and reducing production of thromboxane A2 in platelets. Glucocorticoids are immunosuppressive in nature and inhibit IL-2 production and T cell proliferation rather than stimulating them. Glucocorticoids are immunosuppressive and do not facilitate response to cytokines by upregulating cytokine receptors.

18.4 A 12-year-old female with a history of IgE-mediated responses to a variety of common allergens presents with acute bronchial asthma. Which of the following treatment approaches will most likely be used first in her treatment?

A. inhaled β_2-adrenergic receptor agonist
B. injected adjuvants
C. orally administered aspirin
D. subcutaneously injected cytokines
E. systemically administered antihistamines

The correct answer is A. Inhaled β_2-adrenergic receptor agonists (such as albuterol) are used first to treat acute asthma. Adjuvants are used to heighten immune responses, which is not a goal in treating acute asthma, which may result from allergy. NSAIDs such as aspirin have anti-inflammatory properties but are not quick-acting as an inhaled β_2-adrenergic receptor agonist is. Cytokines would not reduce an immune mediated inflammatory process such as acute asthma. Systemically administered corticosteroids are useful in treating chronic inflammation.

18.5 Following a bone marrow transplant, which of the following therapies will be most appropriate to inhibit T cell–mediated immunity and the development of graft-versus-host responses?

A. adjuvants
B. aspirin
C. corticosteroids
D. cyclosporine
E. cytokines

The correct answer is D. Cyclosporine is a specific inhibitor of T cell–mediated immunity and is an immunosuppressive agent with proven efficacy in the treatment of graft-versus-host disease after bone marrow transplantation. Adjuvants heighten immune responses. Aspirin and corticosteroids have broad anti-inflammatory actions. Cytokines are immune mediators that are sometimes used to enhance immunity, against tumors for example.

Tumor Immunity

19

I. OVERVIEW

Cell growth and cell death are normally balanced. Occasionally, cells arise that no longer respond to the usual checks and balances for division and death. These are tumor cells. Development from a normal cell to a cancerous one requires several transformation steps. Transformed tumor cells express characteristic cell surface antigens and these antigens often initiate immune responses. Therapeutic approaches, which attempt to exploit these normal immune responses to tumors, continue to be investigated. However, tumors also evade recognition by the immune system, and at times, tumor growth appears to be enhanced by immune mediators produced against that very tumor.

II. CANCER

A **tumor**, or **neoplasm**, is a collection of the clonal descendants of a cell whose growth has gone unchecked. When a tumor continues to grow and to invade healthy tissue, it is considered to be a **cancer**.

A. Terminology and definitions

Malignant tumors are distinguished from **benign** tumors by their progressive growth and invasiveness. **Metastasis** is a characteristic of many malignant tumors (cancers). Metastatic cells become dislodged from the main tumor, invade blood or lymphatic vessels, and travel to other tissues, where they continue to grow and to invade. In this way, tumors at one site can give rise to secondary tumors at other sites within the body (Fig. 19.1).

Classification of tumors is based on the embryonic origin of the tissue from which the malignant cells are derived. **Carcinomas** develop from endodermal or ectodermal tissues (e.g., skin, glands) and constitute the majority of malignant tumors, including cancers of the breast, colon, and lung. **Sarcomas** develop from bone and cartilage and have a much lower incidence than carcinomas. **Leukemias** are malignant cells of hematopoietic lineage that proliferate as individual cells, while **lymphomas** arise from malignant hematopoietic cells but grow as solid tumors.

B. Malignant transformation

Experiments with cultured cells have allowed researchers to trace the development of tumors. Cells that are infected with certain viruses

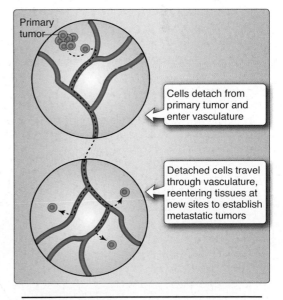

Figure 19.1

Metastasis. Tumor cells can detach from the primary tumor and travel through the vasculature to establish metastatic tumors at other sites.

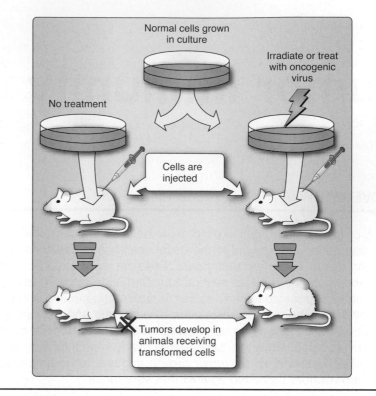

Figure 19.2
Malignant transformation. Transfection or irradiation of normal cultured cells alters them in such as way that they will induce the formation of tumors when injected into experimental animals.

(e.g., SV40 or Rous sarcoma virus), irradiated (ultraviolet light or ionizing radiation), or treated with certain DNA-altering chemicals show altered growth properties and often induce tumors when injected into animals (Fig. 19.2). Such transformed cells can be grown in culture almost indefinitely. In some cases when retroviruses (RNA viruses) induce such growth change in cells, the process is related to the presence of **oncogenes** (cancer-producing genes) of the virus. Change from a normal cell to a tumor cell is known as **malignant transformation.** The process of malignant transformation requires at least two distinct phases. The first phase is **initiation,** which changes the genome of the cell; the second is **promotion**, which results in stimulation of cell division.

C. Tumors of the immune system

Lymphomas and **leukemias** are tumors of immune cells. Lymphomas are solid tumors within lymphoid tissues such as bone marrow and lymph nodes. Hodgkin's and non-Hodgkin's lymphomas are examples. Leukemias are composed of dispersed single cells that arise from the bone marrow and may involve cells from either lymphoid or myeloid lineages. Acute leukemias arise from less mature cells and are found in both children and adults. Chronic leukemias are tumors of more mature cells that develop slowly and are seen only in adults.

D. Oncogenes and cell growth

In some cases, malignant transformation induced by retroviruses (or RNA viruses) has been linked to the presence of cancer-causing or **oncogenes** within the retrovirus. The viral oncogene, *Src* (v-*Src*) from the Rous sarcoma virus is an example of this type of gene. Inserting this virus into normal cells in culture results in malignant transformation. Cells have genes, referred to as proto-oncogenes or cellular oncogenes, that are counterparts of retroviral oncogenes. Conversion of a cellular proto-oncogene (e.g., c-*Src*) into a cancer-promoting oncogene (e.g., v-*Src*) can occur by mutation. This change is generally accompanied by a change in cellular growth because the cellular oncogenes normally code for growth-controlling proteins.

1. **Stimulators of cell division:** Oncogenes that function as stimulators of cell division include those that encode growth factors and growth factor receptors. Oncogenes may also code for proteins involved in signaling pathways, particularly via tyrosine phosphorylation, and those that function as transcription factors. Increased activity of proteins encoded by oncogenes in this category can result in uncontrolled cellular proliferation. Examples include *sis*, which encodes a chain of platelet-derived growth factor, and *erb-b*, which encodes epidermal growth factor receptor (Table 19.1). *Src* and *Abl*, in their proto-oncogenic (cellular) forms encode tyrosine kinases that regulate cell division. In their oncogenic forms, the regulatory function of these proteins has been lost, and affected cells will have unregulated proliferation. *Ras* codes for a GTP-binding protein; continued stimulation of division occurs when the oncogene form of *ras*

Table 19.1
ONCOGENES

Classification	Gene	Function
Stimulators of cell division	Abl	Tyrosine kinase
	erb-b	Receptor for epidermal growth factor
	Fms	Receptor for colony-stimulating factor
	fos	Component of a transcription factor
	Jun	Component of a transcription factor
	Myc	DNA-binding protein
	Ras	GTP-binding protein
	Sis	Altered form of platelet-derived growth factor
	Src	Tyrosine kinase
Inhibitors of cell division: tumor suppressors	NF1	Suppressor of neurofibromatosis
	Rb	Suppressor of retinoblastoma
	p53	Nuclear protein that suppresses tumor growth
Apoptosis regulators	Bax	Stimulator of programmed cell death
	Bcl-2	Inhibitor of programmed cell death

remains active. Transcription factors are encoded by the *fos*, *jun*, and *abl* oncogenes.

2. **Tumor suppressor genes:** Oncogenes that are inhibitors of cell division and are sometimes referred to as *anti-oncogenes* function as tumor suppressor genes. When a tumor suppressor is inactivated through mutation, the ability to suppress cell growth is lost, and uncontrollable cell proliferation can result. Mutated forms of the tumor suppressor *p53* have been found in many human tumor cells. Mutation of the tumor suppressor *Rb* can lead to development of the malignant retinal tumors in children with hereditary retinoblastoma.

3. **Regulators of apoptosis:** A third category of cancer-related genes are those that regulate apoptosis. Some members of this group prevent programmed cell death (apoptosis), while others induce it. *Bcl-2*, an anti-apoptotic oncogene discovered in a B-cell follicular lymphoma, normally regulates cell survival of selected lymphocytes during development. When *Bcl-2* is inappropriately expressed, a cell that would normally die via apoptosis instead survives, resulting in unregulated cell proliferation. One of several proteins related to the prosurvival *Bcl-2* is *Bax*, which is pro-apoptotic. The ratio of Bcl-2 to Bax proteins within a cell determines whether that cell will survive or undergo programmed cell death.

E. Tumor antigens

Tumor cells express antigens on their surfaces that are often the targets of immune responses. Many tumor antigens are cellular peptides presented by MHC molecules that stimulate antigen-specific T cell proliferation (Table 19.2). Some antigenic molecules on tumor cells are variant forms of normal proteins that result from mutation of the gene encoding the protein. Others are normally found only on cells of certain developmental stages or lineages and are antigenic when expressed out of their usual context. Still other tumor antigens are simply molecules found at higher than normal concentration on tumor cells, while a few others are proteins encoded by genes unique to tumors.

1. **Tumor-specific transplantation antigens (TSTAs):** TSTAs are not found on normal somatic cells but result from mutations of genes and the resulting altered proteins that are expressed by the tumor cells. Identification of TSTAs on naturally occurring tumors has proved difficult, most likely because the immune response generally eliminates cells that TSTAs at levels great enough to be antigenic. However, TSTAs have been identified on tumors induced in culture by viral transformation or treatment with carcinogenic chemicals. When introduced into syngeneic mice, TSTAs cell-mediated immune responses that attack the tumor cells (Fig. 19.3).

2. **Tumor-associated transplantation antigens (TATAs):** TATAs are not unique to tumor cells; rather, their expression on tumor

Table 19.2
CANCER ANTIGENS

Gene	Expression
AFP	Serum of fetuses and patients with liver cancer
CEA	Fetal liver and serum of patients with colorectal cancer
BAGE	Melanoma/normal testis
GAGE-1 and 2	Melanoma/normal testis
MAGE-3	Melanoma/normal testis
RAGE	Melanoma/normal testis
P15	Wide expression
PRAME	Wide expression
SART-1	Wide expression

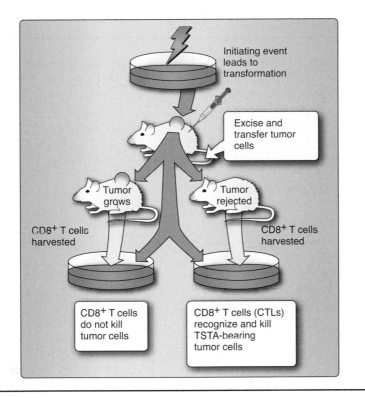

Figure 19.3
Identification of TSTAs. Transformed cells injected into syngeneic mice sometimes induce tumor formation but sometimes do not. When a nontumorigenic line is generated (tumor rejected) and CD8⁺ CTLs are harvested from that animal, those CTL cells can recognize TSTA-bearing tumor cells.

cells is altered. For example, the tumor antigen may be found in excessive amounts or may be expressed on a cell type where it would not normally exist. Human breast cancer cells often have high levels of the growth factor receptor *Neu*, which is found in very small concentrations on normal cells (see Table 19.2). MAGE-1, BAGE, and GAGE-2 are examples of oncofetal antigens because they are expressed on tumors and on normal fetal cells. After the fetal stage of development, normal differentiated cells do not express these oncofetal antigens, except for germline cells of the testis. However, oncofetal antigens are also displayed on human melanomas, gliomas, and breast carcinomas. Another oncofetal antigen, alpha-fetoprotein, is found in fetal liver cells and liver carcinoma cells (and serum of individuals with liver cancer). Other tumor cells may express greater than normal levels of tissue-specific molecules (e.g., MART-1 and gp75 are overexpressed by melanoma cells), while still other tumor cells express aberrant forms of such molecules. An example is MUC-1, a glycosylated (carbohydrate-containing) mucin that is found with decreased glycosylation on pancreatic tumors. Decreased levels of carbohydrates may reveal hidden MUC-1 epitopes.

III. IMMUNE SURVEILLANCE

The immune surveillance theory suggests that cancer cells frequently arise within the body but are normally eliminated before they multiply sufficiently to become clinically detectable. Accordingly, through the workings of an effective immune system that patrols the body and mounts responses against abnormal cells, most transformed cells never become true cancers. Tumors arise only if they are able to escape immune surveillance (Fig. 19.4). Evidence supporting the immune surveillance theory comes from immunosuppressed and immunodeficient individuals who have increased tumor incidence.

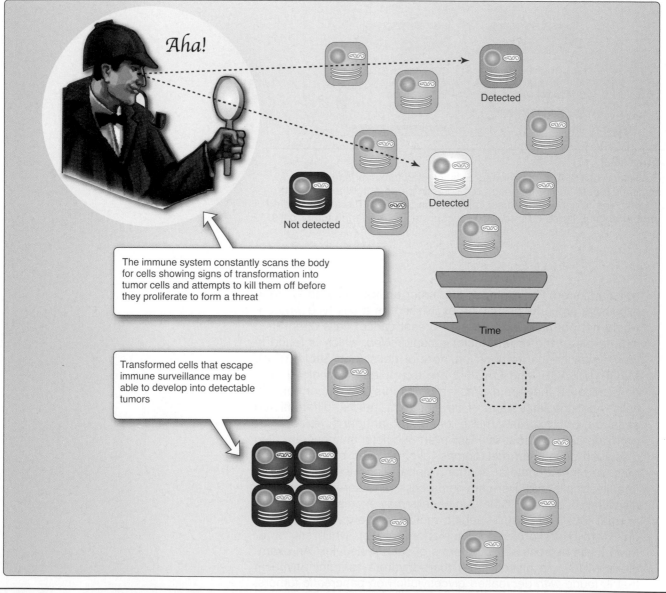

Figure 19.4

Immune surveillance. The immune system is on patrol for abnormal cells, often halting malignant cell growth before tumors arise. Only those malignant cells that escape immune detection become clinical tumors.

A. Innate

The first line of immune defense against tumors comes from the less specific component of the immune response, the innate immune system. These mechanisms to prevent spread of malignant disease are not specific to particular tumor antigens but recognize broad characteristics of tumor cells.

1. **NK cells:** NK cells have a limited ability to discriminate between tumor cells and normal cells. Recall that NK recognition of targets occurs via killer activation receptors (KARs) and killer inhibitory receptors (KIRs) (see Chapter 5). KIRs recognize human MHC class I molecules: HLA-B and HLA-C. Another inhibitory NK receptor, CD94, recognizes another class I molecule called HLA-E. When a KAR is engaged by binding to its carbohydrate ligands on target cells, the "kill" signal to the NK cell is activated (Fig.19.5). However, if the KIR receptors are engaged by binding of ligands

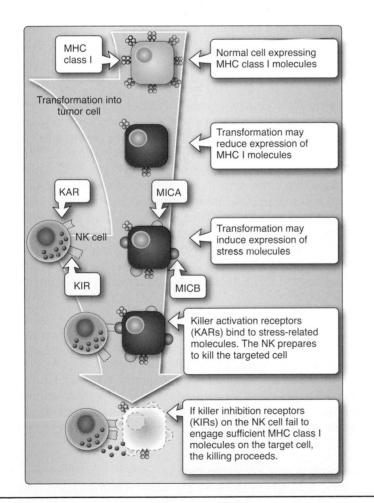

Figure 19.5

NK recognition of tumor cell targets. Transformed cells may have fewer MHC I molecules per cell and express stress molecules that are recognized by KARs on NK cells, allowing the NK cell to kill that target cell. Decreased MHC I expression decreases NK-KIR binding, permitting killing of that target cell.

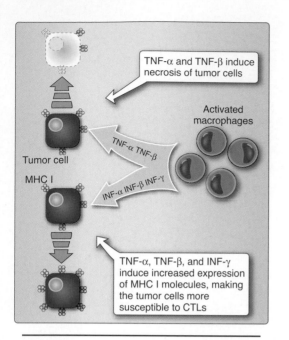

Figure 19.6
Cytokines with antitumor activity. Activated macrophages release TNF-α and TNF-β, which induce tumor cell necrosis and also release IFN-α, -β, and -γ, which increase tumor cell MHC I molecules on tumor cells, allowing them to become targets of CTL killing.

on the surface of a target cell, then the "do not kill" signal is received by the NK cell, and the target cell survives. Failure to engage the KIR will result in NK-induced lysis of the target cell. When expression of MHC I molecules on the cell surface is abnormally low, as is the case in some malignant cells, KIRs might not recognize ligands on the target (malignant) cell and might proceed to kill it. In some cases, Fc receptors on NK cells can bind to antibody present on tumor cells (produced as part of the adaptive response against the tumor cell), leading to antibody-dependent cellular cytotoxicity.

NK cells that are induced to function attack malignant cells are sometimes referred to as **lymphokine-activated killer cells** (LAKs). These cells are generated in the presence of high concentrations of interleukin-2 and are able to kill fresh tumor cells. **Tumor-infiltrating lymphocytes** (**TIL**) are T lymphocytes, often CD8+ CTLs. They may also include some CD4+ T cells and NKT cells. A therapeutic strategy against malignant melanoma involves obtaining tumor-specific TILs from tumor biopsies and expanding the cells by stimulating with interleukin-2. These cells are then injected back into the patient. In some cases, partial regression of the tumors has been observed.

2. **Cytokines:** Cytokines with antitumor activity are secreted by macrophages, which are often found in the vicinity of tumors (Fig. 19.6). **Tumor necrosis factor** (TNF) is one such antitumor cytokine. When injected into animals with tumors, TNF-α and TNF-β can stimulate necrosis of the tumor cells. TNF-α also inhibits angiogenesis, the growth of new blood vessels by decreasing blood flow to the tumor. **Interferons** are another group of cytokines with antitumor activity. IFN-α, -β, and -γ have all been shown to increase MHC I expression on tumor cells (which often downregulate MHC I expression to evade the immune response). Increasing the MHC I expression can increase susceptibility of the tumor cells to CTLs. IFN-γ may also directly inhibit proliferation of tumor cells.

B. Adaptive

Specific antigen-dependent immune responses can develop to antigens that are present on tumor cells. Although they are not always effective in halting progression of a tumor, evidence exists that both humoral and cell-mediated immune responses can be induced in response to the presence of malignant cells (Fig. 19.7).

- **Antibodies** are known to be generated against certain tumor-specific antigens present on the surface of malignant cells.
- **CTLs** can sometimes kill tumor cells by direct contact.
- **DTH** reactions involve Th1 cells recruiting and activating macrophages, which attack and kill tumor cells.

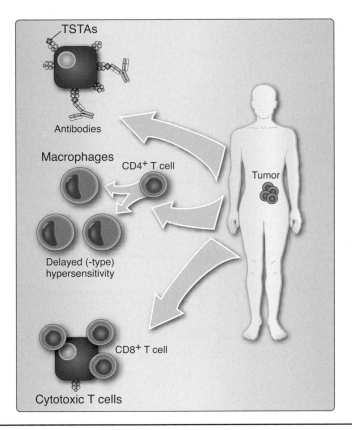

Figure 19.7
Adaptive immune responses against tumor cells. Humoral as well as cell-mediated immune responses are mounted against tumor cells.

IV. IMMUNE EVASION

Although both innate and adaptive immune responses are evoked by the presence of malignant cells, tumor cells often escape the immune system and go on to produce tumors and diseases that are often fatal. Several mechanisms that facilitate evasion of the immune response by tumor cells have been identified.

A. Antibody enhancement of tumor growth

Because attempts to immunize cancer patients by injecting specific antibodies that were developed in culture against their tumor cells often resulted in enhanced tumor growth, studies have been initiated to explore the mechanisms of antibody-induced tumor cell growth. The antitumor antibodies may bind to the antigens on the tumor cells, masking the antigens and blocking the ability of CTL cells to bind and kill the tumor cell. Antibody bound to tumor antigen may inhibit preventing binding of Fc receptors on macrophages and dendritic cells (phagocytosis) and on NK cells.

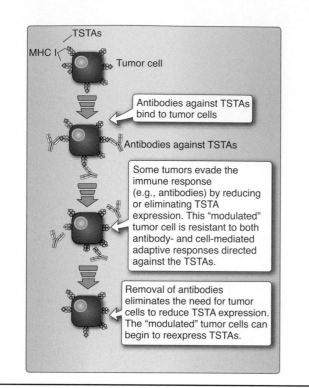

Figure 19.8
Antigenic modulation. Antibodies to tumor antigens may cause the tumor to downregulate antigen expression.

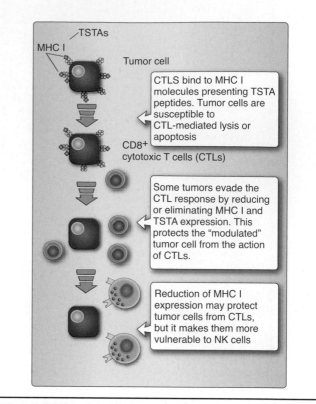

Figure 19.9
Decreased expression of tumor cell MHC I may impair CTL recognition, but increase recognition by and vulnerability to NK cells.

B. Antibody modulation of tumor antigens

In the presence of antibodies directed against tumor antigens, downregulation of expression of certain tumor specific antigens has been demonstrated. In a process known as antigenic modulation, the antigens disappear for a time and then reappear when the antibody is eliminated. Cells that do not express the antigen are no longer targets of other adaptive immune responses (Fig. 19.8).

C. Modulation of MHC I expression

Tumor cells often express reduced levels of MHC I molecules. Malignant transformation may result in a reduction or total loss of MHC I molecules by the transformed cells. If tumor cells express decreased amounts of MHC I, NK cell responses to them may be enhanced while CTL-mediated responses against those tumor cells are decreased (Fig. 19.9).

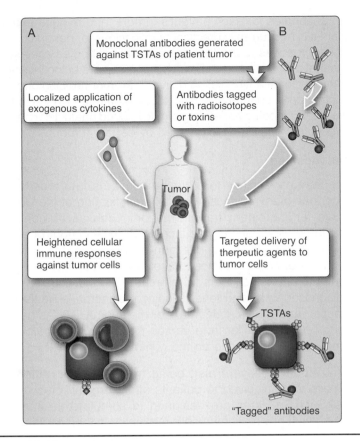

Figure 19.10
Cancer immunotherapies. **A**. Application of exogenous cytokines can heighten immune responses to tumor cells. **B**. Monoclonal antibodies generated against TSTAs of the patient's tumor cells can be "tagged" with toxins or radioactive materials to deliver a therapeutic "magic bullet" to a tumor.

V. CANCER IMMUNOTHERAPY

Cancer immunotherapy is based on enhancement of the natural immune responses that the body mounts against malignant cells.

A. Cytokine therapy

Interleukins and interferons have been used to enhance the immune response to tumors. Because systemic administration of these cytokines can be dangerous, local application is required, complicating the treatment protocols. Although therapeutic benefit is sometimes obtained with cytokine therapy, more research and refinement of protocols are likely necessary before more widespread use and more benefit will be obtained from this approach (Fig. 19.10A).

B. Monoclonal antibodies

Anti-idiotypic monoclonal antibodies have been used to treat B cell lymphomas (Fig. 19.10B). However, the approach is complicated, requires custom antibodies for each patient's tumors, and is quite expensive. Therefore it is not currently practical or efficacious for general use. More general approaches to produce monoclonal antibodies against determinants that are shared by all B cell lymphomas are being investigated. Use of monoclonal antibodies to deliver a toxin or radioisotope directly to the tumor cells, sparing healthy cells, is another promising approach. Monoclonal antibodies are also being developed against certain growth factor receptors commonly expressed by certain tumors.

C. Cancer vaccines

Development of vaccines to protect against the future development of cancer has many obvious benefits. Identification of the viruses responsible for malignant transformation, such as human papillomavirus in cervical cancer, has facilitated development of an immunization protocol to prevent infection by the virus, thus preventing development of cervical cancer. Vaccines are also being developed to attempt to prevent cancers from recurring in individuals who have been diagnosed with conditions including melanoma, a life-threatening skin cancer, and renal carcinoma. For melanoma, TSTAs have been shown to be quite similar from person to person, and vaccines now being developed are based on the common TSTAs.

Customized vaccines are also being made using a patient's own tumor cells and are given to patients after surgical removal of their tumors. Such vaccines are designed to stimulate an immune response against any malignant cells remaining in their bodies. Promising results have been obtained in some clinical trials.

Chapter Summary

- Cancer cells have unregulated rates of cell growth and invade healthy tissue.

- **Metastasis** is a characteristic of many malignant cells as they become dislodged from the main tumor and travel to distant sites in the body.

- **Lymphomas** and **leukemias** are tumors of immune cells that are derived from hematopoietic cells. Lymphomas are solid tumors, while leukemias grow as dispersed, single malignant cells.

- **Malignant transformation** is the process by which a normal cell becomes a cancerous cell.

- **Oncogenes** are sometimes linked to malignant transformation. Mutations of cellular oncogenes often results in a change in cellular growth.

- Tumor antigens include tumor-specific transplantation antigens (TSTAs) that result from altered proteins expressed as a consequence of gene mutations within tumor cells and tumor-associated transplantation antigens (TATAs) that are not unique to tumor cells but have unusual expression on tumor cells.

- The immune surveillance theory suggests that cancer cells frequently arise within the body but are normally eliminated by the immune system before a tumor develops.

- Innate immune responses against tumors include NK cell killing of tumors and macrophage production of antitumor cytokines, including tumor necrosis factor and the interferons.

- Adaptive immune responses against tumors include generation of antitumor antibodies, CTL killing of tumor cells, and DTH reactions.

- Immune evasion by tumor cells facilitates survival of malignant cells. Antitumor antibodies may actually enhance the growth of some tumors and may result in decreased detection of some tumor antigens. In addition, tumor cells often have lower than normal levels of MHC I molecules, helping the tumors to evade immune detection.

- Cancer immunotherapy is designed to increase the immune response against cancer cells. Cytokines and monoclonal antibodies have proven to have some limited effects in treating certain cancers. Vaccination, either to prevent development of a type of cancer or to inhibit recurrence of a tumor within a patient, continues to be explored.

Study Questions

19.1 Which of the following may be expected in cells over expressing *Src*?

   A. enhanced rate of apoptosis
   B. death by necrosis
   C. increased expression of MHC I molecules
   D. senescence (loss of ability to divide)
   E. unregulated cell division

The correct answer is E. A mutation in the oncogene Src results in loss of regulatory function of a tyrosine kinase that normally regulates cell division. *Src* does not regulate cell death by apoptosis or by necrosis, nor would a mutant *Src* induce senescence. Increased MHC I expression would not be linked to a tumor cell with a mutated *Src*; tumor cells often have decreased levels of MHC I expression.

19.2 A bone marrow biopsy from a patient with acute lymphocytic leukemia reveals the presence of a mutated form of p53 within leukemic cells. This mutation is likely responsible for which of the following?

   A. an increase in the Bax-to-Bcl-2 ratio
   B. decreased activity of NK cell KIR function
   C. excess activity of a GTP-binding protein
   D. growth of malignant cells as a solid tumor
   E. loss of suppression of cell growth

The correct answer is E. *P53* is a tumor suppressor gene. When it is mutated, the suppressor action is lost, resulting in unregulated cell growth. An increase in the *Bax*-to-*Bcl-2* ratio would favor apoptosis and not tumor growth that is seen with mutant *p53*. *P53* mutants do not mediate NK cell KIR function. P53 is a tumor suppressor gene and not a GTP-binding protein such as ras. Leukemias grow not as solid tumors but as dispersed, single malignant cells.

19.3 Which of the following is correct regarding tumor-specific transplantation antigens (TSTAs)?

   A. also present in high concentration on normal somatic cells
   B. often found on normal fetal cells as well as on tumor cells
   C. readily identified on most naturally occurring tumors
   D. result from mutant proteins expressed by tumor cells
   E. stimulate apoptosis on cells that express them

The correct answer is D. TSTAs result from mutant proteins expressed by tumor cells. Mutations of genes within the tumor cells lead to altered proteins on the surfaces of the tumor cells. TSTAs are not found on normal somatic cells or on normal fetal cells but are unique to tumors. Although they have been demonstrated on experimentally induced tumors, identification of TSTAs on naturally occurring tumors has proved to be very difficult. Stimulation of apoptosis of tumor cells would result in elimination of tumor cells and would be beneficial to the patient with the tumor. Expression of TSTAs does not appear to stimulate apoptosis.

19.4 According to the immune surveillance theory,

  A. antibodies arise during fetal development that can destroy tumors.
  B. cancer cells rarely arise within a normal individual.
  C. innate immune responses eliminate specific tumor cell antigens.
  D. tumors arise only if malignant cells escape immune detection.
  E. tumor-infiltrating lymphocytes prevent malignant transformations.

The correct answer is D. According to the immune surveillance theory, tumors arise only if malignant cells escape detection by the immune system. This theory suggests that cancer cells frequently arise within the body but are normally eliminated before becoming clinically detectable. This theory does not suggest that germline-encoded antibodies develop to destroy tumors. Innate immune responses against tumors are based on broad characteristics of tumors, not on specific tumor cell antigens. Tumor-infiltrating lymphocytes may induce tumor regression and do not induce a normal cell to become transformed into a cancer cell.

19.5 Which of the following is a cytokine known to have antitumor activity?

  A. epidermal growth factor
  B. interferon-γ
  C. interleukin-2
  D. interleukin-12
  E. platelet-derived growth factor

The correct answer is B. Interferons-α, -β, and -γ have all been shown to increase MHC I expression on tumor cells, and IFN-γ also appears to inhibit tumor cell proliferation. The growth factors and other cytokines listed have growth stimulatory actions.

19.6 Lymphokine-activated killer (LAK) cells are indistinguishable from

  A. B lymphocytes.
  B. macrophages.
  C. malignant somatic cells.
  D. NK cells.
  E. T lymphocytes.

The correct answer is D. LAK cells are NK cells that are generated in the presence of high concentrations of interleukin-2 and are able to kill fresh tumor cells. LAK cells are not B or T lymphocytes, nor are they macrophages. LAK cells can kill tumor cells and are not themselves malignant somatic cells.

19.7 Which of the following provides evidence of immune evasion by tumor cells?

  A. downregulation of MHC I molecules by tumor cells
  B. enhanced production of tumor necrosis factor by macrophages
  C. IFN-γ-mediated inhibition of tumor cell proliferation
  D. generation of antibodies against tumor-specific antigens
  E. stimulation of tumor cell apoptosis by increased Bax expression

The correct answer is A. Downregulation of MHC I molecules is a defense mechanism utilized by many tumor cells to evade recognition by the immune system. The other mechanisms listed all describe immune responses initiated against tumor cells that have the potential to stop tumor growth. TNF and IFN-γ are produced by macrophages and inhibit tumor cell proliferation. Antibodies directed against tumor-specific antigens are part of the humoral immune response aimed at halting tumor progression. Stimulation of apoptosis by increased Bax expression would serve to eliminate tumor cells and is therefore not a mechanism to evade the immune response.

19.8 A new method to reduce the incidence of cervical cancer involves

  A. administration of tumor necrosis factor to the cervix.
  B. injection of antibodies against other patients' cervical tumors.
  C. stimulation of antibody-mediated cell lysis of cervical tumor cells.
  D. use of patient's tumor cells to develop an individualized vaccine.
  E. vaccination against human papillomavirus.

The correct answer is E. Vaccination against human papillomavirus, the causative agent in cervical cancer, may reduce the future incidence of cervical cancer. Neither administration of TNF nor injection of antibodies against other patients' cervical tumors is being done to prevent occurrence of cervical cancer. For certain other cancers, individualized vaccines are being used in clinical trials. However, such a vaccine requires that the patient have a tumor and would therefore not reduce the incidence of a type of cancer.

Measurement of Immune Function

20

I. OVERVIEW

Clinical laboratories provide a wide range of test procedures that are the foundation of modern medicine. Many routine test procedures are antibody-based. These tests rely upon the ability of antibodies to aggregate (agglutination) particulate antigens (e.g., blood typing) or to precipitate soluble antigens (e.g., radial immunodiffusion, Ouchterlony or double diffusion, immunoelectrophoresis). Other assays rely upon chemically modified antibodies to quantitate antigens (e.g., radioimmunoassays and immunosorbent assays) with exquisite specificity and sensitivity. Additional assays (e.g., immunofluorescence and flow cytometry) utilize fluorochrome-labeled antibodies to assess antigen expression both within and on the surface of cells. Immune function may be assessed in the laboratory (e.g., complement fixation, proliferation, and cytotoxic T lymphocyte assay) or in a clinical setting (assessment of hypersensitivity). The variety and range of immune-based clinical assays are well beyond the scope of this book; instead, we offer a few examples of some of the most commonly used assays.

II. EPITOPE DETECTION BY ANTIBODIES

Many clinical lab tests are based upon the specificity of antibodies for antigen and their ability to recognize epitopes, very small portions of an antigen. Antibody-based assays are epitope-detecting tools, and most are based upon the quantitative precipitin curve (Fig. 20.1, see also Fig. 11.2).

A. Particulate antigens

Particulate antigens such as erythrocytes, bacteria, or even antigen-coated latex beads are normally evenly dispersed in suspension. Cross-linking of antigen-bearing particles by antibodies disrupts the homogeneity of the suspension. This cross-linking causes clumping of the particles, also known as **agglutination** (Fig. 20.2). The reaction goes by several different names based upon whether the particulate antigen is an erythrocyte (hemagglutination), whether IgM antibodies efficiently cross-link the particles (direct agglutination), or whether an anti-immunoglobulin (indirect or passive agglutination) is used to cross-link antigen-bound antibodies.

1. **Direct agglutination:** This reaction usually involves IgM antibodies that cross-link epitopes on cells or particles. IgM is the

311

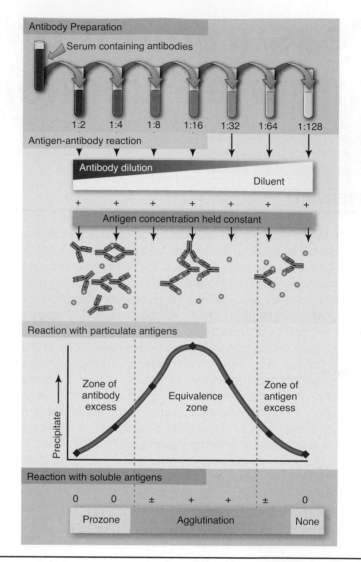

Figure 20.1

Quantitative precipitin curve. **Antibody preparation:** antibody-containing serum is usually serially diluted, producing "half" concentrations of antibodies (expressed as 1:2. 1:4, 1:8 . . . etc.). **Antigen-antibody reaction:** antigen (containing multiple epitopes) in equal concentrations is added to the antibody dilutions resulting in differing degrees of antigen-antibody complex formation. **Reaction with soluble antigens:** antigen-antibody complexes are formed in three zones. In the *equivalence zone*, both antigen and antibody are at concentrations that result in maximal lattice formation, causing precipitation of antigen-antibody complexes. In the *zone of antibody excess*, antibody molecules outnumber available epitopes, and precipitating complexes are not formed due to insufficient lattice formation. In the *zone of antigen excess*, available epitopes outnumber antibody-binding sites, and precipitating complexes are not formed due to insufficient lattice formation. **Reaction with particulate antigens:** maximal clumping or agglutination occurs when epitopes on particles or cells are maximally bound by antibody, similar to the equivalence zone for soluble antigens. Excessive amounts of antibody prevent cross-linking between particles; this is called the *prozone*. The point at which cross-linking of the particulate antigen is no longer observed is called the *titer*.

largest immunoglobulin (~10^6 Da) and has 10 epitope-binding sites (valence). Its relatively large span and valence make it very efficient at cross-linking epitopes on adjacent particles (see Figs. 20.1 and 20.2). Other isotypes, because of their smaller size and lesser valence, are less efficient in direct agglutination. The same rules that govern the quantitative precipitin reaction apply to agglutination reactions (see Fig. 11.2 and Fig. 20.1). Too much antibody inhibits agglutination (equivalent to the zone of antibody excess). Inhibition of agglutination by antibody is known as the **prozone**. To circumvent the prozone effect, dilutions of antibody are added to identical concentrations of particulate antigen. Typically, twofold or serial dilutions of antibody are prepared; each dilution is half as concentrated as the preceding one (see Fig. 20.1). The lowest concentration of antibody that causes agglutination is called the **titer**. Titers are relative measures of antibody activity and are often expressed as the reciprocal of the dilution (e.g., 1:16, 1:32, 1:64).

2. **Indirect or passive agglutination:** This technique is often used to detect non-IgM antibodies or antibodies in concentrations too low to be detected by direct agglutination. Human antibodies may not directly agglutinate antigen-bearing particles (e.g., bacteria, erythrocytes, latex particles) or show agglutination of very low titer. The sensitivity of the agglutination test may be enhanced by the addition of an anti-immunoglobulin reagent (e.g., rabbit anti-human immunoglobulin) in the so-called indirect or passive agglutination technique. Addition of these **second-step antibodies** is used to increase binding over a greater span and to increase valence by virtue of their ability to bind to the primary antibody (Fig. 20.3).

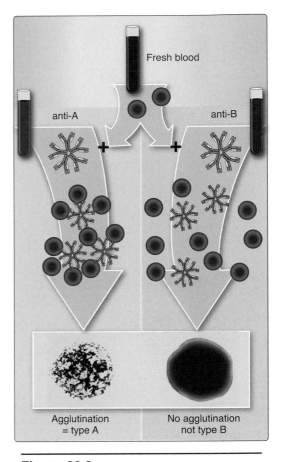

Figure 20.2

Agglutination. Agglutination tests have direct application in a number of serological tests, such as ABO blood typing. A small quantity of freshly drawn blood is admixed with pool of monoclonal anti-A or anti-B human blood group antibodies. The agglutination reaction typically occurs within 15 to 30 seconds. In this figure, blood from one of the authors shows agglutination with antibodies to blood group A, but not with antibodies against blood group B.

CLINICAL APPLICATION
Coombs' test

Antibodies against self blood group antigens occur in some autoimmune hemolytic anemias. Afflicted individuals produce antibodies to their own erythrocytes but in isotypes or quantities that do not directly agglutinate their erythrocytes. In the **direct Coombs'** test, autoantibodies are detected by the addition of antihuman immunoglobulin (secondary antibody). For the **indirect Coombs'** assay, erythrocytes are incubated with the serum to be tested and then washed; antihuman immunoglobulin is then added.

B. Soluble antigens

Often, epitopes present on soluble molecules will precipitate from solution upon reaction with the "right" amount of antibody. The quantitative precipitin reaction (Fig. 20.1; see also Fig. 11.2) requires the preparation of a number of antigen-antibody samples and is too cumbersome and time-consuming to find application in the clinical

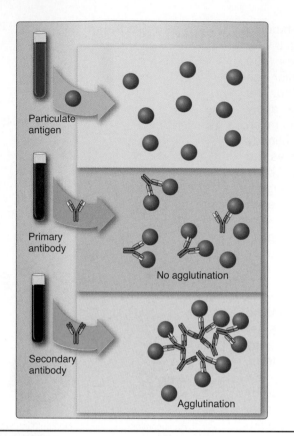

Figure 20.3
Indirect or passive agglutination. This technique is used to detect IgG antibody binding to particulate antigens or to detect low levels of antibody binding. Particulate antigen is incubated with a primary antibody; in some cases, this primary antibody may be preexisting antibody in the individual. A secondary antibody, also called an antiglobulin or anti-immunoglobulin, is added to react with the primary antibody to cause cross-linking or agglutination.

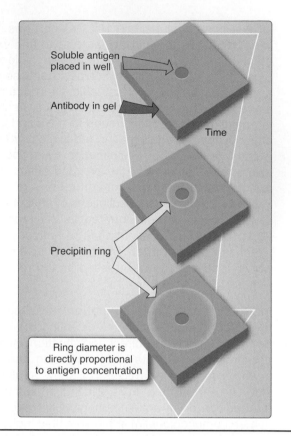

Figure 20.4
Radial immunodiffusion. This technique relies upon the diffusion of soluble antigen through an antibody-impregnated agar gel. A layer of antibody-containing liquefied agar is poured onto a glass slide and allowed to cool (gel). Soluble antigen is loaded into a well cut into the gel and radially diffuses into the gel matrix. A precipitin ring forms at the *equivalence zone* (see Fig. 20.1), the area within the ring closest to the well represents the *zone of antigen excess*, and the area outside the precipitin ring represents the *zone of antibody excess*. The diameter of the precipitin ring is directly proportional to the initial antigen concentration, and by comparing the diameter with a standard curve, the precise concentration of antigen loaded into the well may be determined.

laboratory. Several simple modifications allow visualization of immune precipitates in agar, a semisolid growth medium.

1. **Radial immunodiffusion:** Also called the **Mancini technique**, this test is based upon the diffusion of soluble antigen within an agar gel that contains a uniform concentration of antibody. Antibody-containing molten agar is poured onto a glass slide or plastic dish. When the agar cools and solidifies, wells are cut into the gel matrix, and soluble antigen is placed into the well (Fig. 20.4). Antigen diffuses radially from the well, forming a precipitin ring at equivalence. The diameter of the ring is directly proportional to the amount of antigen loaded into the well. The concentration of antigen in a test sample can be accurately determined by comparing its diameter with a standard calibration curve. This technique allows for the rapid and precise determination of the quantity of antigen loaded into the well.

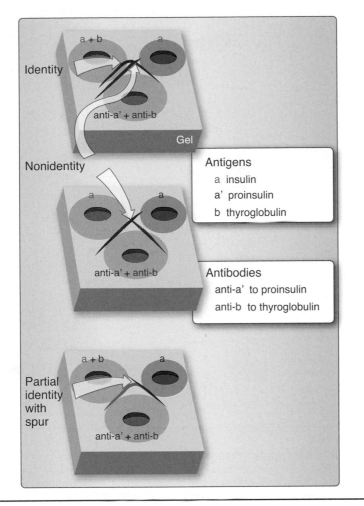

Figure 20.5
Double-diffusion or Ouchterlony technique. This test is a modification of
the radial immunodiffusion technique (see Fig. 20.4). Wells are cut into a
solidified agar gel. Soluble antigen(s) are loaded into one or more wells,
and antibodies are loaded into another well(s), from which they diffuse
through the gel. **Top panel.** A precipitin band is formed at the *equivalence
zone.* For example, antibodies to thyroglobulin (anti-b) react with thyroglobulin (b) to form a precipitin band (depicted in red). Antibodies to proinsulin
(anti-a') react with insulin (a) in adjacent wells to form a precipitin arc (depicted in blue) showing *identity.* **Middle panel.** Antigen-antibody reactions
to insulin (a) and thyroglobulin (b) occur independently of one another
(anti-a' + anti-b) to form crossing, nonidentity precipitin bands. **Bottom
panel.** Antibodies to proinsulin (anti-a') react with both insulin (a) and
proinsulin (a'). Proinsulin is the precursor of insulin containing insulin A
and B chains as well as a 30 to 35 amino acid connecting peptide (C peptide). Antibodies contained within anti-a' react with this "extra" peptide to
form a spur off the identity arc to indicate partial identity.

2. **Double-diffusion (or the Ouchterlony technique):** This test is
   based upon the diffusion of both antigen (loaded in one well) and
   antibody (loaded in another well) through an agar gel. A precipitin line forms at equivalence (Fig. 20.5). Solubility, molecular size
   of the antibody, and detection of epitopes on antigens of different
   molecular size all influence precipitin formation such that multiple
   precipitin lines often develop. An advantage of this technique is
   that several antigens or antibodies can be compared to determine

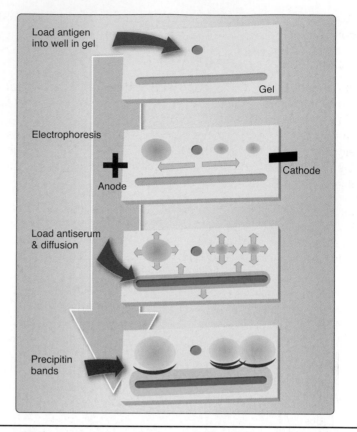

Figure 20.6
Immunoelectrophoresis. This technique is a variation on the double diffusion technique. Antigen is loaded into a well in an agar gel. A current is
applied to the gel and antigens migrate according to charge and size.
A trough is then cut into the gel and loaded with antiserum against one
or more antigens. Both the antigen(s) (blue) and antibodies (red) diffuse
through the gel to form precipitin bands (purple).

identity, partial identity, and nonidentity of antigens and/or antibodies. In contrast to radial immunodiffusion, this is a qualitative
technique.

3. **Immunoelectrophoresis (IEP):** This technique is a modification
   of double diffusion. Antigens are loaded into a well within the
   agar, an electrical current is applied, and antigens migrate according to both their size and their electrical charge (Fig. 20.6).
   The electrical current is removed, a trough is cut into the agar,
   and antiserum is placed in the trough. IEP is qualitative but not
   quantitative.

III. EPITOPE QUANTITATION BY ANTIBODIES

The specificity of antibody molecules makes them ideal probes for detection of a wide variety of epitopes. Antibodies or the antigens they detect
(sometimes referred to as ligands) may be labeled with radioactive

molecules, fluorescent molecules, enzymes, or heavy metals. Antibody or antigen binding is then readily detectable and quantifiable.

A. Radioimmunoassay

Radioimmunoassay (RIA) has been widely used in clinical diagnostic laboratories. Antigens of primary antibodies may be directly labeled with a radionuclide and form the basis for direct RIA. Alternatively, anti-immunoglobulin antibody (secondary antibody) is radiolabeled and used in the indirect RIA. RIA is sensitive but presents problems owing to the potential exposure of laboratory personnel to radioactivity and radioactive waste disposal.

1. **Direct RIA:** This technique utilizes radiolabeled antibody or its ligand (antigen). Antibody is incubated with ligand, and unbound reactants are removed (phase separation) from the system (Fig. 20.7A). Phase separation may utilize precipitation of bound

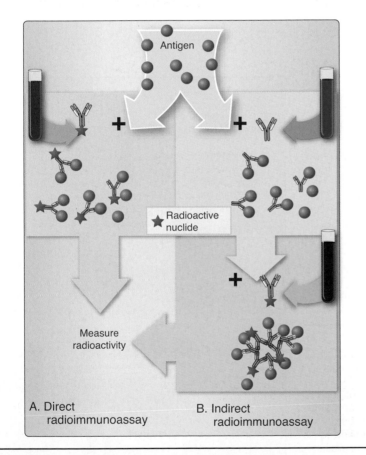

A. Direct radioimmunoassay

B. Indirect radioimmunoassay

Figure 20.7
Radioimmunoassay. As its name suggests, a radionuclide such as I^{125} is used to label a primary or secondary antibody or antigen. **A.** In the direct radioimmunoassay, primary antibody is radiolabeled and incubated with antigen. Unbound antibody is washed away, and bound radioactivity is determined. **B.** In the indirect radioimmunoassay, primary antibody that has bound to antigen is detected with a radiolabeled, anti-immunoglobulin (secondary antibody), the antibody-antigen complex is washed free of unbound antibodies, and bound radioactivity is determined.

reactants (quantitative precipitin reaction), particulate antigens (such as bacteria that may be separated by centrifugation), the immobilization of the nonradioactive reactant onto a solid matrix (such as plastic), and so on.

2. **Indirect RIA:** This technique uses radiolabeled secondary antibody (anti-immunoglobulin) to detect the binding of a primary antibody (Fig. 20.7B). As with direct RIA, a phase separation method must be employed to remove unbound radiolabeled secondary antibody.

B. Enzyme-linked immunosorbent assay

Enzyme-linked immunosorbent assay [ELISA, also called enzyme immunoassay (EIA)] has replaced RIA in a number of tests. ELISA offers the advantage of safety and speed. Because there is no radioactive decay, the reagents that are used are relatively stable. Its sensitivity is often equal to or greater than that of RIA or fluorescent immunosorbent assay, because an enzyme-labeled reactant is used to turn a chromogenic substrate from colorless to a color

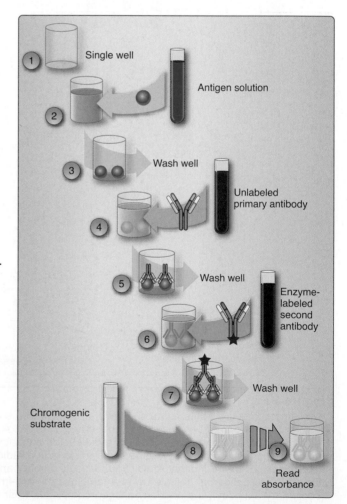

Figure 20.8
Enzyme-linked immunosorbent assay (**ELISA**). Enzyme-labeled antibody is used for epitope detection in this technique. **1.** The assay is generally performed in protein-adsorbing, 96-well polystyrene plates (a single well is shown here). **2.** Soluble antigen is added and non-covalently binds to the plastic. **3.** Unbound antigen is washed from the well. **4.** Unlabeled (often sera to be tested) primary antibodies are added to the well and allowed to bind. **5.** Unbound primary antibodies are washed from the well. **6.** Enzyme-labeled anti-immunoglobulin antibodies are added and allowed to bind. **7.** Unbound enzyme-labeled antibodies are washed from the well. **8.** An enzyme-cleavable, chromogenic substrate is added to the well and allowed to incubate. **9.** Color change indicates the presence of enzyme-labeled secondary antibody. Because the second antibody only binds to the primary antibody and the primary antibody only binds to the epitope, the degree of color change indicates the amount of epitope detected.

(Fig. 20.8). Color change of the substrate indicates that an enzyme-labeled reactant has bound. Increasing substrate incubation time allows low-concentration enzyme to convert more substrate to enhance test sensitivity (within limits). ELISAs are both specific and quantitative.

C. Fluorescent immunosorbent assay

Fluorescent immunosorbent assay (FIA) relies upon antibodies or their ligands labeled with a variety of fluorescent dyes such as fluorescein isothiocyanate (FITC) or phycoerythrin (PE). This technique does not have the concomitant hazards associated with radionuclides. Phase separation of antibody and ligand (antigen) is accomplished by the immobilization of one reactant onto polystyrene prior to the addition of the fluorochrome-labeled reactant. Bound fluorochrome-labeled reactant is retained by virtue of its binding to the immobilized reactant or, if unbound, is removed by washing (Fig. 20.9). Retained fluorescence indicates binding. FIA is specific and relatively sensitive.

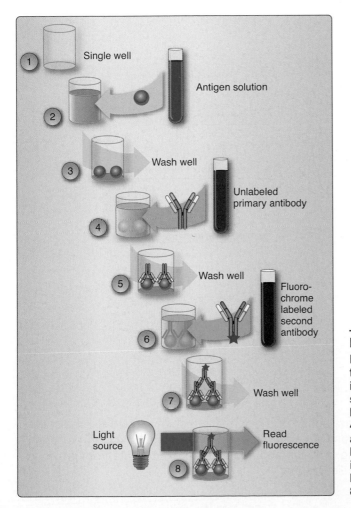

Figure 20.9
Fluorescent immunosorbent assay (FIA). The FIA design is similar to the ELISA design (Fig. 20.8). **1.** The assay may be performed in protein-adsorbing, 96-well polystyrene plates (a single well is shown here). **2.** Soluble antigen is added and noncovalently binds to the plastic. **3.** Unbound antigen is washed from the well. **4.** Unlabeled (often sera to be tested) primary antibodies are added to the well and allowed to bind. **5.** Unbound primary antibodies are washed from the well. **6.** Fluorochrome-labeled anti-immunoglobulin antibodies are added to the well and allowed to bind. **7.** Unbound labeled antibodies are washed from the well. **8.** Fluorescence indicates the presence of epitopes.

CLINICAL APPLICATION
Sensitivity and specificity:
How reliable is the test?

Interpretation of test results requires an understanding of the test's reliability prior to diagnosis or treatment. No test is perfect; every testing method produces a number of false-positive and false-negative results. How much emphasis should be placed on a particular test result requires a knowledge of the probability that the test will be positive in a patient who has the disease in question (this is termed **sensitivity**) and the probability that the result will be negative in a patient who does not have the disease (termed **specificity**).

Reverend Thomas Bayes (1702–1761) developed the mathematical foundation for inferring whether a hypothesis may be true. When applied to medicine, Bayesian mathematics predicts the probability that a patient has a particular disease based upon a particular diagnostic test. In its simplest form, the sensitivity and specificity of a test can be determined by using a 2 × 2 table in which data from previous experience is laid out as follows (a, b, c, and d are actual numbers of observations, not proportions):

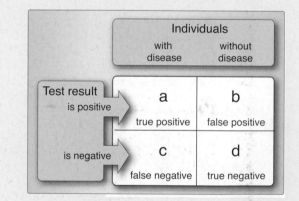

where

$$Sensitivity = \frac{a}{(a + c)}$$

$$Specificity = \frac{d}{(b + d)}$$

Imagine the evaluation of a diagnostic test developed to predict the dreaded disease *Examinus paralysis*, commonly known as "brain freeze," among students about to take an exam. Data from previous experience indicates that

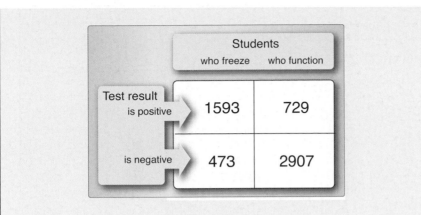

	Students	
	who freeze	who function
Test result is positive	1593	729
is negative	473	2907

Sensitivity and specificity of this diagnostic test may be calculated as

$$Sensitivity = \frac{a}{(a+c)} = \frac{1593}{(1593+473)} = .77 \ or \ 77\%$$

$$Specificity = \frac{d}{(b+d)} = \frac{2907}{(729+2907)} = .8 \ or \ 80\%$$

Thus this test would fail to identify nearly a quarter of the students who would actually suffer brain freeze during the exam (false negatives). About a fifth of the functional students would also be incorrectly identified as likely to freeze (false positives).

IV. EPITOPE DETECTION IN AND ON CELLS

Epitopes expressed both within and on the surface of cells may be detected by using radio-, enzyme-, or fluorochrome-labeled antibodies. Again, the extent and variation in these methodologies are beyond the scope of this book. We briefly outline two techniques that have extensive application in a clinical setting: immunofluorescence and flow cytometry.

A. Immunofluorescence

Immunofluorescence (IF) utilizes fluorescent dyes (e.g., FITC) that are covalently coupled to antibody. A thin, frozen section of tissue is prepared and mounted on a glass slide. The frozen section is then bathed in a solution containing FITC-labeled antibody (direct IF, Fig. 20.10B) or a solution containing a primary antibody and is then washed. An FITC-labeled anti-immunoglobulin is added (indirect IF, Fig. 20.10A). The presence of epitopes is visualized with a fluorescent microscope.

B. Monoclonal antibodies

Antibody responses normally derive from multiple B cells or plasma cells; their antibodies often differ in epitopes that are recognized,

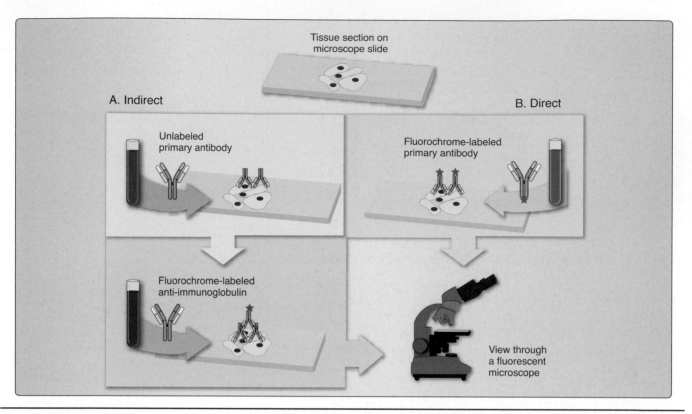

Figure 20.10

Immunofluorescence (IF). Fluorochrome-labeled antibodies are used to visualize epitopes on cells and tissues by microscopy. Tissue sections or cells are affixed to glass microscope slides. **A**. In **indirect IF**, slide-mounted tissues or cells are bathed with an unlabeled primary antibody, then unbound antibody is washed from the slide. A fluorochrome-labeled secondary antibody is then incubated with the preparation, unbound secondary antibodies are washed from the slide, and the epitopes, marked by fluorescence, are visualized in a fluorescent microscope. **B**. In **direct IF**, fluorochrome-labeled primary antibodies are incubated with the slide-mounted tissues, unbound antibodies are washed from the slide, and epitopes are identified with a fluorescent microscope.

affinity, and isotype. Antibody responses that arise from multiple cells are termed **polyclonal** antibody responses. Antibody responses to antigens differ among individuals. This antibody diversity is very important in combating microbial infection. Although polyclonal antibodies can be used in the clinical laboratory, their specificity varies somewhat between batches. In 1975, Georges Köhler and César Milstein fused antibody-secreting plasma cells with myeloid-origin tumor (myeloma) cells. The resulting immortalized cells, or **hybridomas**, secreted antibodies of single specificity and isotype and were termed **monoclonal antibodies** because of their origin from a single antibody-producing cell. Vast quantities of monoclonal antibodies can be produced with no variation between batches. Because monoclonal antibodies produced by any given hybridoma are unique, they can be used together with fluorescent dyes or other markers to distinguish individual epitopes on an antigen or cell.

C. Flow cytometry

A powerful modification of IF is flow cytometry, in which leukocytes or other cells are stained with fluorochrome-labeled antibodies. In our example, peripheral blood leukocytes are stained with fluorochrome-

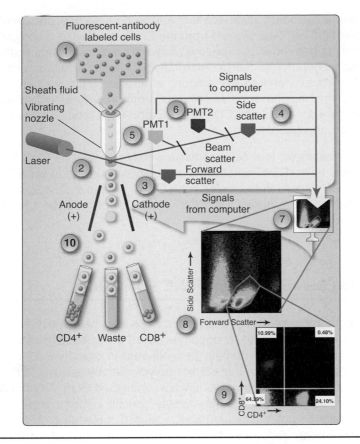

Figure 20.11

Flow cytometry. **1.** Single-cell suspensions of leukocytes or other cells are prepared and stained with the appropriate fluorescent dye-labeled antibodies. **2.** Labeled cells contained within a sheath fluid pass single file through a vibrating nozzle, where a laser beam passes through the stream before droplets are formed. Cells contained within the stream both refract and reflect the light. **3.** A photodetector measures refracted light or forward scatter and is a measure of cell volume. **4.** Reflected light or side scatter, measured at right angles to the laser beam, is an indication of cellular granularity. Beam splitters pass the reflected light through filters to photomultiplier tubes (PMTs) to measure green **(5)** or red **(6)** fluorescence. **7.** Signals generated are analyzed by a computer and represented graphically on the screen. **8.** Forward and side scatter data allow the flow cytometer operator to distinguish cells on the basis of their morphology and electronically "gate" populations for further analysis. **9.** Analysis of a "lymphocyte-gated" population shows a green-stained CD4$^+$ population (24.10%), a red-stained CD8$^+$ population (10.99%), a CD4$^+$CD8$^+$ population (0.48%), and an unstained population (64.29%). **10.** Identified populations can then be isolated or sorted. The computer signals the flow cytometer to apply a positive or negative charge to the sheath fluid before droplet formation. Droplets carrying a negative charge will be attracted to the anode, and those with a positive charge will be attracted to the cathode deflection plate and are collected in a test tube. Uncharged droplets and the cells they contain are consigned to waste.

labeled monoclonal antibodies (in our example, FITC-labeled anti-CD4 and PE-labeled anti-CD8). Single-cell suspensions containing both labeled and unlabeled cells flow through a vibrating chamber (flow cell) in an aqueous stream (sheath fluid), so they pass single-file through a laser beam (Fig. 20.11). Each cell refracts the laser light (forward scatter) and scatters light at approximately right angles to the laser beam (side scatter) and is detected by photomultiplier tubes (PMTs). Data signals from the PMTs are fed to a computer for real-time data analysis. Together, forward scatter and side scatter are used to determine cellular morphology. Additional filters and PMTs are used to measure the amount of fluorescence per cell. Signals from lymphocytes or other cells are electronically identified (gated), and data for FITC-anti-CD4 and PE-anti-CD8 labeled cells may be plotted and quantified.

In our example, four cell populations may possibly be identified. Unstained cells (CD4$^-$ and CD8$^-$) are displayed in the lower left quadrant, CD4$^+$ cells in the lower right, CD8$^+$ cells in the upper left, and, if present, immature CD4$^+$CD8$^+$ would display in the upper right quadrant.

V. ASSESSMENT OF IMMUNE FUNCTION

The functional capacity of phagocytic cells can be assessed by their ability in ingest antibody- or opsonin-coated particles. Stimulating lymphocytes to increase in number or proliferate in response to a specific antigen or to a substance that causes polyclonal mitogenesis (a mitogen) is often used to assess immune function. Activated CD8$^+$ T lymphocytes may recognize and kill cells that display specific peptide + major histocompatibility complex class I (pMHC class I) molecules on their cells surfaces. These cells—cytotoxic T lymphocytes (CTLs)—are able to specifically kill target cells.

A. Phagocyte function

Phagocyte function can be assessed by incubating phagocytic cells with coated particles (e.g., latex beads or antibody-bound cells) or with bacteria for 30 to 120 minutes (Fig. 20.12). Particle inclusion within the cell is assessed by microscopy. Enzymatic activity of phagocytes can be assessed by measuring the levels of individual degradative or oxidative enzymes (e.g., NADPH oxidase) produced by these cells.

B. Proliferation

Peripheral blood mononuclear cells (lymphocytes, monocytes, and dendritic cells) are isolated and placed in tissue culture for 48 to 72 hours. A specific stimulator (antigen) to which the individual may have been previously exposed is added to the culture. Alternatively, a nonspecific stimulant (mitogen) is added to assess the ability of a particular subpopulation of leukocytes to respond. A radionuclide (such as ^{3}H-thymidine) is added for the final 18 to 24 hours of cultures (Fig. 20.13). Incorporation of ^{3}H-thymidine into nascent DNA is taken as a measure of proliferative ability.

C. Cytotoxic T lymphocyte assay

CD8$^+$ T cell function (CTL activity) is assessed by the ability of these cells to induce the lysis and by the number of radiolabeled target cells that are killed. Radioactive sodium chromate (Na$_2$^{51}CrO$_4$)

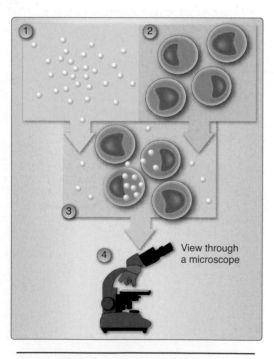

View through a microscope

Figure 20.12

Assessment of phagocyte function. Phagocytes are assessed by incubation of optically visible particles, such as antigen or antibody-coated (i.e., opsonin-coated) particles (e.g., latex beads, bacteria, erythrocytes), with phagocytes **(1)**. Particle uptake **(2)** and phagocytosis **(3)** are visualized with a microscope **(4)**.

readily crosses the cell membrane in live cells and binds to cytoplasmic proteins. Radiolabeled target cells are washed to remove unbound sodium chromate and the target cells are then incubated with CD8$^+$ T cells in a test tube. Within four hours, CD8$^+$ T cells lyse ^{51}Cr-labeled cells bearing the appropriate pMHC class I, releasing ^{51}Cr-protein complexes into the culture medium. Intact cells and cellular debris are removed by centrifugation and radioactivity in the cell-free medium is used to quantify cytotoxic activity (Fig. 20.14). Similar methodology is used to measure NK or NKT activity to lyse NK(T)-sensitive target cells.

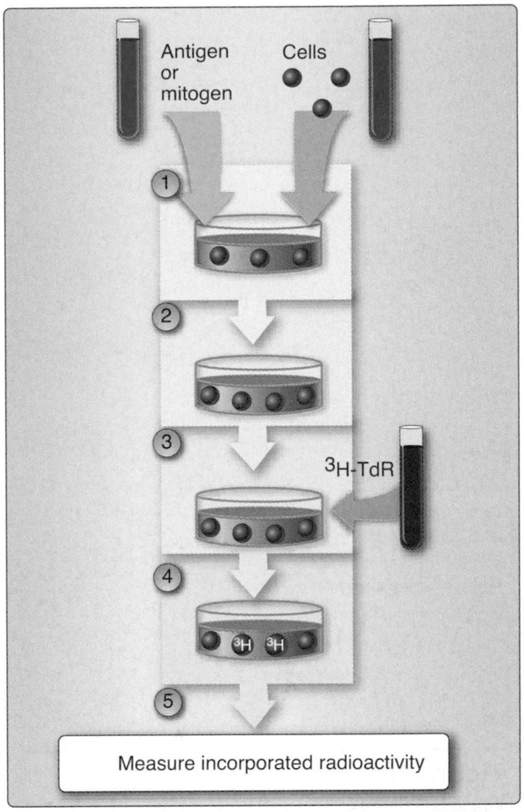

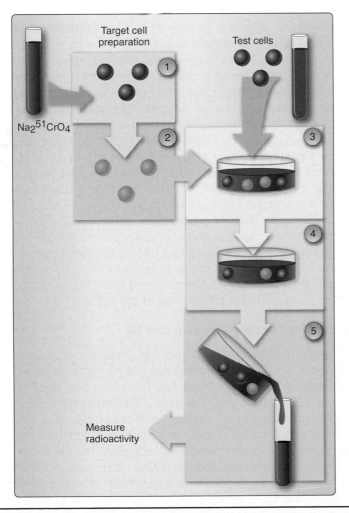

Figure 20.13

Proliferation assays. These tests are used to determine the ability of lymphocytes to respond to a stimulus. **(1)** Antigen or mitogen are added to freshly-established leukocyte cultures and **(2)** allowed to incubate 24 to 72 hours. **(3)** Tritiated thymidine (^{3}H-TdR) or other nucleic acid precursor molecule is then added and the cells incubated for an additional 18 to 24 hours during which time the radioactive molecule is incorporated into newly synthesized DNA. **(5)** Radioactivity incorporated into extracted DNA is used as a measure of proliferation.

Figure 20.14

Chromium release assay. This test assesses the functions of cytotoxic T lymphocyte (CTL), natural killer (NK), and NK-like T (NKT) cells. **1.** Target cells are incubated with radioactive heavy metal (e.g., Na$_2$^{51}CrO$_4$), which strongly binds **(2)** to cytosolic proteins within the cells. **3.** Test or effector cells are coincubated with radiolabeled target cells at different effector-to-target cell ratios. **4.** If present, CTL, NK, or NKT activity causes lysis of the target cells and release of radioactivity into the medium. **5.** Cells are separated, and the amount of radioactivity released into the medium is measured to indicate lytic activity.

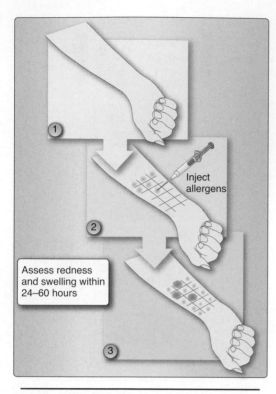

Figure 20.15
Allergy testing. These tests assess Type I hypersensitivities to a variety of potential allergens. **1.** Testing is often performed on the ventral side of the arm. **2.** A grid is marked and small quantities of substances to be tested are injected into the dermis. **3.** Positive reactions are indicated as redness and swelling within one 20 to 30 minutes after re-exposure to the allergen.

VI. ASSESSMENT OF HYPERSENSITIVITY

Immune-mediated damage to host tissues is called hypersensitivity (see Chapter 14). There are four categories of hypersensitivity reactions. Type I reactions are called immediate hypersensitivity reactions because they occur within minutes to hours of antigen exposure. Type II reactions involve complement activation in response to immunoglobulin binding to membranes or the intracellular matrix. Type III reactions involve complement activation in response to "soluble" antigen-antibody complexes. Both type II and type III reactions occur within hours to days. Type IV reactions are "delayed," occurring two to four days after antigen exposure.

A. Allergy skin testing (type I hypersensitivity)

Sensitivities to allergens (antigens) [e.g., pet dander, mold and pollens ("hay fever"), or certain foods] are common allergic disorders. Sensitivity arises from the development of allergen-specific IgE antibodies that decorate the surfaces of tissue mast cells (see Chapter 14). Intradermal injection of a small amount of diluted allergen tests an individual's reaction to an allergen. In some cases, a scratch test can be used where the diluted allergen is administered by scratching the skin surface (percutaneous) rather than being injected into the dermis. Sensitive (atopic) individuals develop a wheal-and-flare (redness and swelling) reaction within 20 minutes after re-exposure to a specific allergen (Fig. 20.15). The test relies upon inflammation caused by allergen-IgE induced degranulation of mast cells in the dermis. Because there is a possibility of the occurrence of a severe allergic reaction, antihistamine or epinephrine should be available during testing. An alternative test, the radioallergosorbent test, is a modified RIA in which allergen is bound to a solid support, serum IgE antibody binds to the allergen, and a radiolabeled anti-IgE antibody is used to detect the binding of the IgE.

B. Complement fixation (types II and III)

Complement fixation tests detect the presence of antigen-antibody complexes on cells or intracellular matrix (type II) or as "soluble" complexes in the serum (type III). There are two parts to this test: the indicator system and the assay. The indicator system contains complement, sheep erythrocytes, and antibodies specific for sheep erythrocytes. Antibodies bind to sheep erythrocytes, forming cell-bound antigen-antibody complexes; complement is activated ("fixed"), causing erythrocyte lysis and the release of hemoglobulin (Fig. 20.16). The amount of hemoglobin is determined spectrophotometrically. To assay for the presence of antigen-antibody complexes in the serum (type III) or tissue-bound antibody (type II) requires that the serum or tissue is incubated with complement. The presence of complement-fixing antigen-antibody complexes depletes the limited amount of complement so that antibody-coated erythrocytes, when added to the reaction mixture, are not lysed, and hemoglobulin is not released.

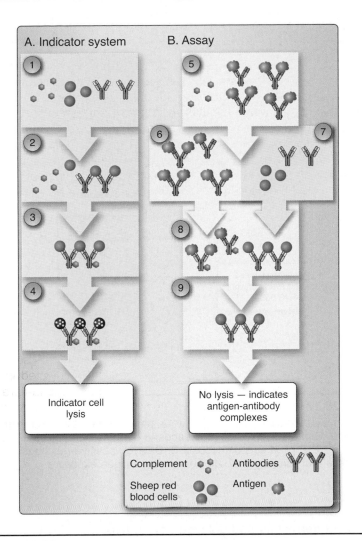

Figure 20.16

Complement fixation. Used to determine the presence of circulating antigen-antibody complexes, this two-part test consists of both an indicator system and the assay. **A.** In the indicator system, antibodies to sheep red blood cells (SRBC), complement, and SRBC are combined in a test tube **1.** SRBC are bound by anti-SRBC antibodies **(2)**. The antigen-antibody complex binds and activates the classical complement pathway **(3)**, resulting in indicator cell (SRBC) lysis **(4)**. **B.** In the assay, serum is collected from an individual **(5)** and heated to 56° C for 30 minutes to inactivate endogenous complement, and a predetermined amount of complement (same amount as used in the indicator system) is added **(6)**. The mixture is incubated to allow complement to bind to antigen-antibody complexes, if present **(7)**. SRBC and anti-SRBC antibodies are added and allowed to incubate **(8)**. The presence of antigen-antibody complexes in the test serum will have depleted the added complement, and the SRBC will not be lysed **(9)**. Absence of antigen-antibody complexes in the test serum will result in a failure to deplete complement, and the indicator cells (SRBC) will be lysed, releasing hemoglobulin into the supernatant that can be measured in a spectrophotometer.

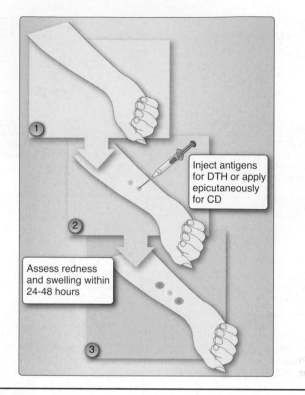

Figure 20.17
Type IV hypersensitivity. **1.** Testing may be performed on the ventral side of the arm. **2.** Small quantities of substances to be tested are injected into the dermis or are applied subcutaneously. **3.** Delayed positive reactions appear as redness and swelling 24 to 48 hours after antigen exposure.

C. Contact dermatitis and delayed (-type) hypersensitivity (type IV)

Application of antigen to the surface of the skin (contact dermatitis) or injected intradermally [delayed (-type) hypersensitivity, DTH] is used to measure type IV hypersensitivity. In this test, antigen is applied to the surface of the skin under a nonabrasive dermal patch. These tests evaluate whether an individual has had prior exposure to a specific antigen. In contrast to immediate hypersensitivity reactions (see Section VI.A above), type IV hypersensitivity reactions are delayed; wheal-and-flare reactions are evident only 24 to 72 hours after antigen challenge (Fig. 20.17).

Credits

Figures 4.1A, 4.1B, 4.1C, 4.1F, 4.1E. From Anderson SC, Poulsen KB. *Anderson's Atlas of Hematology*. Philadelphia: Lippincott Williams & Wilkins, 2003, pp. IA2-44, IA2-65, IA4-8, IA2-17, IIB1-12.

Figure 4.1D. Rubin E MD and Farber JL MD. *Pathology*, 3rd ed. Philadelphia: Lippincott Williams & Wilkins, 1999, pp. 20–35.

Figure 4.1E. Reprinted with permission from Cohen BJ, Wood DL. *Memmler's The Human Body in Health and Disease*, 9th ed. Philadelphia: Lippincott Williams & Wilkins, 2000, p. unn10-1.

Figures 7.1 and 7.2. From Anderson SC, Poulsen KB. *Anderson's Atlas of Hematology*. Philadelphia: Lippincott Williams & Wilkins, 2003, p. IIB1-08.

Figure 7.3. From Anderson SC, Poulsen KB. *Anderson's Atlas of Hematology*. Philadelphia: Lippincott Williams & Wilkins, 2003, p. IA2-44.

Figure 7.4. From Anderson SC, Poulsen KB. *Anderson's Atlas of Hematology*. Philadelphia: Lippincott Williams & Wilkins, 2003, pp. IA2-44 and IA2-68.

Figure 7.5. From Anderson SC, Poulsen KB. *Anderson's Atlas of Hematology*. Philadelphia: Lippincott Williams & Wilkins, 2003, p. IA2-48.

Figures 7.10A, 7.10B, 7.10C, 7.10D, and 9-1A. Reprinted with permission From Ross MH, Pawlina W. *Histology: A Text and Atlas*, 5th ed. Baltimore: Lippincott Williams & Wilkins, 2005, p. 14-16a, 14-17, 17-19, 17-18b, 14-25a.

Figure 13.8. From Sun T. *Parasitic Disorders: Pathology, Diagnosis, and Management*, 2nd ed. Baltimore: Lippincott Williams & Wilkins, 1999, p. 16-20.

Figure 18.3A. Image provided by Anatomical Chart Co/Lippincott Williams & Wilkins.

Figure 18.4B. From Cagle PT. *Color Atlas and Text of Pulmonary Pathology*. Philadelphia: Lippincott Williams & Wilkins, 2005, p. 133.01.

Figure 18.5. Courtesy of Dr. Terry Barrett, Department of Medicine, Feinberg School of Medicine, Northwestern University, Chicago, IL.

Index